AF478728

A Clinical Handbook in
Adolescent Medicine

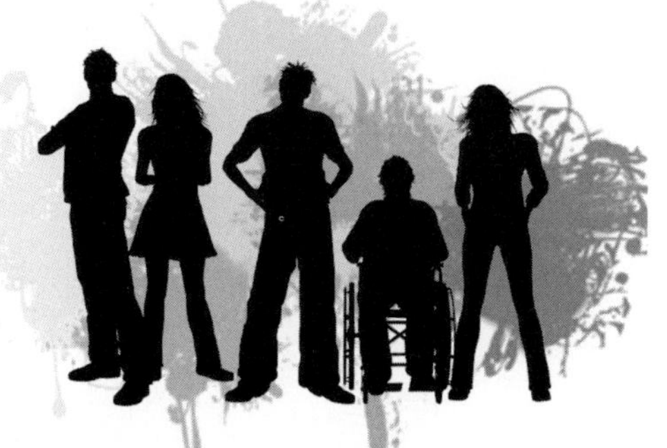

A Guide for Health Professionals Who Work with Adolescents and Young Adults

A Clinical Handbook in Adolescent Medicine

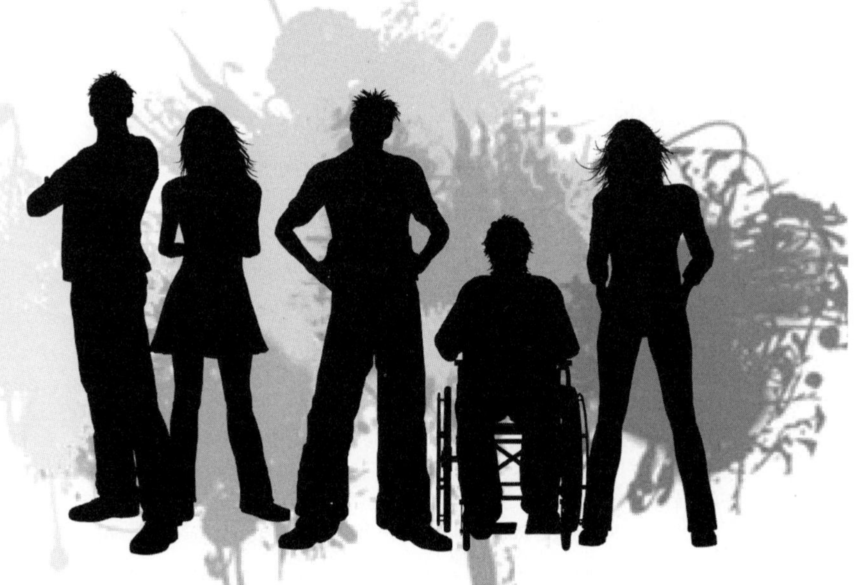

A Guide for Health Professionals Who Work with Adolescents and Young Adults

Kate Steinbeck
University of Sydney, Australia

Michael Kohn
Sydney Children's Hospital Network (Westmead), Australia

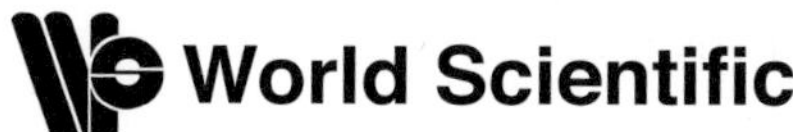

World Scientific

NEW JERSEY · LONDON · SINGAPORE · BEIJING · SHANGHAI · HONG KONG · TAIPEI · CHENNAI

Published by

World Scientific Publishing Co. Pte. Ltd.

5 Toh Tuck Link, Singapore 596224

USA office: 27 Warren Street, Suite 401-402, Hackensack, NJ 07601

UK office: 57 Shelton Street, Covent Garden, London WC2H 9HE

Library of Congress Cataloging-in-Publication Data
A clinical handbook in adolescent medicine : a guide for health professionals who work with
adolescents and young adults / [edited by] Kate Steinbeck, Michael Kohn.
    p. ; cm.
  Includes bibliographical references and index.
  ISBN 978-9814374033 (hardcover : alk. paper)
  I. Steinbeck, Kate. II. Kohn, Michael (Michael R.)
  [DNLM: 1. Adolescent Medicine--methods. 2. Adolescent--physiology.   3. Adolescent Health
Services. 4. Adolescent Psychology--methods.   5. Young Adult. WS 460]

  616.00835--dc23

                     2012051673

British Library Cataloguing-in-Publication Data
A catalogue record for this book is available from the British Library.

In-house Editor: Veronica Low

Typeset by Stallion Press
Email: enquiries@stallionpress.com

Printed by FuIsland Offset Printing (S) Pte Ltd Singapore

Contents

FOREWORD

I am delighted to have the opportunity to introduce this Clinical Handbook of Adolescent Medicine. Adolescents and young people have always been an important part of my professional life, particularly through my work over the years in adolescent psychiatry and Indigenous health. It has been a privilege to work with young people, to appreciate the world as it is seen through their eyes and to marvel at their creativity, despite the challenges of mental and physical health many of them may face.

Professor Kate Steinbeck has been known to me since the early days of her career in Adolescent Medicine and I have watched her progress to her current appointment to the inaugural Medical Foundation Chair in Adolescent Medicine at the University of Sydney. She is a fine researcher and a dedicated clinician who has a comprehensive understanding of the health challenges so many young people face, including mental health and chronic illness. She is also sensitive to the tremendous responsibility that all the health professionals who come in contact with young people bear to advocate for young people in health services.

Dr Michael Kohn is also a leader in the field of Adolescent Medicine. He has established and driven specialist adolescent medical services and played a major role in the translation of adolescent research into the best of clinical practice. These two editors have assembled an internationally respected team of authors for this Clinical Handbook and guided the creation of a comprehensive resource for all health professionals who look after young people around the world.

The subtitle of this handbook is "A Guide for Health Professionals Who Work with Adolescents and Young Adults". Adolescents and young people often feel invisible in both the worlds of paediatric and adult healthcare. They have specific developmental and psychosocial needs which significantly impact on their mental and physical health. They require clinicians who can treat them in context and who understand what is psychologically important to them and in their immediate environment. This Handbook provides clear and concise guidance for such clinicians and I was delighted to see the breadth of coverage and the practical detail which is presented.

As Governor of the State of New South Wales, Australia and Chancellor of the University of Sydney, I recognise that one of the greatest challenges is to ensure that the young people of Australia and the world are equipped, happy and healthy to face life, its challenges and their aspirations. Good healthcare is a fundamental right for all young people. A Clinical Handbook in Adolescent Medicine is a major and significant addition to the medical literature, for it recognises that the health care of young adults is closely related to and represents an extension of the health care of adolescents.

Professor Marie Bashir AC, CVO
Governor of New South Wales
December 2012

ACKNOWLEDGEMENTS

The Editors would like to thank all of our authors who gave their time and expertise to write the individual chapters. The information in this adolescent clinical handbook contains a wealth of up to date and practical information for all clinicians who care for the health of adolescents and young adults.

The Editors acknowledge most gratefully their assistant editors. Ms Tina Cunningham played an invaluable role in the co-ordination of the chapter writing, assisting authors in layout and formatting and keeping to timelines, together with tireless proof reading. Dr Vanessa Shrewsbury provided intensive high quality proof reading and a review of content. The handbook would not have been possible without them.

Contributors

Dr Shirley Alexander, MB ChB MRCPCH FRACP MPH
Staff Specialist, Weight Management Services,
Director, Prevocational Education and Training *and*
Director, Paediatric Physician Education
Sydney Children's Hospital Network (Westmead)
Sydney, Australia

Margaret Allan
Principal (EX)
Sydney Children's Hospital Network (Westmead)
The Children's Hospital School
Sydney, Australia

Professor Geoffrey Ambler, MBBS MD FRACP
Paediatric Endocrinologist
Co-Head of Department, Institute of Endocrinology and Diabetes
The Children Hospital at Westmead,
Section Head, Clinical Endocrinology and Growth
Information Systems and Technology *and*
Clinical Professor, University of Sydney
Sydney, Australia

Gail Anderson, RN RM MN Adolescent Mental Health Cert MACN
Clinical Nurse Consultant
Adolescent Health
Westmead Hospital
Sydney, Australia

Dr Deborah Bateson, MA(oxon) MSc MBBS
Medical Director
Family Planning New South Wales
Ashfield, Sydney *and*
Clinical Lecturer
Discipline of Obstetrics Gynaecology and Neonatology
University of Sydney
Sydney, Australia

Professor Louise Baur, AM BSc(Med) PhD FRACP
Discipline of Paediatrics and Child Health, Sydney Medical School,
Professor, Sydney School of Public Health, University of Sydney *and*
Director, Weight Management Services
Sydney Children's Hospital Network (Westmead)
Sydney, Australia

Dr Richard E Bélanger, MD FRCPC
Paediatrician — Adolescent Medicine Physician
Assistant Professor, Department of Pediatrics
Centre Hospitalier Universitaire de Québec, Université Laval
Quebec City, Canada

Clinical Professor David Bennett, AO MBBS FRACP FSAHM
Senior Staff Specialist, Department of Adolescent Medicine *and*
Head, NSW Centre for the Advancement of Adolescent Health
Sydney Children's Hospital Network (Westmead) and University
    of Sydney
Sydney, Australia

Dr Peter Benny, MB ChB FRCOG FRANZCOG CREI
Medical Director
Next Generation Fertility and Gynaecologist
Sydney, Australia

Helen Bibby, BSc(Psychol) MPsych(Clin) MAPS
Clinical Psychologist/Researcher
Department of Adolescent Medicine
Sydney Children's Hospital Network (Westmead)
Sydney, Australia

Clinical Associate Professor Yvonne Bonomo, MBBS FRACP PhD
  FAChAM
Physician in Adolescent Medicine and Addiction Medicine
Department of Medicine, University of Melbourne *and*
Departments of Addiction Medicine
St. Vincent's Hospital and Western Hospital
Melbourne, Victoria, Australia

Professor Robert Booy, MBBS(Hons) MSc MD FRACP FRCPCH
National Centre for Immunisation Research and
  Surveillance of Vaccine Preventable Disease
Kids Research Institute
Sydney Children's Hospital Network (Westmead)
Sydney, Australia

Dr Carolyn Broderick, MBBS FACSP
Staff Specialist
Children's Hospital Institute of Sports Medicine (CHISM)
Sydney Children's Hospital Network (Westmead)
Sydney, Australia

Lynne Brodie, BA RN PaedCert
Network Manager, Transition Care
NSW Agency for Clinical Innovation (ACI)
Sydney, Australia

Dr Andrew J Campbell, PhD MAPS
Bachelor of Health Sciences Co-Director
Senior Lecturer in Psychology
Faculty of Health Sciences
University of Sydney
Sydney, Australia

Professor Dianne Campbell, MBBS FRACP PhD
Chair of Paediatric Allergy and Clinical Immunology
Sydney Children's Hospital Network (Westmead) *and*
Head of Discipline
Discipline of Paediatrics and Child Health
Sydney Medical School, University of Sydney
Sydney, Australia

Michele Casey, RN ON PICC DipArom GradCert Oncology
Chronic Illness Peer Support Coordinator (Adolescent Nurse)
Department of Adolescent Medicine
Sydney Children's Hospital Network (Westmead)
Sydney, Australia

Clinical Associate Professor Simon D Clarke, MBBS FCP
    FRACP FSAM FACPM
Medical Director, Department of Adolescent Medicine
Westmead Hospital, Sydney, Australia

Clinical Associate Professor John J Collins, AM MBBS
    PhD FRACP
Senior Staff Specialist and Head
Department of Pain Medicine and Palliative Care
Sydney Children's Hospital Network (Westmead)
Sydney, Australia

Dr Julie Curtin, MBBS(Hons) PhD FRACP FRCPA
Head, Department of Haematology
Sydney Children's Hospital Network (Westmead)
Sydney, Australia

Professor Kim C Donaghue, MBBS PhD FRACP
Co-Head, Institute of Endocrinology and Diabetes
Head of Diabetes Services
Senior Staff Endocrinologist
Sydney Children's Hospital Network (Westmead) *and*
Professor, University of Sydney
Sydney, Australia

Dr David R Dossetor, MD(Cantab) MA MB BChir FRCP FRCPsych
    FRANZCP DCH
Area Director for Mental Health
Clinical Associate Professor, University of Sydney *and*
Child Psychiatrist with a special interest in Intellectual Disability
    and Autism
Department of Psychological Medicine
Sydney Children's Hospital Network (Westmead)
Sydney, Australia

Julie C Dunsmore, AM MAPS BSc(Psych) Hons MPH RN
President, National Association for Loss and Grief (NSW) Inc. *and*
Senior Psychologist and Director, Department of Health Promotion
Lower North Shore Northern Sydney Health
The Royal North Shore Hospital
Sydney, Australia

Professor Deborah Erickson, PhD
Provost and Vice President for Academic Affairs
Lock Haven University, Clearfield, PA, USA

Dr Melissa Gabriel, BMBS FRACP
Paediatric Oncologist
Sydney Children's Hospital Network (Westmead)
Sydney, Australia

Dr Anuja Elizabeth George, MD DNB
Assistant Professor
Department of Dermatology and Venereology
Government Medical College Trivandrum, Kerala, India

Dr Melina Georgousakis, PhD
National Centre for Immunisation Research and Surveillance
Sydney Children's Hospital Network (Westmead)
Sydney, Australia

Dr Helena Gleeson, MBBS MRCP(UK) MD
Consultant Endocrinologist
Leicester Royal Infirmary, Leicester, UK

Dr Deirdre Hahn, MBChB(UCT) MMed(Paeds)
Department of Nephrology
Sydney Children's Hospital Network (Westmead)
Sydney, Australia

Professor David J Handelsman, MB BS PhD FRACP
Director, Anzac Research Institute
University of Sydney *and*
Head, Andrology Department, Concord Hospital
Sydney, Australia

Nuala Harkin, RN CDE
Nurse Practitioner
Paediatric Diabetes
Sydney Children's Hospital Network (Westmead)
Sydney, Australia

Dr Anthony Harris, MB BS PhD FRANZCP
Discipline of Psychiatry
Sydney Medical School (Westmead) *and*
Brain Dynamics Centre, Westmead Millennium Institute
University of Sydney
Sydney, Austraila

Dr Catherine Hawke, MBBS FFPH
Senior Lecturer in Rural Medicine
School of Rural Health
Sydney Medical School (Orange)
University of Sydney
Orange, New South Wales, Australia

Dr Philip Hazell, BMedSc MBChB PhD FRANZCP
Conjoint Professor of Child and Adolescent Psychiatry
Discipline of Psychiatry
Sydney Medical School, the University of Sydney *and*
Director, Rivendell Child, Adolescent and Family Mental
    Health Services
Thomas Walker Hospital, Sydney, Australia

Kristine Heels, RN CDE
Manager, Diabetes Clinical Services
Institute of Endocrinology and Diabetes
Sydney Children's Hospital Network (Westmead)
Sydney, Australia

Dr Anne Honey, PhD
Course Director and Senior Lecturer
Discipline of Occupational Therapy
Faculty of Health Sciences
University of Sydney
Sydney, Australia

Dr Alison G Hoppin, MD
Associate Director for Pediatric Programs
Massachusetts General Hospital Weight Center *and*
Instructor in Pediatrics, Harvard Medical School
Boston, MA, USA

Dr Lee Hudson, MBChB MRCPCH FRACP
Honorary Consultant Paediatrician
University College London Hospital *and*
Research Fellow in Adolescent Medicine
UCL Insitute of Child Health, London, UK

Dr Marc S Jacobson, MD
Director, Pediatric Metabolic Medicine
Prohealth Associates, LLP
Lake Success, NY, USA

Clinical Associate Professor Alyson Kakakios, MBBS FRACP
Head, Department of Allergy and Immunology
Sydney Children's Hospital Network (Westmead)
Sydney, Australia

Dr Melissa Kang, MB BS MCH
Senior Lecturer
Department of General Practice
Sydney Medical School
University of Sydney
Sydney, Australia

Patricia Kasengele, MSP BASW
Transition Coordinator
Western Area
Transition Network
NSW Agency for Clinical Innovation (ACI)
Sydney, Australia

Dr Andrew Kennedy, MB BS FRACP
Paediatrician and Adolescent Physician
Department of Paediatric and Adolescent Medicine
Princess Margaret Hospital for Children
Perth, Australia

Dr Siah Kim, MBBS BSc(Hons)
Department of Nephrology
Sydney Children's Hospital Network (Westmead)
Sydney, Australia

Dr Emily Klineberg, BPsych PhD
Marie Bashir Clinical Research Fellow
Academic Department of Adolescent Medicine
Sydney Children's Hospital Network (Westmead)
Sydney, Australia

Clinical Associate Professor Michael R Kohn, FRACP FACPM
Senior Staff Specialist, Department of Adolescent Medicine
Sydney Children's Hospital Network (Westmead) *and*
Clinical Associate Professor, Faculty of Medicine
University of Sydney, Sydney, Australia

Professor Gwynnyth Llewellyn, PhD MEd BA GradDip ContEdDip OT
Director, Centre for Disability Research and Policy
Faculty of Health Sciences
University of Sydney
Sydney, Australia

Dr Cameron Ly, MBBS MM(RES) FAFRM(RACP)
Director, Adolescent Medicine
Sydney LHD and South Western Sydney LHD *and*
Department of Adolescent and Transition Medicine
Royal Prince Alfred Hospital
Sydney, Australia

Dr Richard G MacKenzie, MD CM FAAP FSAHM
Associate Professor, Pediatrics and Medicine
Keck School of Medicine, University of Southern California *and*
Deputy Director, Division Adolescent Medicine
Children's Hospital Los Angeles, Los Angeles, CA, USA

Dr Sloane Madden, MB BS FRANZCP
Head, Department of Psychological Medicine
Sydney Children's Hospital Network (Westmead)
Sydney, Australia

Dr Annabel Magoffin, MBBS MMed(Clin Epi) FRACP
Staff Specialist in Gastroenterology
Department of Gastroenterology
Sydney Children's Hospital Network (Westmead)
Sydney, Australia

Dr Ann Maguire, MB BaO BCH MRCP(UK) GradDip(Clin Epid)
    FRACP PhD
Staff Specialist Paediatric Endocrinologist
Institute of Endrocrinology and Diabetes
Sydney Children's Hospital Network (Westmead)
Sydney, Australia

Dr Kim Matthews, BPharm MBBS FRANZCOG CREI MRM
Fertility Specialist
Next Generation Fertility
Paediatric and Adolescent Gynaecology
Sydney Children's Hospital Network (Westmead)
Sydney, Australia

Dr Damien McKay, MBBS BAppSC(Physiotherapy)
    MSpMEd FRACP
Staff Specialist Paediatrician, Emergency Department
Paediatric Sports Medicine Fellow, CHISM
Sydney Children's Hospital Network (Westmead)
Sydney, Australia

Dr Bronwyn Milne, BSc(Med) MBBS FRACP MPH
Staff Specialist, Service of Addiction Medicine for Youth
Department of Adolescent Medicine
Sydney Children's Hospital Network (Westmead) *and*
Staff Specialist, Youth Drug and Alcohol Service Centre
  for Addiction Medicine
Nepean Blue Mountains Local Health District
Sydney, Australia

Dr Siobhain Mulrennan, MBChB MRCP(UK) MD FRACP
Cystic Fibrosis and Respiratory Medicine Consultant
Adjunct Clinical Senior Lecturer UWA
Sir Charles Gairdner Hospital
Nedlands, Perth, Australia

Associate Professor Craig F Munns, MBBS PhD FRACP
Senior Staff Specialist, Bone, and Mineral Medicine and Endocrinology
Institute of Endocrinology and Diabetes
Sydney Children's Hospital Network (Westmead)
Sydney, Australia

Dr Mugur Nicolae, MD FRACP
Cardiologist Adult Congenital Heart Unit
The Prince Charles Hospital
Brisbane, Australia

Professor Jennifer O'Dea, BA GradDipNutr&Diet MPH PhD
Professor in Health Education and Nutrition
Faculty of Education and Social Work
University of Sydney
Sydney, Australia

Dr Bhavna Padhye, FRACP
Senior Fellow of Oncology
Sydney Children's Hospital Network (Westmead)
Sydney, Australia

Dr Donna M Palmer, BA(Hons) PhD
Research Affiliate
Westmead Millennium Institute *and*
University of Sydney (Westmead)
Sydney, Australia

Associate Professor Donald Payne, MD FRACP FRCPCH
Consultant Paediatrician and Adolescent Physician
Department of Paediatric and Adolescent Medicine
Princess Margaret Hospital School of Paediatrics and Child Health
University of Western Australia
Perth, Australia

Dr Jorge L Pinzon, MD FRCPC FAAP FSAHM
Paediatrician — Adolescent Medicine
Alberta Children's Hospital *and*
Clinical Associate Professor
University of Calgary, Calgary, Canada

Associate Professor Dorothy Radford, AM MBBS MD FRCPE
    FRACP DDU FCSANZ
Director of Adult Congenital Heart Unit
The Prince Charles Hospital
Brisbane, Australia

Fiona Robards, BSc MA MAATH MHA MPH
Manager, NSW Centre for the Advancement of Adolescent Health
Sydney Children's Hospital Network (Westmead) *and*
Clinical Senior Lecturer, General Practice
University of Sydney, Sydney, Australia

Professor David Sillence, MBBS MD FRACP FRCPA FAFPHM FAFRM
Professor of Medical Genetics
Head, Discipline of Genetic Medicine
Sydney Medical School, University of Sydney
Consultant Clinical Geneticist
Sydney Children's Hospital Network (Westmead) *and*
Department of Genetic Medicine, Westmead Hospital
Sydney, Australia

Dr Davinder Singh-Grewal, MBBS FRACP MMedSci(ClinEpi) PhD
Staff Specialist Paediatric Rheumatologist
Sydney Children's Hospital Network (Randwick and Westmead) and
    John Hunter Children's Hospital *and*
Senior Clinical Lecturer, University of Sydney, University
    of New South Wales and University of Western Sydney
Sydney, Australia

Associate Professor Rachel Skinner, MBBS PhD FRACP
Deputy Postgraduate Coordinator
Discipline of Paediatric and Child Health
University of Sydney *and*
Adolescent Physician
Sydney Children's Hospital Network (Westmead)
Sydney, Australia

Grahame H H Smith, FRACS
Lecturer, Discipline of Paediatrics and Child Health
University of Sydney *and*
Head of Urology
Sydney Children's Hospitals Network (Westmead)
Sydney, Australia

Dr Helen Somerville, MBBS Master of Paediatrics (UNSW)
Senior Lecturer, Diploma of Child Health
University of Sydney *and*
Developmental and Disability Physician
Sydney Children's Hospital Network (Westmead)
Sydney, Australia

Dr Shubha Srinivasan, BSc(Med) MBBS PhD MRCP(UK) FRACP
Paediatric Endocrinologist
Institute of Endocrinology and Diabetes
Sydney Children's Hospital Network (Westmead)
Sydney, Australia

Dr Jean Starling
Child and Adolescent Psychiatrist
Director, the Walker Unit, Concord Centre for Mental Health *and*
Clinical Senior Lecturer, Discipline of Psychiatry
Sydney Medical School, University of Sydney
Sydney, Australia

Associate Professor Stephen Stathis, MBBS FRACP FRANZCPCert
ChildAdolPsych DTM&H MSc
Director, Child and Family Therapy Unit
Royal Children's Hospital
Melbourne, Victoria, Australia

Professor Kate Steinbeck, MBBS PhD FRACP
Medical Foundation Chair in Adolescent Medicine
University of Sydney *and*
Academic Department of Adolescent Medicine
Sydney Children's Hospital Network (Westmead)
Sydney, Australia

Dr Michael Stevens, AM MBBS FRACP
Senior Staff Specialist
Oncology Unit
Sydney Children's Hospital Network (Westmead)
Sydney, Australia

Tegan Sturrock, RN BN MPH
Clinical Nurse Consultant
Department of Adolescent and Transition Medicine
Royal Prince Alfred Hospital
Sydney, Australia

Dr Joan-Carles Suris, MD PhD
Research Group on Adolescent Health
Institute of Social and Preventive Medicine
Centre Hospitalier Universitaire Vaudois
University of Lausanne
Lausanne, Switzerland

Dr John Wei-Liang Tan, BSc MBBS FRACP DcH
Fellow, Department of Immunology and Allergy
Sydney Children's Hospital Network (Westmead)
Sydney, Australia

Clinical Professor Susan J Towns, MBBS FRACP MMH
Adolescent Physician, Paediatrician
Head, Department of Adolescent Medicine
Sydney Children's Hospital Network (Westmead)
Sydney, Australia

Dr Paul Turner, BM BCh MRCPCH FRACP PhD
Clinical Lecturer in Immunology
Institute of Child Health, London, UK

Dr Rameswaran (Ramesh) Vannitamby, BMBS(Flind) FRANZCP MPH
Clinical Lecturer, Discipline of Psychiatry
Sydney Medical School, University of Sydney *and*
Staff Specialist, Mental Health Service
Liverpool Hospital, Sydney, Australia

Professor Karen Waters, MBBS FRACP PhD GCCM
Head, Sleep Medicine (Respiratory Support Service)
Sydney Children's Hospital Network (Westmead) *and*
Conjoint Professor of Paediatrics
University of Sydney, Sydney, Australia

Dr Richard Webster, MBBS MSc FRACP
Paediatric Neurologist
Sydney Children's Hospital Network (Westmead)
Sydney, Australia

Dr Eric C Weiselberg, MD
Assistant Professor of Pediatrics
Division of Adolescent Medicine
Hosfstra North Shore-LIJ School of Medicine *and*
Director, Deaf Health Services
Steven and Alexandra Cohen Children's Medical Center of NY
North Shore-LIJ Health System
New Hyde Park, NY, USA

Dr Sandra Whitehouse, MBBS MD FRCPC MALS
Clinical Associate Professor
Division of Adolescent Health
Department of Paediatrics
University of British Columbia
Vancouver, Canada

Professor Leanne M Williams, PhD
Professor in Cognitive Neuropsychiatry
Director, Brain Dynamics Centre
Westmead Millennium Institute and
University of Sydney (Westmead)
Sydney, Australia

Dr Michelle Yeo, MBBS FRACP PhD
Paediatrician and Consultant in Adolescent Medicine
Centre for Adolescent Health
Royal Children's Hospital
Melbourne, Victoria, Australia

Chapter 1

Normal Physical Development
and Growth at Puberty

Geoffrey Ambler

1. Introduction

Puberty is the biological process in which children undergo physical and sexual maturation with the ultimate attainment of adult body characteristics and reproductive capability. It includes primary sexual development (gonadal and genital growth and maturation), secondary sexual development (such as sexual hair development, female breast development, and male voice changes), accelerated height and weight growth and changes in the body composition. Crucially, these biological changes occur in the context of a complex process of psychosocial and cognitive maturation. As well as the hypothalamic–pituitary–gonadal axis, puberty involves a coordinated response from other hormonal systems including the growth hormone and adrenal axes.

The following terms are often encountered in the description of puberty and related processes:

- Thelarche — the onset of breast development in girls.
- Pubarche — the onset of sexual hair development in boys or girls.
- Menarche — the onset of the first menstrual period in girls.
- Gonadarche — the onset of mature gonadal function (sperm production in boys or ovulation in girls).
- Adrenarche — the onset of adrenal androgen production in boys or girls.

2. The Physiology of Puberty

2.1. *Activation of the Hypothalamic–Pituitary–Gonadal Axis*

The onset of puberty is activated through the central nervous system and requires pulsatile secretion of the hypothalamic hormone gonadotropin releasing hormone. GnRH secretion is controlled by the GnRH 'pulse generator' which has been localised to the arcuate nucleus. Pubertal activation of the GnRH pulse generator is through the effects of the neuropeptide kisspeptin and its G-protein coupled receptor. Other gene products and receptors involved include GnRH, GnRH receptor, FGFR1, leptin, and the leptin receptor.

With the onset of puberty, pulsatile GnRH secretion increases in frequency and amplitude, at first during the night. With progression through puberty, there is a relatively greater rise in luteinising hormone pulses and levels than follicle stimulating hormone levels in both sexes as a result of GnRH stimulation.

Sex steroid secretion rises progressively in puberty in association with the rise in gonadotropin secretion. In girls, LH secretion induces the production of androstenedione and testosterone in the ovarian theca cells and FSH induces the aromatase enzyme in follicular cells to produce oestradiol. Oestradiol induces breast development, changes in body shape and composition, a growth spurt, and then growth plate fusion through its effects on growth plates (epiphyses). In early puberty, oestradiol secretion is greatest at night, but subsequently increases during the daytime hours with menarche usually occurring after a year-long rise in daily oestradiol secretion. From late puberty, a series of negative and positive feedback loops that alter gonadotropin secretion are responsible for the mature reproductive cycle. This includes oocyte development, ovulation, and menses, which continues cyclically unless pregnancy occurs (Chapter 50).

In boys, pulsatile gonadotropin secretion induces testicular enlargement and function. LH stimulates the Leydig cells to produce testosterone and maintain spermatogenesis, while FSH stimulates the Sertoli cells and initiates and regulates spermatogenesis, although there is integration of these two systems at several levels. Testosterone (itself and through local tissue conversion to dihydrotestosterone) is the predominant hormone responsible for male virilisation, body composition changes and growth spurt. Oestradiol production (through aromatisation of testosterone and androstenedione) is still responsible for growth plate closure. The hormone Inhibin B progressively rises in boys also, indicating integrity of seminiferous tubule function.

2.2. *Adrenarche*

The word adrenarche describes the increase in the secretion of the relatively weak adrenal androgens (predominantly DHEA, DHEAS and androstenedione) that commonly precede the true onset of puberty. Adrenarche is frequently the cause of the first signs of secondary sex characteristics (in particular pubic hair, axillary hair, oiliness of skin, mild acne and apocrine body odour). Adrenal androgens continue to rise through late puberty. Premature adrenarche is a normal variant condition (Chapter 20). Adrenarche (premature or normal) merges into the processes of true central puberty as the gonads become the predominant source of androgens. The control of the onset of adrenal androgen production remains poorly understood although it is believed to be independent of and not required for gonadarche.

2.3. *The Growth Hormone Axis*

In addition to activation of the gonadal and adrenal axes, puberty involves a coordinated increase in the activity of the growth hormone axis. There is a 2–4 fold increase in GH secretion during puberty and this parallels the growth spurt and hence occurs earlier in girls than boys. The increase in GH secretion is mediated by sex steroids. Increased secretion of GH stimulates increased production of insulin-like growth factor-1, mainly from the liver. Serum IGF-1 levels peak markedly with puberty and parallel sexual development and growth velocity. Levels are also significantly influenced by nutrition, general health, and liver function (lower in under-nutrition and ill-health). IGF-1 production is also directly stimulated by sex steroids in some tissues, especially cartilage. Growth hormone as well has direct effects on some tissues that are not mediated via IGF-1. Thus, the growth axis, in coordination with sex steroids, acts through endocrine, autocrine, and paracrine mechanisms.

Leptin, a hormone secreted mainly by adipose tissue, also increases during puberty and is known to have a role in regulation of weight gain, initiation of puberty, sexual development and changes in body composition. Leptin levels are strongly correlated with body mass index; its role in the initiation of puberty is thought to be permissive rather than primary.

3. Timing of Puberty and Secular Trends

It has been estimated that 50%–80% of the timing of puberty is determined by genetic factors, although the specific genetic factors responsible are not well characterised. In a number of countries the age of menarche declined from approximately 15.5 years in the mid-19th century and plateaued at approximately 12.7 years in the mid-20th century, although there are suggestions that it has risen again slightly in recent years. Suggested recent trends in earlier onset of puberty and menarche are likely to be related to overweight, but in females only. It should be noted that all such data analyses are limited by methodological issues and that no adequate data exist to assess secular trends for boys. There is also evidence for chronic family stress being associated with earlier menarche. Several studies have shown that girls who are adopted internationally into Western countries have significantly early puberty and an increased incidence of precocious puberty, compared to those immigrating with their families. In boys, excess weight gain in childhood may have the opposite effect with a relatively later onset of puberty. Endocrine-disrupting chemicals have also been proposed as being associated with earlier puberty (for example phthalates, phytoestrogens and polychlorinated biphenyls) although evidence is limited. Ethnic differences are well recognised in the timing of puberty; for example African American girls have earlier pubertal onset than white American girls.

4. Physical Changes of Puberty

Although wide variations occur in the timing of onset and tempo of puberty, the sequence of pubertal events is usually fairly orderly and predictable in both males and females. The stages of progression of secondary sexual characteristics in males and females were first comprehensively described by Tanner. Tanner staging descriptions and charts exist for pubic hair in males and females, breast staging in females and genital staging in males (Figs. 1 and 2). For the purposes of describing the timing and sequence of physical changes in puberty in the next sections, composite data are described from Tanner and other studies that reflect those widely used in clinical practice.

In addition to Tanner staging, there are other useful measures of pubertal progress. Measurement of testicular size in males is particularly useful to assess the onset and progression of puberty. This is best performed using an orchidometer. Stretched penile length can also be measured, if there is a concern, and compared to available standards, although this is not

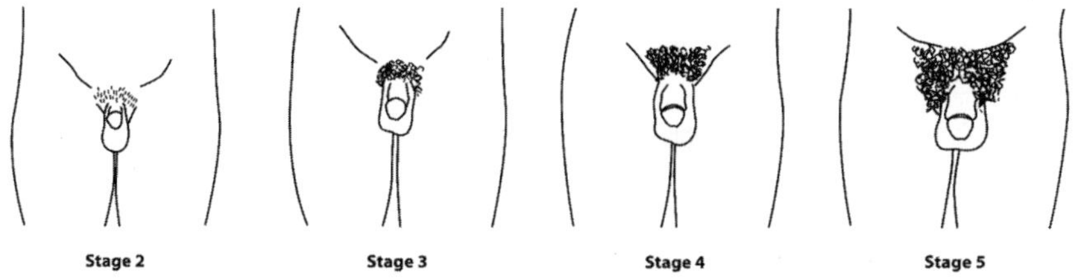

Genital Staging
Stage 1: Pre-adolescent. Testes, scrotum and penis are of about the same size and proportion as in early childhood.
Stage 2: Enlargement of scrotum and testes. The skin of the scrotum reddens and changes in texture. Little or no enlargement of the penis at this stage.
Stage 3: Enlargement of the penis, which occurs at first mainly in length. Further growth of testes and scrotum.
Stage 4: Increased size of the penis with growth in breadth and development of glans. Further enlargement of testes and scrotum; increased darkening of scrotal skin.
Stage 5: Genitalia adult in size and shape.

Pubic Hair Staging:
Stage 1: Pre-adolescent. The vellus over the pubes is not further developed than that over the abdominal wall, i.e. no pubic hair.
Stage 2: Sparse growth of long, slightly pigmented, downy hair, straight or slightly curled at the base of the penis.
Stage 3: Considerably darker, coarser and more curled. The hair spreads sparsely over the junction of the pubes.
Stage 4: Hair now resembles adult in type, but the area covered by it is still considerably smaller than in the adult. No spread to the medial surface of the thighs.
Stage 5: Adult in quantity and type. Spread to the medial surface of the thighs but not up the linea alba or elsewhere above the base of the inverse triangle.
Stage 6: Spread up the linea alba (80% of males)

Fig. 1: Genital and pubic hair staging in males (Tanner staging). Normal data on pubertal timing in boys are relatively few, however the mean age of achieving a testicular volume of 4 ml is reported to be 11.5–12 years (normal range 9.5–13.5 years). While the tempo of puberty can vary considerably, the average time for the completion of genital development is three years (range 2–4.7 years), although growth of the testes to adult volumes occurs over 5–7 years. The average adult testis is an ellipsoid with a volume of 18 ml (range 12–30 ml) and mean adult penile length is approximately 13 cm (range 10.5–15.3 cm).

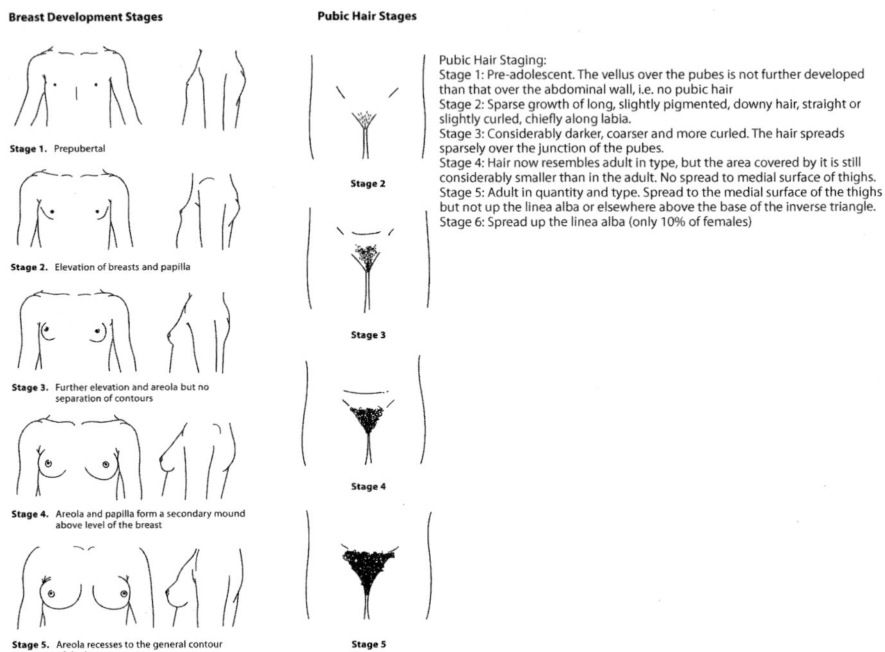

Fig. 2:   Genital and pubic hair staging in females (Tanner staging).

routine. In girls, ovarian ultrasound is a relatively simple and accurate measure of ovarian size when needed to evaluate gonadal development. Axillary hair is staged as (1) no hair, preadolescent; (2) scanty growth of slightly pigmented hair; or (3) hair, adult, in quantity and quality.

4.1. *Physical Changes in Boys (see Fig. 1 and Table 1)*

The earliest sign of puberty in boys is generally defined as testicular enlargement to ≥3 ml volume, although achieving 4 ml or longitudinal axis measurement of 2.5 cm is used by others. Testicular enlargement is an indicator of pulsatile gonadotropin secretion. Most of the increase in volume (approximately 70%) relates to development of seminiferous tubules and Sertoli cells, with Leydig cells occupying only a small volume. Testicular enlargement usually precedes significant pubic hair or genital growth. Pubic hair is less reliable as a marker of onset of puberty, since this may

Table 1: Approximate timing of key pubertal events in males (composite data).

Event	Mean age (years)	Normal age range
Onset of testicular enlargement to ≥3 ml	11.8	9.5–13.5
Genital stage 2	11.8	9.0–14.0
Pubic hair stage 2	12.2	10.2–14.2
Gynaecomastia (occurs in 75%)	13.2	11.7–14.8
Genital stage 3	13.3	11.8–15.0
Spermarche (first detection of sperm in centrifuged morning urine samples)	13.5	11.7–15.3
First enlargement of larynx/voice beginning to break	13.5	11.6–15.7
Maximum height velocity and weight gain	13.5	11.6–15.2
Testes volume 10–12 ml	13.5	11.5–15.5
Pubic hair stage 3	13.9	12.1–15.8
Onset of axillary hair	14.0	11.8–16.2
Deepening of voice	14.1	12.3–15.8
Pubic hair stage 4	14.7	13.9–16.5
Onset of facial hair growth	14.9	12.7–17.0
Genital stage 5	15.1	13.0–17.5
Pubic hair stage 5	15.3	13.9–17.0
Onset of chest hair	16.5	15.0–18.0
Peak muscle strength	22.0	18.0–25.0
Peak bone mass	24.0	20.0–25.0

result from the normal (or early normal variant) physiological rise in adrenal androgen secretion (adrenarche) which may precede true puberty. Tanner described the typical succession of changes in genital and pubic hair staging in male puberty as shown in Fig. 1.

In the male breast, the areola enlarges and darkens in puberty. Transient pubertal gynaecomastia starting in early to mid puberty is reported to some degree in up to 75% of boys and usually regresses within two years (Chapter 20). Other changes of puberty continue into the late teenage years, including increasing facial, chest and body hair as well as increases in muscle bulk and strength. Typical chronology of key pubertal events in males is summarised in Table 1.

4.2. *Physical Changes in Girls (see Fig. 2 and Table 2)*

The appearance of the breast bud (Tanner stage 2) is usually the first sign of female puberty, reported to occur at a mean age of 10.9 years (normal range 8.0–13.5 years). However, appearance of pubic hair may sometimes precede this, presumably of adrenal origin. Early breast changes can be asymmetrical and this may be a source of concern to girls and parents, but is a common normal variant. The changes in breast and pubic hair staging as described by Tanner are shown in Fig. 2.

During puberty, under pulsatile gonadotropin stimulation, the ovaries enlarge from an individual pre-pubertal volume of less than 1.5 ml to reach mean post-menarchal volumes of 8 ml (range 2.5–20 ml) when measured by ultrasound. The uterus also matures with the body of the uterus enlarging and endometrium forming in late puberty. The first menstrual period is reported to occur at a mean of 12.7 years, although there is wide variability. The time from onset of breast development to menarche in girls is variable, but averages approximately two years. The typical chronology of key events of pubertal development in girls is shown in Table 2.

4.3. *Growth and Body Composition at Puberty*

The pubertal growth spurt is a major physical change of puberty. Up until the commencement of puberty, there are minimal differences in height or weight between boys and girls. Girls commence puberty on an average two years earlier than boys and also achieve peak height velocity and final height approximately two years earlier. Peak growth velocity in girls occurs early in puberty (Stage 2–3), on average at 11.5 years (range 9.5–13.5 years), with a peak whole year height velocity averaging 8.2 cm/year (range 6.1–10.4 cm/year). In boys, peak growth velocity occurs in mid to late puberty (Stage 3–4, testicular volume 10–12 ml), on average at 13.5 years (range 11.5–15.2 years) with a peak averaging 9.6 cm/year (range 7.2–12.0 cm/year). This means that for a short period,

Table 2: Approximate timing of key pubertal events in females (composite data).

Event	Mean age (years)	Normal age range
Onset of breast development stage 2 (breast budding)	10.9	8.0–13.5
Pubic hair stage 2	11.2	8.0–13.5
Maximum height velocity	11.5	9.5–13.5
Breast stage 3	12.0	9.8–13.9
Pubic hair stage 3	12.0	9.5–14.0
Maximum weight velocity	12.5	9.5–15.0
Onset of axillary hair	12.7	11.5–14.5
Menarche	12.7	10.0–16.0
Breast stage 4	12.8	10.5–15.5
Pubic hair stage 4	13.2	11.0–15.6
Regular menstrual cycles	14.0	12.0–18.0
Breast stage 5	14.9	12.0–17.0
Pubic hair stage 5	14.5	12.5–17.0
Peak muscle strength	20.0	16.0–22.0
Peak bone mass	22.0	20.0–25.0

girls are taller and heavier than boys, but on average by 13.5 years, boys are passing girls in height and weight (Fig. 3). On average, boys gain 28 cm in puberty and girls 20 cm. The average mean difference between adult male and female height is approximately 13 cm. These are indicative data only and there is clearly population and ethnic variation.

Body composition in childhood varies minimally between the sexes. Female infants have slightly more body fat and less fat-free (lean) mass than males, but these become comparable in early and mid-childhood. By late childhood (10 years), girls again have slightly more fat mass and slightly less fat-free mass. Marked changes in body composition develop during puberty, with major sex differences. During puberty, males gain greater amounts of fat-free mass and skeletal mass, whereas females acquire significantly more fat mass. Total fat-free mass is stable by 15–16 years in females and 17–19 years in males, reflecting the time of final height attainment and the majority of bone mineral accretion. In early adulthood, males have an average of 20 kg greater fat-free mass than females and 5–6 kg more absolute fat mass. Body proportions and fat

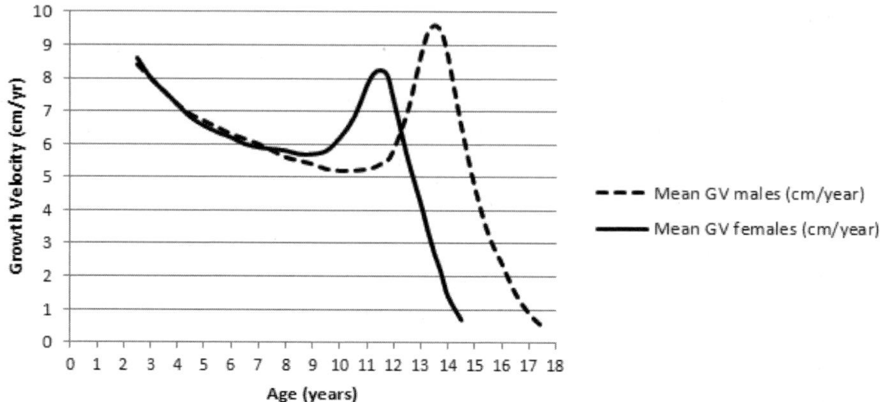

Fig. 3:   Mean growth velocity in males and females.

distribution change during the pubertal years as well, with males assuming a more android body shape and females assuming a more gynaecoid shape.

Bone mass is acquired steadily in childhood and rapidly in adolescence, proportional to increases in fat-free mass. Pre-pubertal males have slightly greater total body bone mineral content and bone mineral density than pre-pubertal females. Approximately 25% of total adult bone mass is laid down in the two years spanning peak growth velocity in boys and girls. Bone mineral status correlates with pubertal staging and with sex steroid levels. By the end of puberty, 90% of peak bone mineral density has been achieved, with the remainder gained in the late teens and early twenties. Delayed puberty is associated with delayed acquisition of bone mass (Chapter 37).

4.4. *Practical Clinical Assessment of Puberty*

There is frequently a need to assess the progress of puberty in the context of concerns about the progress or timing of growth or puberty or in the evaluation of syndromes and chronic disease.

4.4.1. *History*

The history should include the timing of onset of any pubertal signs, any observations about growth pattern, parents' and siblings' heights, family history of timing of puberty and fertility, any exogenous hormone exposure, and history of any chronic disease symptoms (including neurological or visual symptoms and sense of smell). Information on pubertal timing is more accurate in mothers who recall the events of onset of breast development and particularly onset of menarche. There is no reliable event that is recalled to time male puberty; fathers tend to recall pubertal progression more vaguely and usually their strongest recollection is if they had delayed puberty or growth spurt. Age of first shaving regularly or of the voice breaking may be recalled.

4.4.2. *Physical examination*

Available growth data for the adolescent (and parents) should be plotted on the appropriate growth charts. The approach to further physical examination needs to be sensitive. The clinician should ensure as best possible that there has been an appropriate explanation to the young person with agreement and understanding of why puberty staging is needed in their medical care. The general examination and puberty staging is generally performed with parents or caregivers in the room, with the curtain drawn if that additional privacy is requested. Sometimes young people may request that their parents wait outside or request another chaperone.

For puberty staging, the standard Tanner staging system is used as described in the previous sections. Additionally in boys, testicular volume should be measured using an orchidometer or alternatively measuring the longitudinal axis of the testes. The left testis usually hangs lower than the right after puberty and the consistency of the testes should also be noted, since small testes which are unusually firm or soft are abnormal. A minor degree of asymmetry of the testes in boys is relatively common during normal puberty (with the right testis often being slightly larger). Also, in girls, breast development may start asymmetrically, but persistent major asymmetry is uncommon.

Other secondary sexual characteristics or signs of androgenisation (normal or abnormal) should be noted in both sexes. In males, assess for facial and body hair, acne, voice quality, musculature, body shape, and gynaecomastia. Similarly in females, assess for facial and body hair (which may indicate virilisation), acne and body shape. In both males and females, palpation of breast tissue assists in the assessment of the relative amounts of glandular tissue and adipose tissue, with glandular tissue having a firmer texture than adipose tissue.

Puberty staging can usually be performed quickly and easily in the context of a general examination. The usual practice is to talk to the young person through each step of any examination so that they feel comfortable and they know what is happening and with the aim of minimising any embarrassment or other concern. In situations where young people decline pubertal examination, self-staging can be performed by having the subject compare with Tanner charts, although this has limited reliability.

References

Auchus RJ. (2011) The physiology and biochemistry of adrenarche. *Endocr Dev* **20**: 20–27.

Biro FM, Lucky AW, Huster GA, Morrison JA. (1995) Pubertal staging in boys. *J Pediatr* **127**(1): 100–102.

Buckler JM. (2007) Growth at adolescence. In: Kelnar CJH, Savage M, Saenger P, Cowell C (eds), *Growth Disorders*, pp. 150–164. Hodder Arnold, London.

Desmangles J-C, Lappe JM, Lipaczewski G, Haynatzki G. (2006) Accuracy of pubertal tanner staging self-reporting. *J Pediatr Endocrinol* **19**(3): 213–221.

Divall SA, Radovick S. (2009) Endocrinology of female puberty. *Curr Opin Endocrinol Diabetes Obes* **16**(1): 1–4.

Gajdos ZK, Hirschhorn JN, Palmert MR. (2009) What controls the timing of puberty? An update on progress from genetic investigation. *Curr Opin Endocrinol Diabetes Obes* **16**(1): 16–24.

Lewis K, Lee PA. (2009) Endocrinology of male puberty. *Curr Opin Endocrinol Diabetes Obes* **16**(1): 5–9.

Loomba-Albrecht LA, Styne DM. (2009) Effect of puberty on body composition. *Curr Opin Endocrinol Diabetes Obes* **16**(1): 10–15.

Marshall WA, Tanner JM. (1969) Variations in pattern of pubertal changes in girls. *Arch Dis Child* **44**(235): 291–303.

Marshall WA, Tanner JM. (1970) Variations in the pattern of pubertal changes in boys. *Arch Dis Child* **45**(239): 13–23.

Rogol AD. (2010) Sex steroids, growth hormone, leptin and the pubertal growth spurt. *Endocr Dev* **17**: 77–85.

Tanner JM. (1962) *Growth at Adolescence.* Oxford Blackwell Scientific.

Zachmann M, Prader A, Kind HP, Hafliger H, Budliger H. (1974) Testicular volume during adolescence. Cross-sectional and longitudinal studies. *Helv Paediatr Acta* **29**(1): 61–72.

Chapter 2

The Normal Development
of the Adolescent Brain

Donna M Palmer and Leanne M Williams

1. Introduction

Adolescence is a time of intensive change and reorganisation of brain networks as these develop from childhood, through adolescence and into young adulthood. Those networks involved in emotion processing undergo a particularly pronounced degree of change. A hallmark of many psychological and psychiatric disorders is their onset in adolescence. These disorders are typically characterised by emotional problems, with core dysfunctions in the interpretation and regulation of emotion, and flow on effects to social functioning. This chapter will focus on the brain changes that continue to take place across adolescence and the implications of these changes for understanding healthy emotional functioning and dysfunction disorders.

2. Brain Development

The brain develops at different rates according to the region of the brain involved. Some regions reach an adult level of maturity by late childhood, while others continue to develop across adolescence and into young adulthood.

15

Even though there are different rates of change throughout the brain, all brain regions follow a similar progression of phases: an initial rapid formation of synaptic connections in early childhood, which stabilises for a period of time and is then followed by the loss (or 'pruning') of synapses that are redundant or unnecessary. Brain development is also characterised by the parallel formation of a myelin sheath coating around the external layer of connective tracts throughout the brain.

In combination, these changes give rise to a greater efficiency of cognitive processing. Initial synaptic generation in childhood is thought to support rapid learning and accumulation of knowledge. The subsequent pruning of redundant synaptic connections enables cognitive processes to then become more focused, by eliminating excess neural activity and competing responses, and thereby allowing the remaining connections to be reinforced and to operate faster and more efficiently. The parallel increase in myelin enables faster communication along brain pathways, by improving the conduction speed of electrical signals that travel along connective tracts, and this further boosts the efficiency of cognitive processes.

The following sections provide more details about the pruning and myelination that occur in adolescence.

2.1. *Synaptic Pruning*

The process of initial synaptic generation and subsequent synaptic pruning takes place at different rates for different brain regions, following a posterior to anterior (back to front) and ventral to dorsal (lower to higher) trajectory. Primary sensory cortices located in the posterior region mature the fastest, and support basic processes of hearing, vision, and touch. One of the fastest developing regions is the primary visual cortex, reaching an adult level of maturity by around 10–11 years of age. Frontal and parietal association cortical regions follow a slower developmental course, continuing to mature well into young adulthood.

Functionally, cortical synaptic loss gives rise to a shift in brain organisation and the way that incoming information is processed. In middle to late childhood, electrical brain activity in response to external stimuli is characterised by an excitatory and simple mode of processing, with comparatively little inhibition. In early adolescence, this mode of processing shifts to becoming relatively more inhibitory, complex, and also faster, reflecting a mode of cognitive processing that is more focused and efficient.

2.2. *Myelination*

The trajectory of myelin sheath development has some similarities with synaptic generation and pruning. The majority of subcortical regions cease myelination within infancy and early childhood, supporting automatic relaying of sensory input. By contrast, myelin thickness for short-range axonal connections within the cortex increases steadily from early childhood until young adulthood. Some long-range connections between cortical and subcortical regions also continue myelination across adolescence and early adulthood. These include long-range thalamo–cortical tracts, particularly those projecting to frontal and posterior association areas critical for efficient cognitive processing. These connections also include tracts from the brainstem reticular formation that have extensive direct connections to the thalamus and cortex, which allow rapid 'alerting' of the cortex when significant sensory input is detected.

The functional impact of this myelination of thalamo–cortical tracts is an improved speed of communication between subcortical and cortical regions that mediate a wide range of information processing. The speed with which communication between subcortical and cortical regions is cycling can be directly measured by the electroencephalograph. In the EEG trace there is a prominent peak of activity that occurs in the EEG power spectrum within the alpha frequency band (around 8–12 Hz; 10 Hz is 10 cycles a second). This measure is called 'alpha peak frequency', and faster cycling is indicative of more rapid communication and better performance during cognitive tasks. The alpha peak frequency speeds up with maturation until middle to late adolescence, arguably reflecting the contribution of myelination of long-range thalamo–cortical connective tracts across this period.

3. The Influence of Brain Changes on Cognitive Development in Adolescence

Neuroscience is increasingly demonstrating that cognitive abilities continue to develop throughout adolescence and into early adulthood, reflecting the ongoing brain development that also occurs across this period. This evidence challenges presumptions from several decades ago that the brain was fully formed by early adolescence.

Throughout adolescence and into early adulthood, synaptic pruning and myelination give rise to a shift in the way that brain activity is organised — from a childhood pattern of 'localised' activity to an adult pattern of more 'integrative' global networks for cognitive processing. This shift in brain organisation contributes to a corresponding shift in cognitive development. In younger childhood, cognitive development primarily involves the *acquisition* of new knowledge and skills (via the generation of new synaptic connections). In adolescence, cognitive development is about an efficient *integration* of previously acquired skills and knowledge with new learning and behaviour, by engaging a more network-driven mode of processing (via the more rapid engagement of the frontal cortex in cognitive processing, enabled by myelination of connective tracts), and more specialised processing within each of the focal regions that form these networks (via the elimination of excess synaptic connections).

Cognitive functions that continue to develop throughout adolescence include information processing efficiency, inhibitory control of impulsivity and emotional functioning.

3.1. *Rapid Engagement of Frontal Regions*

This shift to an integrative network-driven mode of cognitive processing, and the corresponding late development of these cognitive functions, have largely been attributed to the ongoing development of the frontal cortex from both synaptic pruning and myelination. It is expected that this continued development of the frontal cortex has the greatest impact on shifting to a network-driven mode of processing in early adolescence, followed by a refining of this system throughout middle to late adolescence.

The effects of frontal development on integrative processing are most effectively demonstrated for inhibition of impulsive responses. Children show an impulsive style of responding with a lack of inhibition, relying mostly on localised posterior parietal regions for this task. Across adolescence there is a shift away from this localised processing towards increasingly greater engagement of the frontal cortex, and by adulthood we mainly recruit frontal regions (particularly the dorsolateral prefrontal area) and can more effectively inhibit impulsive responses.

This shift to more rapid engagement of the frontal cortex is also evident in changes in emotion processing. Frontal inhibition has a widespread effect on the way that threat-related and other emotionally significant information is processed, in that automatic 'alerting' activity can be contextualised and dampened down more rapidly when needed.

Similarly, ongoing myelination of frontal connective tracts is linked to specific aspects of late cognitive development. Maturational increases in myelin thickness of fronto–striatal tracts are directly associated with faster reaction times for a variety of cognitive tasks that engage the same frontal regions. Improvements in spatial working memory (where multiple pieces of information can be deployed and manipulated) are also linked to the myelin thickness of fronto–parietal fibre tracts connecting the specific cortical regions engaged by this task. Enhanced memory abilities and executive functioning are associated with greater myelin in frontal and temporal association areas.

4. Development of the Emotional Brain in Adolescence

Emotional functions are a prominent domain of cognition that show continued development across adolescence. The ongoing development of these functions involves the same brain changes (frontal cortex and long range connections) that are implicated in other domains of adolescent cognitive development. Emotional functioning plays a key role in most psychological and psychiatric disorders of childhood and adolescence, particularly for those that typically first emerge during the adolescent period. The onset and course of these disorders may be influenced by the developmental brain changes underlying emotional functioning across this time.

4.1. *The Emotional Brain*

The concept of emotional function used here extends beyond traditional concepts focused on feeling states and their regulation. It considers emotion as the spectrum of perceptions, reactions, feelings, and regulatory mechanisms that all involve the same underlying brain networks. From this view, emotional functions are defined as those that are core to our most fundamental motivational goals — to minimise exposure to danger or threat, and to maximise exposure to reward or pleasure.

This spectrum also considers a time scale of emotional functions, from those that occur automatically, to those that rely on feedback about experienced feelings, and ultimately those that require decisions over time about how to regulate reactions and feelings.

Three aspects of emotion-related brain function are considered here:

- Nonconscious: automatic aspects of emotion-related processing (very early processing of emotionally significant information that occurs without conscious awareness).
- Conscious: controlled or explicit aspects of emotion-related processing (the way that emotionally significant information is used to interpret perception and experience, and to make decisions that require conscious awareness and feedback).
- Self-regulation: regulation of emotion processes over longer time scales (the capacity to manage emotional reactions in order to find a balance between reacting to automatic input and engaging controlled functions).

4.1.1. *The nonconscious emotional brain in adolescence*

Myelination of long-range tracts contribute to changes in nonconscious emotional brain functions across adolescence, such as the automatic functions of perception and reaction to emotionally significant information.

These automatic functions are mediated by very early activation of emotional brain networks, within a fifth of a second (200 milliseconds). Brain activity within this time frame reflects a combination of the early perception of significant emotion cues, and the brain's hardwired reaction to these. Within 200 ms the brain can detect low level cues that are significant indicators of potential threat, such as a sudden sound or wide-open eyes in fearful facial expressions. Some cues are innate to humans, while others are created as a result of experience or repetition over time to act like innate cues. Detecting these cues trigger automatic reactions in the brain, starting in subcortical regions and rapidly travelling to the cortex along long-range connective tracts. Developmental changes in early automatic processing in adolescence reflect both the development of the brain networks themselves and the contribution of the adoloscent's experiences.

Development of the connections from the brainstem's ascending reticular activating system to the cortex, and particularly the frontal cortex, most likely contribute to the changes in automatic emotion processing over adolescence. The greatest impact of this shift arguably occurs at the onset of adolescence. In late childhood it takes longer than 300 ms for the frontal cortex to be engaged by this rapid alerting system, whereas by early adolescence the frontal cortex is engaged by this rapid alerting system within 150 ms. This earlier frontal engagement is understood to enable automatic 'alerting' activity to be contextualised and dampened down more rapidly when needed, or acted upon more quickly in the presence of immediate threat.

4.1.2. *The conscious emotional brain in adolescence*

Conscious processing of emotion relies on feedback from the cortex and on the strength of long-range cortical–subcortical connections. Development of the frontal cortex and myelination of these connective tracts almost certainly influence this stage of emotion processing, to enhance efficiency and accuracy of processing.

Conscious processing of emotional input extends from 200 ms onwards, and encompasses the initial conscious evaluation of significant information and any associated cognitive decisions and/or behavioural responses, as well as any consciously experienced emotion states. Conscious processing involves feedback from cortical activation back to subcortical regions, and lateral feedback within the cortex, enabling conscious awareness and the capacity for conscious thinking and feeling processes. These feedback processes allow individuals to be aware of their emotional reactions, and to register the context of emotion input in order to make conscious decisions about how to respond. These processes are highly important for response inhibition, and for contextualising felt emotions.

Perceptual improvements have been observed between adolescence and young adulthood in brain activity related to the processing of facial expressions of emotion. Young adults engage prefrontal cortical regions in this task more than do adolescents, as well as engaging the hippocampus to a greater extent, reflecting the process of integrating contextual information from previous learning experiences. These improvements are likely due to continued myelination of both long-range thalamo-cortical fibre tracts and connections within the hippocampus itself. Corresponding improvements also occur in both the speed with which this brain activity occurs, and the accuracy with which the facial emotions are identified.

4.1.3. *Self regulation and the emotional brain in adolescence*

Developmental changes in myelination of long-range fibre tracts, and within the frontal cortex itself, also contribute to improvements in self-regulation of emotion across adolescence and into young adulthood.

Self regulation acts to evaluate and contextualise aspects of thoughts and feelings in terms of a person's self-concept and place in time, and to take consequent action (cognitive or behavioural) to satisfy motivational needs associated with the minimisation of danger and maximisation of reward. These actions may be changes in the way that an individual behaves or plans for the future, or more subtle changes on the cognitive level such as the way that an individual thinks about issues or events.

Self regulation involves ongoing interactions between subcortical and cortical (primarily frontal) regions, as well as communication between separate regions within the frontal cortex. This ongoing activity particularly involves interactions between frontal areas for significance processing, such as the medial prefrontal cortex and orbital frontal cortex (for danger and reward, respectively), and memory updating areas such as the hippocampus and dorsolateral prefrontal cortex.

Successful self regulation relies upon a concept of self identity and a comprehensive understanding of place in time, both of which develop considerably across late childhood and adolescence. An important aspect of the development of self identity in this period is the additional development of specific memory abilities. For example, comprehensive autobiographical memory, which develops around mid-adolescence, enables the self to be compared with others across multiple experiences. At the level of brain structural changes, increased connectivity between the subcortical hippocampus and frontal cortical regions would support this ability to integrate and evaluate new information in the context of long term situations, relative to current place in time and sense of self. This enhanced memory ability also enables aspects of thoughts and feelings to be evaluated over a longer period of time, in greater depth and within a wider context. The impact of these emerging memory abilities during adolescence has been proposed to influence the emergence of psychological disorders during this maturational period.

Increased connectivity between the frontal cortex and subcortical regions also enables greater inhibitory control of cognition and behaviour. In combination with the development of a greater awareness of sense of self and place in time, this allows short term rewards to be sacrificed for the attainment of larger long term rewards, such as the attainment of material objects, or the inhibition of short term behaviours in order to maintain relationships or to align with aspects of self-concept. This development of inhibitory control continues throughout adolescence, and does not reach maturity until early adulthood.

More localised changes within the frontal cortex, such as synaptic elimination, further contribute to the development of other cognitive tools necessary for the consideration and fulfilment of emotional needs over longer periods of time, such as executive abilities of goal setting and planning.

5. Summary

There are two main causes of structural change in the brain that take place during adolescence — loss of unnecessary excess short connections and greater speed of communication along long connective pathways. These changes mean that the brain becomes a much more efficient and global network for processing information, giving rise to a shift in the way that incoming information is processed, evaluated and responded to, as well as the way that longer term decisions are made.

These pathways of normal adolescent brain development are clearly variable between individuals and contribute to the diversity of developmental stage seen during adolescence. These progressive stages of brain development are associated with the ability to assess risk and to make decisions which impact on safety. There is still much to be learnt about how environmental exposures such as alcohol and other drugs and chronic illness affect brain development during adolescence and whether these trajectories of brain development can be substantially altered by specific therapeutic manipulation.

References

Benes FM. (1998) Brain development, VII. Human brain growth spans decades. *Am J Psychiatry* **155**(11): 1489.

Bohn A, Berntsen D. (2008) Life story development in childhood: The development of life story abilities and the acquisition of cultural life scripts from late middle childhood to adolescence. *Dev Psychol* **44**(4): 1135–1147.

Casey BJ, Giedd JN, Thomas KM. (2000) Structural and functional brain development and its relation to cognitive development. *Biol Psychol* **54**(1–3): 241–257.

Clark CR, Paul RH, Williams LM, Arns M, Fallahpour K, Handmer C, Gordon E. (2006) Standardized assessment of cognitive functioning during development and ageing using an automated touch screen battery. *Arch Clin Neuropsychol* **21**(5): 449–467.

Gordon E, Barnett KJ, Cooper NJ, Tran N, Williams LM. (2008) An "integrative neuroscience" platform: Application to profiles of negativity and positivity bias. *J Integr Neurosci* **7**(3): 345–366.

Huttenlocher PR. (1990) Morphometric study of human cerebral cortex development. *Neuro-psychologia* **28**(6): 517–527.

Klimesch W. (1999) EEG alpha and theta oscillations reflect cognitive and memory performance: A review and analysis. *Brain Res Brain Res Rev* **29**(2–3): 169–195.

Luna B, Sweeney JA. (2004) The emergence of collaborative brain function: FMRI studies of the development of response inhibition. *Ann N Y Acad Sci* **1021**: 296–309.

Luna B, Thulborn KR, Munoz DP, Merriam EP, Garver KE, Minshew NJ, Keshavan MS, Genovese CR, Eddy WF, Sweeney JA. (2001) Maturation of widely distributed brain function subserves cognitive development. *Neuroimage* **13**(5): 786–793.

Sowell ER, Delis D, Stiles J, Jernigan TL. (2001) Improved memory functioning and frontal lobe maturation between childhood and adolescence: A structural MRI study. *J Int Neuropsychol Soc* **7**(3): 312–322.

Williams LM, Gatt JM, Hatch A, Palmer DM, Nagy M, Rennie C, Cooper NJ, Morris C, Grieve S, Dobson-Stone C, Schofield P, Clark CR, Gordon E, Arns M, Paul RH. (2008) The integrate model of emotion, thinking and self regulation: An application to the "paradox of ageing". *J Integr Neurosci* **7**(3): 367–404.

Williams LM, Mathersul D, Palmer DM, Gur RC, Gur RE, Gordon E. (2009) Explicit identification and implicit recognition of facial emotions: I. Age effects in males and females across 10 decades. *J Clin Exp Neuropsychol: Official J Int Neuropsychol Soc* **31**(3): 257–277.

Yakovlev PI, Lecours AR. (1967) The myelogenetic cycles of regional maturation of the brain. In: Minkowski A (ed.), *Regional development of the brain in early life*, pp. 3–70. Blackwell Scientific Publications, Oxford.

Chapter 3

Normal Psychosocial Development in Adolescence

David Bennett and Richard G MacKenzie

1. Introduction

Adolescence is the period of transition from childhood to adulthood, of variable duration and with variable rates of change. Variably synchronised development occurs in the following domains:

- Physical — puberty (physical growth, secondary sexual characteristics, and reproductive capability).
- Psychological — development of independence and autonomy.
- Cognitive — moving from concrete to abstract thought.
- Emotional — shifting from narcissistic to mutually caring relationships.
- Social — peer group influences, formation of intimate relationships, decisions about future vocation.

It is the adaptation and integration of these attributes into a sense of self that generates the tasks of adolescence. In an age of rapidly evolving technology, however, the challenges of adolescent development have become more complex and traditional models may no longer be totally valid. Powerful underlying forces influenced by the speed of communication, exposure to a diversity of lifestyle choices, along with a significant consumer role, have greatly influenced the trajectory to adulthood.

New insights from research in brain development (Chapter 2) also challenge our old models and intellectual complacency. Knowing and recognising the 'anatomy' of development is integral to the understanding of the bio–psychosocial model of adolescent development.

2. Modern Concepts of Adolescence

The modern understanding of youth in terms of 'adolescence' is a comparatively recent phenomenon, emerging only at the beginning of the 20th century. In most societies, perceptions of 'adolescence' are evolving and not all societies view young people in the same way, some not even seeing the need to define anybody as 'youth' or 'adolescent'. Adolescence, as a psychosocial process, is usually viewed as being triggered by the apparent and measurable biological onset of puberty, leading to highly variable social transitions that mark its completion. In more recent times, the period of transition from childhood to adulthood has become prolonged for both males and females, allowing for broader influences and trends, with subsequent implications for emotional and social well-being. For instance, in pre-industrial societies, the duration of adolescent transition between puberty and the assumption of adult roles, as defined by marriage and/or parenthood, ranged from approximately two years in females to four years in males. In today's developed economies, with extended periods in education, greater affluence and the availability of effective contraception, adolescence may persist for well over a decade. Maturation of reproductive capacity may precede role transitions into parenthood and marriage by more than a decade. This is not only exceptional in human history, but also may lead to risky behaviours, disease or other unwanted outcomes.

3. Normal Adolescent Development

Adolescence, a distinct and significant period of life, has been formally described by Ingersoll as the beginning of

> *. . . a period of personal development during which a young person must establish a sense of individual identity and feelings of self-worth which include an alteration of his or her body image, adaptation to more*

mature intellectual abilities, adjustments to society's demands for behavioural maturity, internalising a personal value system, and preparing for adult roles.

In short it is an experience that is biologically driven, behaviourally expressed, and socially defined. Theoretically, the ebb and flow of the developmental progression typical of adolescence are replaced by the relative consistency and assumption of responsibility generally characteristic of young adulthood onwards. That is to say, within the context of the existing social ecology, the young person in transition variably seeks stability (settling down) through a stable relationship, career preparation, and (hopefully) employment.

3.1. *Developmental Stages*

Psychosocial development can also be highly variable in terms of progression from one stage to the next or the order in which these stages occur. Physical, cognitive, and psychological changes may be 'out of sync'. For example, an early-developing, physically mature girl may be psychologically/emotionally unprepared for the social and sexual attention directed at her, leaving her vulnerable to relationships and behaviours that may put her at risk. Adolescence is usually seen as spanning three periods.

3.1.1. *Early adolescence (10–13 years)*

Predominant issues are the new bodily sensations during puberty and a preoccupation with defining a personal normal self. Same sex peers then become all-important for comparison and validation. Opposite sex peers generally become the indicator and litmus tests of success. High levels of physical activity and out-of-the-ordinary behaviours are common. Illness may lead to a distortion of body image and perceived imperfection leading to isolation from peers. Transitional behaviours often become impulsive and exaggerated. Comparing self with others, real or imagined, may lead to unacknowledged anxieties or moods.

3.1.2. *Mid-adolescence (14–16 years)*

The major focus is on validating oneself and developing a sense of well-being separate from parents and family (individuation). Peers become all important as individuation begins to be expressed as independence. Validation of self as a worthwhile person now becomes the driving force behind behaviours, motivation, and social comfort. Continuing brain maturation expresses itself in a growing ability to reason and think 'outside the box', often with a self-centred quality. Onset of illness during adolescence may bring about enforced dependency or result in less acceptance by peers, experiences that may be especially difficult to handle.

3.1.3. *Later adolescence and young adulthood (17–26 years)*

Orientation is towards defining one's functional role in terms of ongoing education, work, lifestyle, and relationship plans. There is a degree of psychological autonomy, a realistic body image, and a more comfortable sense of one's sexual identity. Relationships increasingly demonstrate mutual caring and responsibility. Illness may result in reduced vocational options, and an increasing dependence with a growing sense of inadequacy, often expressed through anger and non-compliance. Concerns about relationships in the present and future and potential for child-bearing may predominate.

3.2. *Psychosocial Development and Behaviour*

As adults are required to have certain competencies, the successful completion of developmental tasks is a universal process for adolescents and young adults in our society. These tasks include:

- The formation of self-identity and affirmation of a growing self esteem.
- Actualisation of self as a sexual and gender-affirmed being.
- Accomplishing autonomy embedded in an interdependent lifestyle and, ultimately, independent living.
- The achievement of a healthy sense of self.
- The ability to form healthy relationships with same sex and opposite sex peers.

- The development of a personal ethos and a set of moral beliefs and standards.
- The acquisition of a life purpose or vocation that supports assumed responsibilities.

Of all these developmental tasks, of paramount importance is the evolution of a sense of identity and self-worth. Essentially, the adolescent must gain a sense of who they are as a validated and acknowledged, effective individual, separate from the family. Young people need to become aware of their strengths and weaknesses, their likes and dislikes, a sense of personal values, and a consistent projection of self to others. Erik Erikson described adolescent development as a conflict between identity formation and identity confusion. He suggested the process as one of active searching and experimenting with identities. This focus on selfish experimentation in pursuit of self-definition often leads to conflict with parents, challenging of authority, a need for privacy, emotional outbursts, intense interest in peer activities, and the taking of risks. The successful achievement of identity brings autonomy, better control over impulses (largely related to neurobiological development), a decrease in self-absorption, resistance to peer conformity, and more harmonious relationships within the family.

Young people typically experiment with new activities and challenges, testing their limits, exploring yet unproven skills, and taking pleasure in the associated excitement and freedom. Learning to appreciate the normal highs and transcend the lows of life is also part of growing up. Moodiness is a common feature of adolescence, but is normally short lived and forgotten easily. Other behaviours, as listed in Table 1, justify greater concern.

3.3. *Neurocognitive Development*

Based on observational studies, the Swiss psychologist Piaget proposed the classic accepted theory of cognitive development. He proposed four stages that are qualitatively different from each other, culminating in what he called 'formal operational thinking' or, put simply, the ability to think abstractly. He suggested that for most adolescents, neurocognitive

Table 1: Adolescent behaviours.

Normal adolescent behaviours	**Worrying behaviours**
Moodiness, flare ups, open and talkative with friends, monosyllabic with family, active striving for independence, trying new experiences, need to be like peers, sleeping in, critical, and argumentative.	Wild mood swings, dramatic and/or persistent behaviour change, self-neglect, isolation from peers or healthy peer activities, failing school performance or dropout, violent or aggressive behaviour, dangerous drug and/or alcohol use, loss of routine, excessive sleeping or difficulty getting to sleep, being withdrawn or secretive.

changes occur that allow them to now think beyond the real world. They are thus able to embrace concepts and ideas and to reason and hypothesise in a more sophisticated manner than younger children whose thinking is more here-and-now, 'show me', concrete thinking. However, our own experience tells us that not all individuals pass through these stages in the way Piaget precisely described them. With some children, abstract thinking may develop and be expressed during the pre-adolescent years. And interestingly, up to 15% of adults remain predominately concrete thinkers leaving them at somewhat of a loss to grasp theoretical concepts or base present decisions on possible future risk.

Adolescents also come to enjoy thinking about their own thoughts, or thinking about thinking. This can make them at times appear pensive and self-centred. Elkind described this self-focus as the 'personal fable' — the tendency to think of themselves as unique, with special qualities that make them indestructible. They sense an 'imaginary audience' — the belief that everybody is watching them — which often manifests as an excruciating self-consciousness. Over time, with increasing security around their own sense of self, often gained through life experience, these beliefs abate.

More recently, findings of brain magnetic resonance imaging have increased our understanding of how behaviours may relate to brain development (Chapter 2). The longitudinal effects of puberty hormones, and the importance of biological windows in which behaviours can most effectively develop, still need to be researched.

The development and maturation of executive function is interdependent with evolving impulse control, emotional regulation, and motivation. In other words, the adolescent brain is a 'work in progress' — the highest-level areas may not be completely mature until the mid to late twenties. Clinically, this means that while teenage brains may be developing in a way that makes their owners more open to ideas and more amenable to change (and increased opportunity), it also makes young people more likely to experiment, seek high excitement activities, and take risks (with possible increased danger).

The prefrontal cortex has been called 'the area of sober second thought' (or reasoning) with resultant better judgments and behavioural control. Continuing maturation processes provide insight into some of the erratic and otherwise 'infuriatingly normal' behaviour typical of early adolescence. Since adolescence tends to be a time of demand for increased freedoms and decreased parental monitoring, these findings may also suggest that at times young people may be given more freedom than they can handle. It is important to realise that the relationship between functional neurobiological findings and changes in thinking and functioning have not been fully elucidated. Clearly, major changes in cognitive abilities occur throughout the adolescent years that are quantitative and that lead to improvements in memory, inductive reasoning, and information processing.

3.4. *Moral Development*

Stages of adolescent moral development grew out of Piaget's concepts (page 31). Most would agree that moral development is a product of cognitive and social development. A young person's moral development involves an increasing sense of their own values, thinking, life challenges, and sense of self. As adolescents mature, they acquire an increased sense of empathy and the ability to see things from another's perspective. This assists them in making moral judgements. Stanrock describes young people's moral development as involving their thoughts, behaviours, and feelings. A young person's reasoning or discerning right and wrong helps them to determine: the right thing to do; their behaviour or how they actually act in a given situation (especially one that holds a moral dilemma); how they feel about moral issues; and is the anticipation of feeling guilty about doing 'the wrong thing' acting as a deterrent. Adolescents may also develop an interest in broader community values and societal issues, often enjoying the process of being politically active or environmentally aware, volunteering, or showing an interest in religion. This may reflect an advanced stage of moral development — one that values society as a whole with a desire for betterment.

4. Adolescence in Broader Contexts

Young people are not a homogeneous group — there is enormous diversity, regardless of where they happen to live. The needs of boys and girls differ throughout adolescence, and gender inequity continues as a cultural–religious reality in most countries, including Australia. The periods of early, middle, and late adolescence, as described previously, are widely recognised in Western countries as corresponding roughly with phases in physical, psychological, and social development.

An individual's personal potential, immediate environment, and the presence of risk and protective factors create obvious differences. For example, the lives of young people of lower socio–economic status are different from those of wealthy communities. The same can be said for the lives of indigenous young people, those living in remote areas, youth surviving on the streets of major urban centres, youth seeking asylum from countries in social or political unrest, sexual minority youth, young people with chronic and disabling conditions, or those deprived of their liberty.

As noted by Bennett & Eisenstein, maturation rates vary among young people and there may be 'maturational asynchrony' with chronological age, biological age, affective/emotional age, academic age, or social/survival age differing radically among individual youths.

- A 14 year old boy living on the streets is likely to be short, thin, pubertally delayed, and possibly illiterate, but with natural smartness and well-developed survival and social skills.

- A 15 year old female of privileged background might be overweight, emotionally dependent, and academically and socially underachieving in a private school.

Notwithstanding such examples of diversity, the core experiences of adolescence are remarkably similar, with major commonalities transcending individual, cultural, and social diversity. All young people, for example, have to negotiate a path between pressure to conform and achieve and the need to establish a separate, individual identity. Adolescence highlights the inevitable struggle between inner drives, their social ecology, and outside expectations.

4.1. *Family, School, and Peers*

4.1.1. *Family and parenting*

While young people want close relationships with their parents, there is often tension related to their struggle for individuation, independence, freedom, control, and privacy. The rules and limits that parents need to negotiate require ongoing review and refinement as a young person matures. Teenagers need the sense of security that comes from structure as well as sufficient room to move as they stretch their wings and develop. Evidence suggests that knowing what parents require and expect of them (mature and responsible behaviour, for example) does provide some protection against risky behaviour.

Styles of parenting have been identified and researched in terms of outcomes. An *authoritative style* where a parent is nurturing, attentive, empathic, and affectionate, sets fair and consistent limits in negotiation with their adolescent, and monitors the young person's behaviour (high warmth, high regulation), is the most effective. This warm, firm, and confident approach also accepts the young person's evolving need for psychological autonomy. As Steinberg describes, adolescents from authoritative homes achieve more in school, report less depression and anxiety, score higher on measures of self-reliance and self-esteem, and are less likely to engage in anti-social behaviour, including delinquency and drug use. They also show more positive social behaviour, self-control, cheerfulness, and confidence. Other parenting styles, including *laissez-faire/permissive* (high warmth, low regulation), *chaotic/neglectful* (low warmth, low regulation), or *authoritarian* (low warmth, high regulation) are less effective. Authoritarian parenting with its inconsistency, predominant focus on discipline and punishment but with a lack of care and warmth, has been shown to actually drive adolescents to behave in anti-social and self-destructive ways. Certain factors may influence a parent's ability to provide a supportive relationship. These include such things as poverty, marital conflict, mental health problems, and substance use issues.

4.1.2. *School*

Young people are keen to have experiences that allow them to develop mastery, control, and confidence. Schools provide such opportunities and contribute to a young person's resilience and safety through fostering a sense of achievement and self-efficacy in the context of a positive school ethos. Research shows that, together with parent–family connectedness, perceived school-connectedness (having a sense of belonging at school, feeling recognised and respected) is protective against nearly all risky behaviours (except pregnancy). The most effective interventions around adolescent well-being are those where parents and educators work together.

4.1.3. *Peer group*

For young people, belonging to a peer group provides a sense of identity and feelings of social acceptance, with peer pressure providing a powerful impetus to behave in certain ways. Peer consensus is powerful, sometimes the primary authority for teenagers, rather than traditional authority figures such as doctors. Communication with the young person should aim to empower them and, as much as possible, give them control (Chapter 5). Given the intrinsic altruism of young people, providing opportunities for them to participate in community activities where they are making a true contribution to support and change, adds much to their sense of value, personal power, and self-concept.

4.2. *Impact of Cultural Background*

Puberty is a biologically universal phenomenon, but the broader concepts of adolescence differ between cultures. The expectations, roles, and duration of adolescence may differ significantly. Cultural norms and life experiences (such as being a refugee or migrant, having a chronic illness or disability) will affect the timing of developmental milestones and significantly shape expectations of what is considered 'normal'. The nature of the fundamental psychosocial tasks which the young person must negotiate in their progression towards maturity, and the importance placed upon their achievement, can vary greatly between Western and non-Western cultures.

- In Western culture, the individual is generally paramount and young people are encouraged to develop independence from an early age.
- In non-Western collective cultures, ethnic identity and allegiance to the family and community are more greatly valued as a rule, and play a central role in shaping the development of the adolescent's identity.

In Australia, adolescents from non-English speaking backgrounds face the challenge of dealing with the tasks of adolescence while growing up between two cultures. This involves not only two languages, but also different behavioural and social expectations. Subtle stressors (personal, peer, family and social) influence decisions about ethnic identity and working out how they can remain connected to their culture of origin and also determine their place within the new culture. The adolescent may be torn between the family's expectations about maintaining the values and customs of their 'old' culture, and experience 'extreme' parental restrictions and close monitoring, while striving to adopt the norms of the new culture in order to fit in with their peers. Young women in particular may be subject to stricter controls, especially if parents feel threatened by their exposure to the more hedonistic values of the new culture.

Those young people who manage to retain the most important elements of their ethnic culture, while developing the skills to adapt to the new culture, appear to cope best in their psychosocial adjustment. Often these young people may be seen as having a dual identity — the one they present to their family and community, and the other to their peers and others they relate to in the new society. Health practitioners also need to be aware of the health issues and needs of indigenous young people and the impact of culture on the presentation, diagnosis, and treatment of their health problems.

4.3. *Growing Up in a Rapidly Changing World*

The past 50 years have seen technological, social, and political changes unparalleled in human history. Through the global spread of telecommunications and its associated portable technology, along with travel, tourism, and migration, the world has shrunk, and the rate of change continues to accelerate. More than ever before, young people know a great deal about the concerns and aspirations of their peers wherever they happen to live in the world, particularly through music, television, mobile phone technology, and the internet.

The impact of new media on young people growing up today has generated much interest and concern. Many have drawn a link between the media, body image, and significant health effects. At the same time, there is an increasing digital divide between parents, teachers, and young people as they struggle to negotiate appropriate access to and supervision of new media. Parents and health professionals need to play a more active role in facilitating conversations about new media to help young people develop media literacy skills.

5. Conclusion

The clinician is in the unique position to engage trust, establish meaningful relationships, and have a positive influence on the health behaviours of young people. Experience has taught us that transitions facilitate behaviour change. Adolescence is one of those transitions. Understanding normal psychosocial development or 'anatomy' and the impact of the new social ecology on its universal processes and challenges affords a golden opportunity to provide integrative care. One needs, then, to ideally address all domains of health in a manner that focuses not only on treatment but also on prevention and health promotion.

References

Bennett DL, Eisenstein E. (2001) Adolescent health in a globalised world: A picture of health inequalities. In: Alderman EM, Brown RT (eds.), *Adolescents, families and societies in the new millennium, adolescent medicine: State of the art reviews,* pp. 411–426. Hanley and Belfus Inc., Philadelphia.

Bennett DL, Kang M, Chown P. (2006) Cultural diversity in adolescent health care. In: Greydanus DE (ed.), *Essential adolescent medicine*, pp. 43–50. McGraw-Hill, New York.

Carlson N, Buskist W. (1997) *Psychology: The science of behaviour*, 5th ed. Needham Heights MA, Allyn and Bacon, USA.

Elkind D. (1978) Understanding the young adolescent. *Adolescence* **13**: 127–134.

Giedd JN. (2004) Structural magnetic resonance imaging of the adolescent brain. *Ann N Y Acad Sci* **1021**: 77–85.

Ingersoll GM. (1989) *Adolescence,* 2nd ed. Englewood Cliffs, Prentice-Hall, NJ.

Marsella AJ, Yamada AM. (1999) An introduction and overview of foundations, concepts and issues. In: Cuellar I, Paniagua F (eds.), *Handbook of Multicultural Mental Health Assessment and Treatment of Diverse Populations.* Academic Press, New York.

Patton GC, Viner R. (2007) Pubertal transitions in health. *Lancet* **369**(9567) 1130–1139.

Piaget J. (1970) *Science of Education and the Psychology of the Child* (translated by Coltman D). Orion Press, New York.

Rowe L, Bennett DL, Tonge B. (2009) *I Just Want You to be Happy: Preventing and Tackling Teenage Depression.* Crows Nest, Allen & Unwin, Australia.

Schmitt KL, Dayanim S, Matthias S. (2008) Personal homepage construction as an expression of social development. *Dev Psychol* **44**(2): 496–506.

Stanrock JW. (2007) *Adolescence,* 11th ed., McGraw Hill, Boston.

Steinberg L. (2001) We know some things: Parent–adolescent relationships in retrospect and prospect. *J Res Adolesc,* **11**(1), 1–19.

Chapter 4

Body Image Issues in Adolescents

Jennifer O'Dea

1. Introduction

Body image and self-esteem are prominent issues for young people, particularly during adolescence as they experience the physical changes associated with puberty. Westernised societies are known to produce an unhealthy pursuit of the 'perfect' slim or muscular body. This unrealistic ideal creates unnecessary pressure on young males and females to engage in social comparison and can lead to profoundly negative effects on well-being, via the development of poor body image, high body dissatisfaction, and low self-esteem. These changes are linked to both the development of eating disturbances and physical health problems.

2. Definition of Body Image

Body image encompasses the mental picture we have of our bodies and how we feel about our bodies. Body image incorporates a concept or scheme including a collection of feelings and perceptions such as awareness of the body, perception of body boundaries, attention to various parts of the body as well as the whole, perception of size of parts and the whole, position in space and gender-related perceptions. Body image thus includes an individual's perception and judgment of the size, shape, weight, and any other aspect of their body that relates to body appearance. Body dissatisfaction is defined as 'a person's negative thoughts and feelings about his or her own body.'

3. Presentation of Body Image Problems in Clinical Practice

3.1. *Concerns in Girls*

In clinical practice, adolescents and/or their parents may present with concerns about recent weight loss or a request for weight loss advice and/or medications. Commonly, the young person with body image concerns is overweight or obese and is seeking weight loss, but normal weight and underweight adolescents present with weight concerns as well. Body image concerns in girls are more common during and after puberty. Menarche is a point at which the clinician can expect body image concerns to arise. The expected weight gain around menarche should be discussed with the adolescent girl, as it is often an area of concern for both adolescents and their parents, who may be unduly alarmed about the normal peri-menarchal weight gain.

3.2. *Concerns in Boys*

Boys may present to the clinician with a request for weight gain information and/or concerns about their growth, height, strength, sports performance, and pubertal development. Boys may also present with weight lifting injuries with the underlying problem being their body image concerns.

Figure 1 describes the range of signs and symptoms of body image problems in both male and female adolescents. The early onset of weight and shape concerns in adolescents may progress to more serious eating disorders, so early identification, intervention, and psychological counselling are recommended.

4. Dieting and Fad Diets

Dietary restraint is one of the strongest predictors of eating disorders in male and female adolescents and it must not go unnoticed in the clinical setting (Fig. 2).

Behavioural (both sexes)
- Fad dieting: cutting out food groups; becoming vegetarian; only consuming fluids; requesting diet pills/request referral to dietician; ritualistic eating (cutting food into tiny pieces; only eating with teaspoon).
- Refusal to eat in public.
- Claims to be 'allergic' to food.
- Compulsive/excessive exercise: more than two hours a day, exercises when injured or sick.

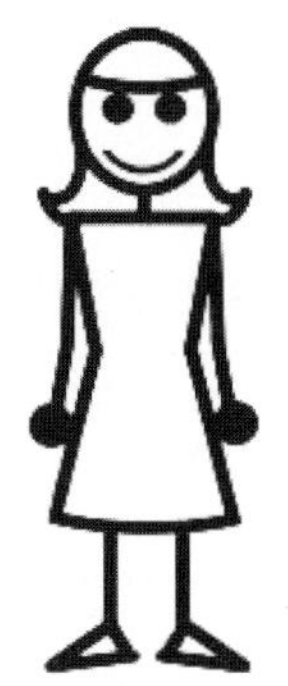

Social (both sexes)
- Avoiding social situations where food is present.
- Social isolation and withdrawal.
- Avoiding previously enjoyed activities such as sport, dance or swimming.

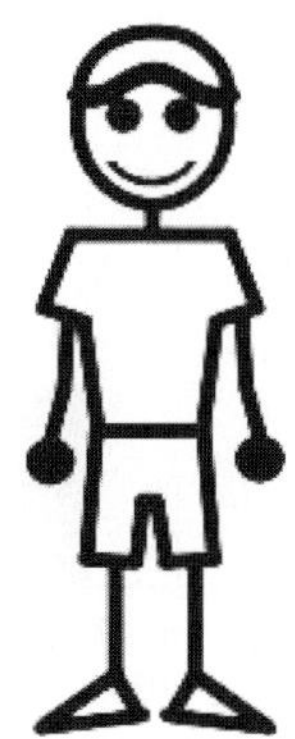

Psychological (both sexes)
- Concerned with weight and shape and appearance.
- Fear of eating and weight gain.
  - Anxiety at meal times.
  - Secretive eating.
- Low self esteem: feelings of worthlessness, guilt, shame, self loathing.
- Fear of puberty.
- Anxiety, depression, moodiness.

Fig. 1: Signs and symptoms of body image problems in male and female adolescents.

4.1. *Fad Weight Loss Methods*

Adolescents engage in a wide array of weight control methods as shown in Table 1. The clinician should ask the adolescent about their use of dangerous weight loss methods such as fasting, vomiting, laxative abuse, diuretics, amphetamines, and cigarette smoking for appetite control. These methods are used by 2%–10% of older adolescent girls and 2% of boys. Amphetamines are also used by young adults in order to prolong exercise sessions for weight loss. Diet pills and diuretics are often surreptitiously

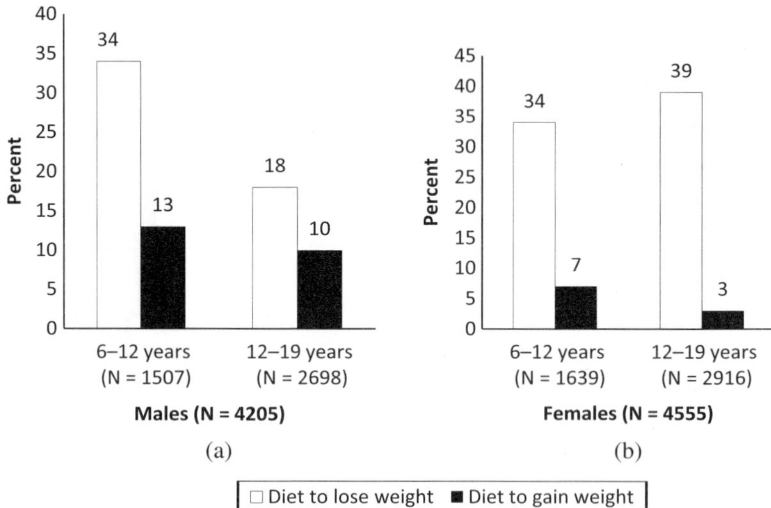

Fig. 2:　Dieting to lose weight or gain weight in a large study of male and female children and adolescents (O'Dea 2010).

obtained from the adolescent's mother, so clinicians should be careful when prescribing these medications to women with adolescents, particularly daughters.

4.2. *Dieting For Weight Gain*

Dieting for weight gain has been identified in studies of adolescent males with the major purpose of increasing strength for sports performance. A discussion with the adolescent will often enable the clinician to identify the major methods employed, including dietary methods (38% of males attempting to gain weight) which include:

- Eating more food.
- Eating protein foods such as meat and eggs, taking protein milk formulas, eating raw egg whites.
- Taking dietary supplements (creatine, amino acids, vitamins, minerals, and zinc).
- Drinking beer and sports drinks.

Table 1: Weight loss practices of male and female adolescents in the previous 12 months.

Weight Loss Method	Females (%) ($N = 2916$)	Males (%) ($N = 2698$)
Exercise	77.3	58.3
Keeping busy to avoid eating	47.2	35.8
Not eating between meals	41.9	18.9
Own diet	36.5	15.7
Drinking water before meals	36.3	27.8
Avoiding/skipping meals	30.1	10.5
Selecting only low calorie foods	16.2	8.3
Avoiding situations where there will be food	15.5	7.8
Fasting/ Starvation for 24 hours or more	15.1	4.8
Taking advantage of illness to avoid eating	14.2	5.3
Excessive exercise	13.0	18.6
Magazine or other diet	11.9	3.0
Becoming vegetarian	8.4	2.5
Vomiting	8.0	2.0
Natural laxatives to lose weight (eg prunes, bran)	6.8	4.2
Smoking to lose weight or suppress appetite	5.0	3.2
Chewing but not swallowing food	2.4	2.3
Laxatives	2.3	2.3
Slimming pills	2.2	1.3

Data are from a national study of 6,000 Australian adolescents in 2006 (O'Dea 2010).

Exercise, particularly weight lifting, is used as another means to gain weight in nearly one third of males. A concerning number of male youth (5%) report using drugs for weight gain and body building, which include 'pills' obtained from the gym, steroids, diuretics, and injecting insulin. This behaviour is additionally dangerous because they may be taking impure or veterinary compounds and because of the increased risk of needle sharing and contact with drug dealers, particularly in gyms. Other concerns for the clinician to be aware of include *Salmonella* poisoning from eating raw eggs, inadvertent fat gain from excessive food, drinks and calories, and adverse reactions to creatine monohydrate (gastrointestinal upsets, arrhythmias, renal damage).

5. Assessment of Body Image Problems in Clinical Practice

Adolescents with body image concerns may also have low self-esteem and/or psychological or psychiatric disorders such as eating disorders, depression, and anxiety. These issues should be clarified by clinical assessment and/or using standardised psychological tests. In the clinical setting, the clinician may use some quick body image assessment questions which have been previously validated against the clinical instruments. One such method is the 'score out of 10' which assesses how the adolescent perceives his or her body. The body image questions ask the adolescent to rate their physical appearance ('How you look' and 'How your body looks') using a score of zero to 10 points, with 10 being perfect. Adolescents can also rate the physical appearance scores they perceive 'other people', 'their best friend', 'the opposite sex', their mother, and their father would give them. A self perceived score of between 0 and 4 correlates well with clinical measures of low self-esteem and high scores on the Eating Disorders Inventory, Beck Junior Depression Inventory and Spielberger State and Trait Anxiety Inventory. The clinician can regularly assess this simple score during ongoing management of the adolescent over several years.

6. The Preventive Role of the Clinician

Measurement and reassurance from the clinician about the adolescent's height and weight growth, and pubertal development (Chapter 1) are helpful, and should be conducted and recorded on an ongoing basis.

Positive feedback from the clinician about gains in height are immeasurably helpful for adolescents and their parents, as is the assessment of familial body shapes and body composition as the body size, height, muscularity, and shape of adolescents is largely genetically determined. Parents and other family members should be reminded to refrain from negative comments about their adolescent's body, and also about their own as this reinforces stereotypes about the importance of physical shape or size.

Advice about a healthy lifestyle, a balanced diet, physical activity, and social/psychological health status is important for adolescents of any shape or size. Often a young person will believe that their life and popularity would be dramatically altered for the better by a change in body shape, when improving social competency, confidence in their ability to deal with issues, and physical fitness have much greater effects.

Often, the young person with body image concerns and their family will also benefit from some counselling from a dietician, as they may be receiving nutrition misinformation and undertaking fad weight loss or body building diets. Sensible nutrition information provides adolescents and their parents with the answers to many ongoing questions about weight control, body composition, pubertal growth trajectories, and what constituties a healthy diet.

References

Ackard DM, Peterson CB. (2001) Association between puberty and disordered eating, body image, and other psychological variables. *Int J Eat Disord* **29**(2): 187–194.

Cash TF, Smolak L. eds. (2011) *Body image: A Handbook of Science, Practice, and Prevention,* Guilford Press, New York.

Neumark-Sztainer D, Hannan PJ, Story M, Perry CL. (2004) Weight-control behaviors among adolescent girls and boys: Implications for dietary intake. *J Am Diet Assoc* **104**(6): 913–920.

O'Dea J. (2009) Self perception score from zero to ten correlates well with standardized scales of adolescent self esteem, body dissatisfaction, eating disorders risk, depression, and anxiety. *Int J Adolesc Med Health* **21**(4): 509–517.

O'Dea J. (2010) Studies of obesity, body image, and related health issues among Australian adolescents: How can programs in schools interact and complement each other? *J Student Wellbeing* **4**(2): 3–16.

O'Dea J, Abraham S. (1995) Should body-mass index be used in young adolescents? *Lancet* **345**(8950): 657.

O'Dea J, Rawstorne PR. (2001) Male adolescents identify their weight gain practices, reasons for desired weight gain, and sources of weight gain information. *J Am Diet Assoc* **101**(1): 105–507.

Persky AM, Brazeau GA. (2001) Clinical pharmacology of the dietary supplement creatine monohydrate. *Pharmacol Rev* **53**(2): 161–176.

Teter CJ, Mccabe SE, Lagrange K, Cranford JA, Boyd CJ. (2006) Illicit use of specific prescription stimulants among college students: Prevalence, motives, and routes of administration. *Pharmacotherapy* **26**(10): 1501–1510.

Thompson JK, Shroff H, Herbozo S, Cafri G, Rodriguez J, Rodriguez M. (2007) Relations among multiple peer influences, body dissatisfaction, eating disturbance, and self-esteem: A comparison of average weight, at risk of overweight, and overweight adolescent girls. *J Pediatr Psychol* **32**(1): 24–29.

Chapter 5

Communicating with Adolescents

Richard G MacKenzie

1. Introduction

In general, physicians are familiar with the various symptoms and medical problems that young people bring to their attention. Where they do find difficulty is in taking a coherent history, interviewing or providing some basic educational counselling to adolescents and young adults. Paediatricians, in particular, who are accustomed to talking to parents or guardians about their child's problems, are at times especially challenged when they have to talk directly to their patients. Learning professional and developmentally appropriate communication skills is one of the most important distinguishing features of incorporating young people into a practice.

It is only through good communication skills that one can obtain the necessary and often situational or contextual information that allows for the discovery of the behavioural and social influences that lead to the important integrative diagnosis. And equally important are the effective communication skills, both in words and delivery, that are needed to give information to educate and influence behavioural change. *Adolescents are naïve health care consumers. Each health care visit is a valuable opportunity to influence future health care behaviours.*

2. Setting the Stage

Some will think that in order to clearly communicate with adolescents, one must understand and almost be part of their social ecology and lifestyle. Such behaviours may actually alienate teenage patients as it may be seen as mimicry and bogus. It is not necessary to talk their language and know their slang, dress like them, or adapt to their trendy lifestyles. Be the professional that you are. That sets a clear boundary for the interaction and encourages the young person to be who they are. Learn a little of current interests and behaviours, especially those that put young people at risk. *Be wary not to act as a surrogate parent through your body positioning, facial expression, or verbal admonitions.* And, of course, if your style of communication begins to fail, be careful not to professionally 'bully' the adolescent into cooperating or being compliant.

There are attitudes and behaviours that will facilitate communication. You must like and enjoy working with this age group and be able to respect them as individuals. Understanding and clinically recognising the bio–psychosocial anatomy of the adolescent will promote objectivity in your observations, define boundaries and add clarity to communication. *Why this sensitivity and emphasis on bio-psychosocial development?* Young people challenge the health professional to think in an integrated fashion. Many of their problems are bio-behavioural in origin. The adolescent's behaviours are being established and the related influences are usually in the present. A golden opportunity exists for affecting positive change within the dynamic setting of puberty and adolescence. *This thinking in two dimensions, development, and behaviour, often challenges the skills of the health professional.*

We all have an 'adolescent within' — our own adolescent experience that we usually have not totally distanced from our present-day functions. Being mindful of this will help avoid dangerous pitfalls in judgment and voice tone that may tell the young patient that you are uncomfortable with their honesty. Your full attention must be on the teenage patient and not on the experience of your own teen years.

3. Making Contact

It is helpful to establish a routine practice on initial contact that empowers the adolescent. Often recognising the young person first, through a handshake, in the presence of a parent, guardian, or others goes a long way in establishing the special nature of the professional relationship. It also helps to separate the young patient from the parent, permitting you to establish through consent/assent a confidential relationship under which the teen can be honest. Without confidentiality, adolescents will avoid disclosure of many of their behaviours that put them at risk for disease and dysfunction.

4. Communication and the Medical Visit

Effective communication has special significance during the medical visit. Information gathering during that time guides the physical examination, and the need for additional tests that will lead to a diagnosis and ultimately treatment. It also provides a wonderful context of that individual's life and thus the perfect opportunity for risk assessment and counselling for prevention. Information gathering whether for alleviation of disease and/or anticipation of behaviour change, should always be done in a climate of empowering the young person while promoting healthy development in all domains of health — physical, psychological, social, and personal. Put simply, there are *four cardinal attributes* that health professionals must have to effectively communicate with adolescents:

- An ability to listen and hear what is being said in the context of that young person's life experience.
- The knowledge and skills to integrate the elicited information into both developmental contexts and diagnostic determinations.
- To be able to effectively summarise and feed back information, findings, diagnosis, and plans for intervention or amelioration of symptoms.
- An ability to integrate brief problem-focused counselling using motivational communication skills.

Review of systems, for example, can be done during the physical exam and appropriate, but relevant and sensitive questions can also be asked. Likewise, with practice, pertinent prevention messages can also be given.

5. Communication for Behaviour Change

Any attempts to affect behaviour are best done during periods of unsettledness, questioning, and change. Adolescence itself is embedded in biological awakening with puberty as its foundation. From the young person's point of view, this awakening leads to the desire to widen life experiences. Not unlike the inherent neuro-endocrine driving forces of puberty, there are associated inherent driving forces of the psychosocial processes of adolescence. Just as growth arrest is well documented at the biological level, similarly growth arrest can occur at the psychosocial level. This failure to move through psychological and social development may be associated with failure of biological change or completely independent of it. Young people may be mature biologically, but immature behaviourally or the converse may be true.

Within the context of the clinical visit and communication with the adolescent, it is important to *recognise the constancy of change and the innate discomfort and restlessness that it can produce*. It is this discomfort and restlessness that is realised in what they say, how they say it, their symptoms, behaviour, and other forms of expression. Blend this with the teenager's inherent increased appreciation and seeking of pleasure, simultaneous with the attainment of reproductive competence, and one can now readily recognise the probable co-occurrence of sexual and other risk behaviours.

To the astute and practiced clinician, communicating with adolescents then becomes a much more complex issue than just asking questions, documenting responses, and giving counsel. Communication becomes an art form, based in understanding the bio-psychosocial anatomy of that unique individual teenager. Understanding bio-psychosocial anatomy is similar to a surgeon understanding human anatomy and its variations in both structure and pathology. It is from this indepth knowledge of both structure and function, that the gifted surgeon is able to assess the circumstance and decide what will work best to relieve disease and dysfunction. Such will also be the experience of the knowledgeable and gifted clinician who cares for young people.

Effective communication for behaviour change is not usually time dependent, but more situation and skill dependent. The power of words and language to motivate or effect change is well known in the world of marketing and business. Success depends on this. The effective clinician who communicates for change must go beyond just education and be aware of the power of language to promote or discourage. This is a learned skill. We must appreciate the unique differences from individual to individual while at the same time recognising their similarities. *The similarities are often based in their development while the differences in their expression are based in the context of their life experience.* It is this convergence of life attributes that often leads to a multidisciplinary focused team approach in adolescent health.

6. Discovering Risk Behaviours

Adolescence is a dynamic state with expression of change through behaviour, emotion, and words — usually in that order. Young people do things for a reason. Subsequent behaviours may communicate their adaptation to or discomfort with new psychosocial demands. Supportive peers or media may further amplify dysfunctional behaviours without being offset by an aware and supportive home or social environment. *It is estimated that over 80% of problems in adolescents, whether expressed through disease or dysfunction, are greatly influenced by family, peer relationships, and school.* This realisation supports a broader view of the chief complaint to one that includes both bio-behavioural and psychosocial issues.

Thus, under most circumstances, the purpose of the interview is to gather information that will help to better understand the presenting complaint, the context in which the complaint developed, the subsequent diagnosis, and the optimal (acceptable) approach to intervention. Occasionally, the interaction may be focused on establishing a rapport or context in which the physician may provide some basic counselling. Whatever the purpose, it is helpful to have a basic understanding of brain development during the teenage and young adult years (Chapter 2). *Therefore with no fault of their own, except the dilemma of their own development, adolescents often are unable to truly understand what is being said.* In other words there may indeed be a neuro-developmentally based communication gap.

7. The Dance of the Professionals

Communication with teenagers may be seen as a dance of professionals — the health professional and the professional adolescent. It is a dance where sometimes the physician leads and sometimes the adolescent leads. The ultimate success of the dance, of course, rests with the professional.

8. Making the Visit More Rewarding

Here are 12 practical suggestions to help make the office visit more productive and rewarding:

- Initially *welcome the adolescent* with a simple gesture such as a handshake or in some way acknowledging them first. This clearly defines who is the patient. It introduces, non-verbally, the importance of collaboration in resolving the issue or problem that prompted the visit. It also highlights and empowers the teenager or young adult.
- Each young person that you see will be unique in their own way although sharing a developmental process with others of the same age. It is important to *show respect for each person and his or her life experience.* This may be quite challenging at times, particularly when their look or behaviour at the time of the visit is so different than yours at that same age.
- In a busy practice, it is helpful to *acknowledge the time limitation of the visit up front.* This minimises the possibility that the young person will feel slighted or their problem minimised or considered unimportant. It also helps you to get to the reason for the visit quickly and efficiently.
- *Be careful not to ask sensitive questions out of the blue.* Create a context if one does not already exist. If the questioning is focused on such issues as sex, drugs or other risk taking behaviours, it is important to state or reiterate confidentiality with its exceptions.

- *Avoid writing especially when asking sensitive questions.* Adolescents are naïve patients and often are unsure as to who has access to their health record. If it is important to write, it is helpful to precede this with a comment such as 'let me just make some notes to myself so I do not keep asking the same questions.'
- When asking questions, counselling or educating, *use language that the young person will understand.* Keep in mind their developmental stage, life experience, and culture. Much of this can be determined from the HEADSS Assessment outlined in Table 1.
- *Always sidestep power struggles.* These may be between the teenager and the parent/guardian, a teacher or a societal carer. Very little is to be gained from taking sides until all the information is elicited. Even then, be judicious and keep focused on what is best for your adolescent patient.
- *Always be an advocate both in words and action.* Sometimes it is so easy to give in to the system despite the unfair and negative impact it will have on the adolescent. Unfortunately, with the more complicated problems, this may take time that you do not have. Ask others, such as a nurse, social worker, front office staff, or school officials to assume responsibility and keep you informed.
- *Outline expectations of the visit.* The adolescent may have heard from friends or read about what a doctor's visit is all about and assume that is going to happen to them. This is particularly true in relation to intrusive or embarrassing aspects of the examination such as a genital or pelvic examination. Letting the young patient know what to expect will help them to focus on the present and enhance cooperation.
- *Many of the symptoms that adolescents have are psycho-physiologic in origin.* That of course is reasonable considering the psycho-biological and physical development that is taking place and the uncertainty that they have regarding what is normal. Although reassurance based upon evidence or lack thereof will help some, others will need a more creative approach. Be very careful not to dismiss the complaint with the impression that 'it is all in your head'.
- *Listen and instil responsibility by highlighting constructive behaviours.* This may be done with words or by a shift to a more attentive position with body posture or a facial expression. Unless this is a part of your everyday behaviour at first this may seem somewhat artificial, but with

Table 1: HEADSS Assessment.

H — Home

- Where do you live?
- Who lives with you?
- Do you have your own bedroom?
- Do you feel safe at home?
- How does each household member get along?
- Who could you go to if you needed help with a problem?
- Parent(s) jobs? Recent moves? Run away? New people at home?

H — Harassment

- Many young people experience bullying or teasing at school. Have you ever had to put up with this?
- Do you get worrying or stalking type emails, text messages, or 'tweets'?

H — History (Family)

- Are there any diseases that run in the family?
- Is there any history of emotional/psychiatric/psychological problems in your family (including alcoholism and substance abuse)?

E — Education/Employment

- What do you like/not like about school/work?
- What is your favourite subject?
- How do you get along with teachers/other students?
- Do you have a lot of friends at school?
- Grades, suspensions? Changes?
- If employed — what kind of work do you do? How long have you worked there?
- Do you have many friends at work? Do you get along with your coworkers?

E — Eating/Exercise

- Sometimes when people are stressed they can over eat/under eat. Have you ever experienced this?
- In general, what do you eat — Breakfast? Lunch? Dinner? Snacks?
- Eating disorders — ask about body image, pursuing thinness, the use of laxatives, diuretics, vomiting or excessive exercise, and rigid dietary restrictions to control weight.

(Continued)

Table 1:   *(Continued)*

A — Activities

- With peers? What do you do for fun? Where? When?
- With family?
- Sports — regular exercise?
- Hobbies? Do you go to many parties? What are they like?
- How much TV do you watch? Favourite music?
- Crimes? Arrests?

A — Affect

- Make a note about how they appear: Forlorn, worried, flat, happy, bright.

A — Accidents

- Do you think you are accident prone?
- Have you had many accidents? Have you been seriously injured?

A — Ambition

- What do you want to do when you have finished high school? College? University?
- How did you get interested in that particular ambition/focus?

D — Drugs/Cigarettes/Alcohol

- Many people at your age are starting to experiment with cigarettes/alcohol. Have any of your friends tried these or maybe other drugs like marijuana, IV drugs, etc.?
- How about you, have you tried any? Under what circumstances do they use? Then ask about the effects of drug taking/smoking or alcohol on them. How much are they taking and how often and has frequency increased recently?

D — Dieting

- How do you feel about your present weight? Have you been on a diet in the past year? For how long? Was it successful? How much would you like to weigh? How will you know when you are the 'right' weight?

D — Dating (This may be an outdated term and you may go to a local equivalent)

- Do you have a girlfriend/boyfriend? (Ask this question carefully so as not to assume heterosexuality). Are any of your friends dating? How do your parents feel about dating? If dating, where do you go and what do you do?

(Continued)

Table 1:   (*Continued*)

D — Driving

- Do you have your driving licence? Do you have your own vehicle? Do you wear your seat belt all of the time? Do your friends also have a car and drive? How do you handle drinking/taking drugs and driving?

S — Sexuality

- Some young people of your age are getting physically involved. Have you had a sexual experience with a guy or girl or both?
- Degree and types of sexual experience?
- Number of partners?
- Contraception?
- Knowledge about sexually transmitted infections?
- Has anyone ever touched you in a way that's made you feel uncomfortable or forced you into a sexual relationship? (History of sexual or physical abuse?)
- How do you feel about relationships in general/about your own sexuality?

S — Suicide/Depression/Mood Screen

- How do you feel right now on a scale of 1–10?
- What sort of things do you do if you are feeling sad/angry/hurt?
- Is there anyone you want to talk to?
- Do you feel this way often?
- Some people who feel really down often feel like hurting themselves or even killing themselves. Have you ever felt this way?
- Have you ever tried to hurt yourself or take your own life? What have you tried?
- What prevented you from doing so? Do you feel the same way now?

S — Safety

- Sun protection, immunisation, bullying, carrying weapons?

S — Spirituality

- Beliefs, religion, music, what helps you to relax, etc.?

---

practice and awareness it will add a rewarding dimension to the interaction between you and your adolescent and young adult patients.

- *Within the limitations of consent and confidentiality and the complexity of the presenting complaint, it may be important to include parents, guardians, and other members of the family right from the very beginning.* This helps in obtaining or expanding information about evolution of the teenager's problem or complaint. Often, parents and sometimes other family members will play a critical role in resolving bio-behaviourally based problems.

9. The HEADSS Risk Profile Assessment

In the context of a busy practice there is an efficient way to evaluate the context of a young person's presenting complaint and also develop a risk profile for present, imminent, and future problems. The HEADSS assessment (Table 1) was developed at the Division of Adolescent Medicine at Children's Hospital Los Angeles to better understand the background and risk behaviours of homeless and runaway youth. It has subsequently proven effective in developing a risk profile for all youth whether in school, employed, living at home, in detention or living alternate lifestyles. Its application fits right into the medical style of gathering information prompted by an easily recalled acronym to remind of relevant and important topical areas. In addition, it structures the assessment such that the interviewer, and the adolescent or young adult, progress from the relatively low charged subjects of home to the more difficult and often disturbing areas of drugs, sex, and suicidal ideation and attempts. This has become known as the HEADSS Risk Profile Assessment. Some typical questions are suggested, but are not all inclusive or necessarily asked of each patient.

10. Conclusion

It is tempting to rush through health care visits by adolescents as they usually have a single problem focus, or present for a general check up with a physical examination. By doing so, we miss the golden opportunity to provide critical prevention and early intervention messages. To provide this guidance does not need to take an excessive amount of time. The outlined communication skills can be integrated into existing practice and personal style. Including the HEADSS Assesment Risk Profile in each clinical contact will do much to identify risk, while at the same time demonstrating a genuine interest and concern. It will add a new dimension and personal satisfaction to each visit to your office by your young patients.

References

Cavanaugh RM Jr. (1986) Obtaining a personal and confidential history from adolescents. An opportunity for prevention. *J Adolesc Health Care* **7**: 118–122.

Ehrman WG, Matson SC. (1998) Approach to assessing adolescents on serious or sensitive issues. *Pediatr Clin North Am* **45**: 189–204.

Goldenring JM, Rosen DS. (2004) Getting into adolescent heads: An essential update. *Contemp Pediatr* **21**: 64–90.

MacKenzie RG. (1990) Approach to the adolescent in the clinical setting. *Med Clin North Am* **74**: 1085–1095.

Ozer EM, Adams SH, Lustig JL, Gee S, Garber AK, Gardner LR, Rehbein M, Addison L, Irwin CE Jr. (2005) Increasing the screening and counseling of adolescents for risky health behaviors: A primary care intervention. *Pediatrics* **115**: 960–968.

Shallice T. (1982) Specific impairments of planning. *Philos Trans R Soc Lon B Biol Sci* **298**: 199–209.

Chapter 6

Consent and Confidentiality

Michelle Yeo

1. Background

During adolescence, clinical care shifts from placing much of the burden of care on parents to involving the young person in the management of their own health. One of the most important aspects of providing care to adolescent patients is balancing the need to respect the young person's growing sense of independence and autonomy whilst continuing to encourage the involvement of parents in the care of their adolescent. It is important for clinicians to have a broad understanding of the law as it applies to adolescents, as well as the ethical principles that govern good practice when working with young people. The principles discussed in this chapter relate to young people's ability to consent to health care decisions, their competence in doing so and the provisions of confidential health care services.

1.1. *Ethical and Legal Principles*

Children were historically regarded as the legal property of their parents and lacked rights in being able to make decisions about their health and their lives. Along with changing socio–cultural and political perspectives on adolescence, legal views too have shifted to recognise the growing autonomy of adolescents. This has been reflected in the United Nations

Convention on the Rights of the Child, which empowers children and young people to make autonomous decisions, taking into account their evolving capacities and their family context.

2. Young People's Capacity to Consent

In Australia, as in many countries of the world, 18 years is the legal age of majority or 'adulthood'. The law assumes that young people aged 18 and above are competent to consent to treatment or refuse treatment, even if this is not regarded to be in their best interests.

A legal precedent to allow adolescent patients to consent to their own medical treatment was set in 1985 by the landmark case of ***Gillick* vs. *W Norfolk and Wisbech Area Health Authority*** in the United Kingdom. In this case, Victoria Gillick sought a court order that it was not lawful for medical practitioners to prescribe contraceptive treatment to minors under 16 years of age without their parents' consent. However, the court established that an adolescent under 18 years (a minor) was capable of providing informed consent when he or she 'achieved a sufficient understanding and intelligence to enable him or her to understand fully what is proposed.' This is known as the 'mature minor principle'. In Australia this was upheld by a case known as Marion's case, where the High Court determined that 'parental power to consent to medical treatment diminishes gradually as the child's capacities and maturity grow.'

Whilst the legal system has paved the way to allow young people to make decisions about their health, there is a lack of guidance about what constitutes 'sufficient understanding and intelligence' or the lower age limit for a mature minor. Thus for young people under the age of 18 years (minor), clinicians are required to make a clinical judgement as to their maturity and their capacity to consent.

2.1. Competence

2.1.1. Assessment of competence

In order to consent to treatment or a medical procedure, the young person needs to be considered competent, that is, to understand the issue being discussed. There are no universally accepted tests used to assess competency in adolescents. Most commonly, clinicians rely on a detailed discussion with the young person. From this discussion, the clinician needs to be satisfied that the young person has sufficient understanding about and is able to express:

- The nature of the clinical problem.
- The purpose of treatment and what it involves.
- The seriousness of the treatment.
- The effects of treatment including possible side effects.
- Other treatment options available.
- The consequences of discovery of treatment by parents or guardian.

2.1.2. *Assessment of cognitive abilities and maturity*

Competence is strongly linked to cognitive ability and social experience. Research has shown that adolescents aged 14 are capable of the same decision-making capacity as adults when given a hypothetical scenario. Notwithstanding this, the capacity for a young person to consent is linked to their cognitive development rather than age alone. The young person's level of schooling, their ability to function in other areas of their life, and additional responsibilities, such as employment, are also important factors to be taken into consideration. A young person living independently of his/her parents may be considered to be more capable of making decisions pertaining to his/her health than one still living with his/her parents.

2.1.3. *Assessment of the family context*

Families from different ethnic, cultural, and religious backgrounds may have different expectations of young people's roles and behaviours, with some families being more 'permissive' than others. Parents themselves may also have expectations of the extent to which they are involved in their child's healthcare decisions. Tensions can arise in the clinician/patient/parent relationship, especially when parents' views oppose those of the patient or clinician. While it is important to continue to engage the family when working with the young person, young people need to be accorded their legal rights to confidentiality.

In certain circumstances, parents may not be able to adequately support their teenager, for example, a parent with drug or alcohol abuse or significant mental illness. Where the young person is not deemed competent, the involvement of protective services may be necessary.

2.1.4. *Complexity of treatment*

Competency is task specific. The degree of competency required of a young person will vary with the level of complexity of the treatment proposed. The mature minor principle was established for the prescription of the oral contraceptive pill, which is considered a low risk procedure. Treatments or procedures that are more complex — for example, an appendectomy or termination of pregnancy will require a higher level of maturity before a young person is judged to be able to consent. Special medical procedures such as sterilisation in an intellectually disabled teenager or gender reassignment may require authorisation from the Family Court. An adolescent assessed as competent for one procedure may not necessarily be assumed to be competent for another.

2.2. When is a Young Person Not Deemed to be Mature Minor?

Young people with a significant intellectual disability or a mental health condition that impair their cognitive abilities such as severe depression or anxiety, low weight anorexia nervosa, or psychosis may not be deemed competent. In such cases consent needs to be obtained from the parent or guardian, who must act in the best interest of the adolescent. Psychiatric conditions can fluctuate over time and the young person's ability to provide consent may also change. The competence of such individuals needs to be assessed in each case and each situation.

2.3. Refusal of Treatment

Do young people have a right to refuse treatment when they are considered competent? Although the court upheld the right of a competent young person to consent to treatment in the case of ***Gillick* vs. *W Norfolk and Wisbech Area Health Authority***, the court did not confer the corresponding right for a competent young person to refuse treatment. The nature and necessity of the treatment is relevant to all considerations.

2.3.1. *Non-essential treatment*

It is not infrequent that young people choose not to undergo certain procedures or treatments, for example refusing to have a venipuncture for laboratory tests, intravenous antibiotics for a non-serious infection, or scar revision surgery.

Putting pressure on the young person to undergo a treatment against their will affects trust and can potentially affect adherence to future treatment. Where the condition does not pose a significant threat to health, it is reasonable to accept the young person's decision if he/she has been judged to be competent. Attempting to understand the reasons behind the refusal, encouraging the young person to think through their decision, and inviting them to review their decision again at a later date or discussion with their parents or a trusted adult will aid the partnership in the decision-making process.

2.3.2. *Treatment for a potentially serious condition, or life saving treatment*

The treating clinician is placed in a difficult situation if a young person refuses treatment, especially when the proposed treatment will prevent death or significant harm. Some examples include refusal of an organ transplant, chemotherapy for leukaemia or psychiatric medication. In such circumstances, despite the young person being competent, parents have the right to override their child's decision. In discussions with the young person, every attempt should be made to encourage the young person to involve his/her parents in the decision. Legal intervention may be required if the decision cannot be reached through negotiation and mediation. However this avenue should remain the last resort.

3. Confidentiality

The principle of confidentiality is one of the central tenets of the practice
of medicine. Confidentiality can be defined as 'an agreement between the
patient and provider that information discussed in the consultation will not
be shared with other parties without the explicit permission of the patient.'
The law recognises that competent adolescents deserve the same rights to
confidentiality as adults. Apart from the legal context, there are other reasons for confidentiality being important in this age group.

3.1. *Confidentiality — The Clinical Context*

Studies in Australia and elsewhere show that young people rate confidentiality as one of the most important factors when seeking health care
services. Concerns about confidentiality influence young people's access
to services, not only general practice, but also sexual and reproductive
health, mental health, and drug and alcohol services.

Over 50% of young women report that they would stop using sexual
health services and delay testing or seeking treatment for sexually transmitted infections if their parents were notified. A third of young people do
not attend healthcare services because they do not want a parent to know.
Those that were foregoing health care tended to be those young people
who were at higher risk of significant health problems.

Confidentiality is also important in gaining the young person's trust
as the clinician tries to build rapport with him/her. It is known that preventable behaviours such as unintentional injury, drug and alcohol misuse,
and unsafe sexual activity as well as mental health problems contribute
significantly to the burden of disease in adolescence. Clinicians are
encouraged to opportunistically screen for risk behaviours and emotional
distress in order to identify risk and intervene early. Confidentiality is
essential for accurately obtaining sensitive information from the young
person and the clinician's assurances of confidentiality encourage the
young person to be honest in disclosing sensitive information as well as
returning for follow-up.

The discussion of confidentiality must be brought up early in the consultation with the young person, with the limits of confidentiality

explained. Spending time alone with the young person, encouraging him/ her to express his/her views, and taking steps to making decisions help increase the young person's sense of responsibility and their ability to be an advocate for their own health.

Many professional organisations have now adopted policy and position statements supporting the provision of confidential care for young people, recognising this as an important indicator of quality health service.

3.2. *Exceptions to the Duty of Confidentiality*

There are a number of exceptions to the duty of confidentiality. These include:

- The young person consenting to disclosure; however the clinician needs to clarify with the young person to whom and what specific information will be disclosed.
- The young person being at risk of serious self-harm or suicide.
- The young person is at risk of harming others.
- The young person is at risk of or is the victim of physical, sexual or emotional abuse. Various countries have federal and state laws regarding the mandatory reporting of child abuse.
- Legal requirements for disclosure which include court proceedings, notifiable diseases and testing for blood alcohol levels or other drugs.
- Necessity for the young person's well-being, such as during an emergency when urgent communication is required, or communication between members of the treating team.

If the clinician feels that a disclosure should be made, it is helpful to inform the young person of this decision and to discuss the reasons for this with them.

3.3. *Communicating with Parents*

Although there are tensions between balancing the young person's right to confidentiality and the parents' rights to be informed, one does not necessarily occur at the expense of the other. Every effort needs to be made to involve the family. The provision of confidential services has been shown not to damage parent–child relations. Parents support clinicians being able to openly communicate with their adolescents; however, they need to be educated about confidentiality for young people. At the same time, clinicians need to be actively encouraging young people to share important information with their parents.

4. Conclusions

The provision of developmentally appropriate care to young people takes into account the young person's growing capacity to make choices and decisions about their own health. A broad understanding of the local law as it relates to young people's capacity to consent to treatment as well as confidentiality is essential in providing good quality health care to this population.

References

Appelbaum PS. (2007) Clinical practice. Assessment of patients' competence to consent to treatment. *N Engl J Med* **357**(18): 1834–1840.

Ford CA, Davenport AF, Meier A, Mcree A-L. (2009) Parents and health care professionals working together to improve adolescent health: The perspectives of parents. *J Adolesc Health* **44**(2): 191–194.

Larcher V. (2005) Consent, competence, and confidentiality. *BMJ* **330**(7487): 353–356.

Larcher V, Hutchinson A. (2010) How should paediatricians assess Gillick competence? *Arch Dis Child* **95**(4): 307–311.

Lehrer JA, Pantell R, Tebb K, Shafer M-A. (2007) Forgone health care among US Adolescents: Associations between risk characteristics and confidentiality concern. *J Adolesc Health* **40**(3): 218–226.

Michaud P-A, Berg-Kelly K, Macfarlane A, Benaroyo L. (2010) Ethics and adolescent care: An international perspective. *Currt Opin in Pediatr* **22**(4): 418–422.

Office of the High Commissioner for Human Rights (1990) *Convention on the rights of the child*. Available online at: http://www2.ohchr.org/english/law/crc.htm (accessed January 2011).

Chapter 7

Communicating with Parents and Carers

Anne Honey and Gwynnyth Llewellyn

1. Introduction

The demands of living with a health condition can complicate developmental tasks of adolescence such as individuation, self-responsibility, and identity consolidation. Young people with health conditions show poorer psychosocial outcomes than their peers, for example, significantly lower overall life satisfaction, poorer mental health, and lower self-efficacy. These outcomes are influenced by environmental factors including social support and importantly, family functioning. Parents play a significant role in facilitating both positive adolescent transitions and illness management.

Clinicians can assist by providing guidance to parents about how best to support their son's or daughter's health management and psychosocial development; and by assisting parents to manage the emotional and practical impacts of caring for an adolescent and/or young adult with a health condition.

For adolescents with ongoing health conditions, the patterns of self-management they establish at this time influence disease outcomes in adulthood and parents can play a significant role in assisting the transition into young adulthood.

This chapter summarises the influence of parents on adolescents with health conditions and addresses ways in which clinicians, through their communication with parents, may assist parents to support their adolescent son or daughter with a health condition to promote optimum health care and facilitate positive social and psychological development.

2. Influence of Parents

Adolescents are able to participate in and make decisions about their treatment. Clinical consultations increasingly involve communicating directly with the adolescent. At the same time, parents continue to play an important part in assisting their son or daughter to manage their ongoing condition and to become autonomous in health care, a role which often continues into young adulthood. Hence, family factors continue to influence adolescent health behaviours and predict a variety of psychological and physical outcomes.

2.1. *General Parent–Adolescent Interactions*

Supportive family environments with high cohesion, connectedness, expressiveness, and low conflict, are associated with positive outcomes for adolescents with health conditions. Beneficial outcomes include higher emotional well-being, treatment adherence, and lower illness severity.

Large-scale and longitudinal studies show that emotional support, from family and other sources, positively influences mental health and well-being for adolescents and young adults.

There is considerable evidence that authoritative parenting, which involves high acceptance/involvement and high strictness/supervision, results in better outcomes for adolescents in terms of their school performance, adjustment and behaviour. Parents who adopt this style are warm but firm. They are accepting of and attuned to the child's needs. They encourage age-appropriate independence, allow the adolescent to develop opinions of their own and consider their viewpoints. They maintain limits and boundaries but are willing to discuss and explain these, and they encourage maturity and responsibility. For adolescents with health conditions, authoritative parenting has also been shown to have a specific positive influence, for example, on self-care behaviours and metabolic control in adolescents with diabetes.

2.2. *Health/Illness Related Interactions*

Parental involvement in adolescents' health care has been associated with better treatment adherence and health outcomes. However, high parental involvement can also lead to illness-related conflict with a negative impact on the adolescent's quality of life. The types of interactions are important.

2.2.1. *Supportive interactions*

Adolescents with health conditions may regard their parents as allies, a safe base, a source of strength, and role models and coaches for information management. Helpful parental involvement includes support, acceptance, understanding, reassurance, working with the adolescent or sharing responsibility, and praising the adolescent's accomplishments. For adolescents with a health condition, a primary concern is to normalise their lives, thus they especially appreciate parents reassuring them about their ability to meet normal life challenges and helping them to fit their health care into everyday life. Better illness management has also been associated with families maintaining traditions and structured family routines in the face of chronic illness. Self-reported regimen adherence has been associated with adolescent reports of parents giving positive feedback, rewarding compliance and jointly planning self-care.

2.2.2. *'Miscarried helping'*

The term 'miscarried helping' is used to describe parental overprotective behaviours which inadvertently foster dependency and low self-efficacy or resentment and rebellion, leading to poor self-care.

Excessive parental control and restrictions have been linked to low self-esteem, depression, and problems with autonomy development. This type of parental behaviour can be seen as infantilising, showing distrust and negating the adolescent's own knowledge and competence.

The relationship between parental and adolescent behaviour is likely to be reciprocal and mutually reinforcing such that, for example, parent's willingness to allow autonomy is also shaped by the competence and responsibility demonstrated by the adolescent. An adolescent's negative and rebellious behaviour may be shaped by parents continuing to maintain overly high levels of control.

2.2.3. *Transition to independence*

As Berntsson noted, adolescents with a health condition experience well-being when they are allowed to prepare for living a normal life integrated into society, including autonomy in health-care and in their everyday lives. Families do not necessarily discuss transfer of health care responsibilities from parents to their adolescent children and problems can result if responsibility is given too early or particular tasks are neglected or overlooked. Parents can be torn between the competing demands of protecting their child's health and supporting their increasing independence and autonomy. The parent–adolescent conflict around health management may be highest in early to mid-adolescence during the transitional self-management phase, when adolescents are responsible for some tasks and decisions but parents are responsible for others. The adolescent-dominant self-management that follows is characterised by reduced conflict.

2.3. *Knowledge, Attitudes, and Beliefs*

Parents' knowledge, attitudes, and beliefs about their adolescent child and the health condition influence their behaviour towards them and can affect treatment outcomes. Parents, the young person, and the health professional may have differences in beliefs about, for example, the seriousness of the condition or management expectations. Any concerns, misapprehensions or differences in perspective related to treatment may lead to treatment drop out or 'adaptive noncompliance'. Ideally, parents will have reasonable expectations and confidence in their young person's overall competence to manage. Parental beliefs that an adolescent is vulnerable have been associated with adolescent anxiety and illness uncertainty.

Similarly parental beliefs serve as an attitudinal role model about the illness and whether this is seen as stigmatising or socially acceptable.

2.4. *Parental Stress and Coping*

Parental levels of stress and distress related to the health conditions predict adolescent outcomes including illness severity, health care use, and psychosocial adjustment. Parents experience a broad range of emotions in providing care and support. They need to manage both the health condition and the conflict and anxiety it generates, including financial strains, loss of privacy and spontaneity, problems with service providers, grief, marital strain, and role conflict. Parents of children with health conditions have more depressive symptoms and families are more likely to develop dysfunctional family patterns. Factors such as socio–economic status play a part in this relationship.

3. How Clinicians Can Help Parents Support Adolescents with Health Conditions

As children move towards adolescence and early adulthood, the parental role in treatment is less clear. There is a repetitive need for renegotiation around the illness, just as there is around many aspects of the adolescent's life. Parents have indicated that they look to clinicians to:

- Include them in treatment decisions.
- Provide them with guidance to foster competence.
- Maintain a positive relationship with them.

3.1. *Involvement in Treatment*

Parents can provide input and corroboration and a complementary perspective. As adolescents become older, this input needs to be judicious and not as a list of negatives.

- Parents may be concerned that they do not receive information if excluded from a consultation. The adolescent's right to keep information from their parents might not be in their best interest and many adolescents and young adults would wish to consult their parents about therapeutic decisions. One clinical approach is to talk with the adolescent by themselves, clarify what information is to be provided to parents and then provide the information to parents with the adolescent present. *This may be time consuming but there are very few clinical indications to see the parent of a teenager without the teenager being present.* Adolescents may not convey information to their parents for many reasons, but may have no objection to the clinician providing the information. Clinicians are in a good position to assess what information is relevant and helpful, to explain why and to encourage the adolescent to allow the information to be provided. Adolescents value parents understanding their situation and may therefore react positively to clinicians seeking to facilitate understanding between parents and their adolescent. From our work, adolescents believed that clinicians could give the information more clearly, calmly, and with authority; as one young person reported: 'Doctors say it well... they're not so emotionally attached to it, and they're not scared of upsetting their mother.'

- Transition to adult care is best performed as a planned and gradual process in which the adolescent becomes more autonomous with health care. The transfer between services does not necessarily coincide with adolescent independence. Clinicians in adult services working with adolescents and young adults need to acknowledge the parental role at the same time as continuing to support the young person to move towards taking responsibility for their own health care. Once the teenage patient is legally recognised as an adult, the clinician has to deal with the competing legal requirements of confidentiality and the wishes of the young person, and the needs of the parents who wish to remain involved and act as reporters. Rather than abruptly terminating a relationship, as often happens in transition to adult care where the clinician is unused to dealing with parents, it may be better if the clinican adopts the approach of 'I will listen, but may not be able to comment'. In this situation the clinician will also experience the dilemma of whether to let the young adult know about the contact. If they do, the approach would be to acknowledge the parent's concern and reiterate that the young person's confidentiality is being kept, except under defined circumstances (Chapter 6). Reminding the parent of these circumstances provides some reassurance.

3.2. *Guidance*

- Parents can benefit from understanding how their parenting style and family interactions influence adolescent well-being. Clinicians can continue to educate the parents with information about their adolescent's health condition and its potential interaction with adolescent development, after gaining permission from the adolescent. A frequently encountered example is the adoloscent's desire to strive for behavioural autonomy which can be an important component of non-adherence to health care regimens. While this non-adherence is clearly undesirable, it should be seen as developmentally normal, rather than as deviant behaviour. Emphasising the normality of such behaviour promotes a more understanding and less critical response by parents. If clinicians can help parents to understand their adolescent's need to learn by doing and from making their own mistakes, parents may be less likely to expect and demand perfection which may have the effect of further alienating the young person.

    There are additional ways for clinicians to support parents in the autonomy/protection dilemma.

- Clinicians can help parents to develop perceptions of their adolescent's abilities that are both realistic and optimistic, for example, by assessing their perceptions of the adolescent's vulnerability and providing education to minimise inaccurate perceptions. Clinicians are often well placed to notice changes in the adolescent that indicate a readiness to take more responsibility for their health care, and then to talk to parents about 'allowing' their young person to be more independent. While parents should show interest in and be involved in their adolescent's self-care, they must be reminded that their input needs to be positive, encouraging, and confident rather than overly strict or critical.

- The clinician can provide reflection about family interactions if they consider that the parenting style and family interactions are influencing adolescent well being. Information and support with regular encouragement and reassurance can assist parents to move, as adolescence progresses, towards a more equal relationship characterised by greater flexibility and respect, and less control. Adolescents identify this as an important strategy. In our study with parents of adolescents with mental illness, parents frequently reported changing their style of interaction with their adolescent based on recommendations made by clinicians, for example, about becoming more accepting and less authoritarian. Clinician's suggestions were better accepted by the parents when these suggestions were presented in response to the parents' voiced concerns, and as parenting strategies appropriate to the current context of their son's or daughter's health condition, rather than as a criticism of their overall parenting.

- Clinicians can assist parents to cope by identifying and appropriately managing parents' emotional responses to the situation. It may be necessary to refer the parent to a counsellor or a carer support group to develop specific coping strategies.
- Tailoring support and guidance, particularly for parents of teenagers with chronic conditions, means ongoing assessment of parents' resources for managing the physical, financial, time, and emotional costs of the condition and to identify their support needs as these change over time. Letting go and allowing the young person increasing freedoms in relation to their health condition may provide much needed respite for parents.

3.3. *Positive Relationships*

A supportive relationship with a clinician whom the parents' trust to take optimum care of their child, to provide them with accurate and helpful guidance, and to understand rather than judge them on the issues they face, can also assist parents to manage their adolescent son's or daughter's health condition. As one father in our study put it: 'That experience and confidence, that's something they can pass on to us.'

- For the older adolescent, the general practitioner or family physician should consider whether they might prefer to see a different doctor in the practice or attend a different practice. The older adolescent and young adult may prefer to start with a 'clean slate' as part of their independence. Often a doctor attached to the young person's tertiary education facility or one who practises closer to work is a better choice. Clinicians can assist parents to see this as a positive step to self-care.

- Parents of adolescents with a chronic health condition must form a new and different relationship with clinicians when the transition to adult care is made. They may seek reassurance that the correct choice of clinician has been made and that the new clinician fully understands their son's or daughter's condition. Just as frequently they may be pleased to see their young person enter a new phase of care in an adult environment.

Whatever the situation, there are important messages that the clinician can communicate:

- They are primarily there to see the young person but acknowledge the experience and expertise that the parents bring. At some time, in the first consultation, take a history from the parent if they are present. The young person is usually relieved to avoid this boring task.
- Unless absolutely necessary, make no major changes to therapy on the first consultation but instead discuss the positives of making a completely new assessment.
- Clearly state expectations about communication, and clarify when it is appropriate to deal with the parent rather than the young person. As an example, young people may not wish to call for results during the day if at school, university or work, and may prefer that a parent continues this role.

4. Conclusion

Adolescence is a time of ongoing negotiation between parents and adolescents about the degree of autonomy that is appropriate. In the context of the adolescent with a health condition, the optimal level will vary depending on the adolescent's age, maturity, and the nature of their illness. By directly communicating with parents as well as adolescents, clinicians provide optimal care, in turn minimising the likelihood of illness related conflict and poor parent–adolescent relationships.

References

Anderson BJ, Wolpert HA. (2004) A developmental perspective on the challenges of diabetes education and care during the young adult period. *Patient Educ Couns* **53**(3): 347–352.

Berntsson L, Berg M, Brydolf M, Hellstrom A-L. (2007) Adolescents' experiences of well-being when living with a long-term illness or disability. *Scand J Caring Sci* **21**(4): 419–425.

Burns JJ, Sadof M, Kamat D. (2006) The adolescent with a chronic illness. *Pediatr Ann* **35**(3): 206–10, 214–6.

Dimatteo MR. (2004) The role of effective communication with children and their families in fostering adherence to pediatric regimens. *Patient Educ Couns* **55**(3): 339–344.

Emerson E, Hatton C, Llewellyn G, Blacher J, Graham H. (2006) Socio-economic position, household composition, health status and indicators of the well-being of mothers of children with and without intellectual disabilities. *J Intellect Disabil Res* **50**(12): 862–873.

Farrant B, Watson PD. (2004) Health care delivery: Perspectives of young people with chronic illness and their parents. *J Paediatr Child Health* **40**(4): 175–179.

Honey A, Boughtwood D, Clarke S, Halse C, Kohn M, Madden S. (2008) Support for parents of children with anorexia: What parents want. *Brunner-Mazel Eat Disord Monogr Ser* **16**(1): 40–51.

Honey A, Emerson E, Llewellyn G. (2011) The mental health of young people with disabilities: Impact of social conditions. *Soc Psychiatry Psychiatr Epidemiol* **46**(1): 1–10.

Lopez WL, Mullins LL, Wolfe-Christensen C, Bourdeau T. (2008) The relation between parental psychological distress and adolescent anxiety in youths with chronic illnesses: The mediating effect of perceived child vulnerability. *Child Health Care* **37**(3): 171–182.

Mullins LL, Wolfe-Christensen C, Pai ALH, Carpentier MY, Gillaspy S, Cheek J, Page M. (2007) The relationship of parental overprotection, perceived child vulnerability, and parenting stress to uncertainty in youth with chronic illness. *J Pediatr Psychol* **32**(8): 973–982.

Reiss JG, Gibson RW, Walker LR. (2005) Health care transition: Youth, family, and provider perspectives. *Pediatrics,* **115**(1): 112–20.

Smetana JG, Campione-Barr N, Metzger A. (2006) Adolescent development in interpersonal and societal contexts. *Ann Rev Psychol* **57**: 255–284.

Steinberg L. (2001) We know some things: Parent–adolescent relationships in retrospect and prospect. *J Res Adolesc* **11**(1): 1–19.

Young B, Dixon-Woods M, Windridge KC, Heney D. (2003) Managing communication with young people who have a potentially life threatening chronic illness: Qualitative study of patients and parents. *BMJ* **326**(7384): 305.

Chapter 8

Communicating Electronically with Adolescents

Fiona Robards and Andrew Campbell

1. Introduction

Young people face many barriers in accessing health and other services. We also know from the work of Rickwood and others that young people are more likely to access support through the internet than via teachers, school counsellors, general practitioners/family doctors or other health professionals. New media presents exciting opportunities to engage young people in the spaces that they frequently inhabit. Technology can be used in a range of ways, including:

- As a tool for organising appointments.
- A clinical platform that enables therapeutic conversations.
- To support promoting access to information or health care services.
- As an opportunity for young people to participate in service delivery, design, and research.

How much time young people spend on the internet, and the ways in which they share information, including online behaviour such as cyber bullying, are topics that can be explored with a young person within a clinical context in order to promote health and safety. However,

81

the focus of this chapter is oriented more towards the use of the internet to engage and effectively communicate with young people using electronic media.

2. Direct Communication

Health practitioners often find that communicating with adolescents can be challenging. Meeting with them in spaces where they are comfortable in communicating can aid in the provision of health care and be a safe and non-threatening way to build rapport and improve dialogue.

2.1. *Text Messaging*

Text messaging is the act of communicating through standard or abbreviated language, sometimes called 'txtspeak', via mobile phones. Text messaging includes Short Message Service and Multimedia Messaging Service. The pros and cons of text messaging with patients are:

- Texts are especially useful for appointment reminders.
- Young people may be able to receive but not send messages if they are out of credit.
- Texts can be used for mood or monitoring.
- MMS can be used to record and send images. There should be a clear protocol regarding their use. In some cases, these can be used as a part of therapy sessions.

Consider how the content of text messages can be recorded in the young person's files. New e-health systems provide client and business software management and include automated SMS to patients for bookings and cancellations.

2.2. *Email*

In contrast to telephone or direct face-to-face contact with a health professional, email is more anonymous. For young people who are often embarrassed about talking with health professionals, this can make help-seeking easier. And while young people are more likely to access telephone counselling for family and relationship problems, Beattie *et al.* found that young people may prefer to disclose information about risk-of-harm issues in seeking help via the more anonymous email and web counselling services. Points to consider with email counselling are:

- Be clear about crisis management. Seek the person's name and telephone number before you begin ongoing communication via email.
- Be clear about expectations, for example, when negotiating time frames for response.
- Emails are deemed legal records of communication and should be printed or saved into patient files.
- Consider your 'out-of-office' reply, not only for days off, but for out-of-work hours in general. Include information about where young people can seek help in a crisis.

2.3. *Chat*

Online chat happens in real time. Thus it is similar in feel to a regular conversation, except that the text is sometimes abbreviated into 'net-speak' (similar to txtspeak). The flow of conversation is important to note when chatting with young people, as they sometimes tend to move quickly and can lose track of responses. Young people tend to multi-task whilst chatting on instant messaging services for example. It is important to note the following:

- Online chat often involves abbreviations or acronyms for fast communication of common phrases (tnx = thank you; brb = be right back). If unsure of online acronym meanings, consult a glossary such as www.noslang.com.
- Emoticons are often used to add expression and communicate about emotions. These visual cues are typically used throughout a chat session. Notably, they have been validated in research to be as important in communicating online as regular sentence and grammar use

- Develop a safety plan and know the name and telephone number of the person with whom you are chatting. Be clear with the young person about the limits of confidentially.

2.4. *Online Peer Support Networks*

Many online communities are emerging in Australia, mostly supported through discussion boards and online chat sites, including Livewire by The Starlight Foundation (www.starlight.org.au), ReachOut from The Inspire Foundation (www.reachout.com) and Kids Help Line run by Boystown (www.kidshelp.com.au). Online peer support networks for young people's physical health or mental health are evolving.

In the context of health, learning, and positive youth development, online web spaces are simply another place where young people can be together and make connections, through a common interest because they belong to similar demographic groups, and have similar types of illnesses, or experience similar challenges. Young people with comparable characteristics can come together in online spaces to support each other. This can be particularly helpful for those who are socially or geographically isolated and are keen to connect with others like themselves. When working with young people seeking communities online:

- Look out for existing communities and consider available mechanisms for connecting young people online.
- Always ensure online group facilitation for 'at risk' support groups (for example, eating disorders, depression, etc.).
- Be aware, as a health professional using social networking or other kinds of technology, of keeping your professional and personal identities separate. For example, one should not 'friend' clients from your personal account. Discuss this with the young people with whom you work.

3. Clinical Tools

Using games can be a fun way to engage a young person clinically, whether via online clinical resources, serious games, or virtual worlds.

3.1. *Online Clinical Resources*

Online surveys and questionnaires, such as psychological tests that give the user immediate feedback and a connection to a professional or expert facilitator (if needed), are useful tools in giving young people basic answers to their concerns. State and trait testing items in personality, mood, anxiety and stress scales, as well as fun tests on temperament and intellect, give young people confidence in asking questions of facilitators about specific results they have received. Therapeutic programs such as Cognitive Behaviour Therapy can be found online and have been rigorously shown to improve mood in adolescents.

3.2. *Online Journals*

Some young people like to keep a reflective journal and may choose to keep this online in the form of a blog. This may be useful as a supportive reflection (bibliotherapy) tool in between contacts with health professionals. When working with blogs in therapy, consider the following:

- Discuss with the young person with whom they would be willing to share their personal information. Are they using an avatar (symbol/picture and name to represent themselves anonymously) or their real name and real picture?
- Discuss the purpose of the journal and how it might supplement the young person's journey to better health and well-being.

3.3. *Serious Games*

Serious games including virtual worlds, rehabilitation games, sand box games, (building or creating scenarios), and biofeedback games, specifically target therapy through ongoing interaction with the game environment which provides psycho-education, mindfulness, cognitive behaviour therapy, or group support.

Games that promote mental health in a variety of ways have been shown to be effective for such conditions as pain management, stress and attention disorders. Other electronic games, made fun by using formats based on physical fitness and weight management programs, can facilitate physical therapies. Such games are common, and include off-the-shelf consoles and software.

- Be aware of the range of games that are available.
- Remember that some games may have content that is only appropriate for adolescents over 15 years old; use the game rating system as a guide.
- Understand that even some serious games can cause potential problems such as headaches, eyestrain, and loss of motivation to sleep or undertake other essential tasks such as homework.

3.4. *Virtual Worlds*

Virtual worlds open up spaces for new clinical contexts. These worlds allow young people to communicate and interact with others online using an avatar (a virtual, animated character) in an environment that is either pre-determined or designed by the users. The virtual world has proven to be a popular online tool in counselling individuals and has been shown to be a potentially effective tool for group therapies related to smoking cessation in young people.

3.5. *Online Health Records*

Health records are increasingly becoming electronic, with a further move for these records to be consumer-owned and managed. It is important to distinguish between an electronic health record and a personal health record. The latter are online spaces where people can store their health information, share it with those to whom they have given consent, and be supported to manage their health.

4. Engaging Young People

Other ways in which technology can be useful when working with adolescents include health promotion, the promotion of social inclusion, access to information and services, and via opportunities for involvement in service design and data-collection in research.

4.1. *Social Inclusion*

Technology provides young people with increased opportunities to participate and contribute to society, enhancing resilience, preventing problems or giving skills to those already facing challenges.

Notwithstanding the many concerns about the potential risks to young people from various social networking sites — cyberbullying, grooming by paedophiles, exposure to inappropriate materials such as pornography — there are many potential benefits. For example, online identity exploration has also been found to be part of normal adolescent development, another way of exploring, 'Who am I?' Social networking can offer opportunities for young people to connect with others via online relationships that complement their face-to-face relationships, as well as other benefits including civic engagement, cultural, creative, educational, self-expression and social development, and health opportunities. Consider the following:

- Do your patients have access to technology?
- How can you enable this?
- Social networking can also be accessed via smart phones and similar wireless technology.

4.2. *Promoting Access to Information and Services*

Many young people access the internet looking for information on sex, sexuality and contraception, particularly because they can do so independently and confidentially. Young people also state that they are more likely to access help via the internet than from professionals or community agencies — an increasing trend.

The internet may provide an effective setting for health promotion activity. New media can reach large numbers of young people through the provision of health education material to increase their knowledge and promote healthier and safer choices. For example, a computerised web-based course on drug prevention, CRUfADschools (www.crufadschools.org), that school teachers can use to teach students about health and well-being, was found effective in reducing drug use and increasing knowledge of harm minimisation skills.

Websites offer new ways of encouraging access to help in several ways, whether through information about various health issues or encouragement of help-seeking. Examples include:

- ReachOut has websites in Australia (www.reachout.com), Ireland (ie.reachout.com) and the United States (www.inspireusafoundation.org/our-work/reachout-com).
- The Australian Kids Helpline which is a telephone counselling service also has a website (www.kidshelp.com.au) with information about their services, a community-based service directory, health information fact-sheets, and a discussion forum.
- In the UK, Centrepoint (www.centrepoint.org.uk) promotes access to services for homeless young people through their website.

Through other websites, young people can email questions anonymously and receive answers from a health professional. This can be especially useful in relation to subjects that can be embarrassing to speak about, such as sexual health.

Social networking, text messaging, and other forms of technology can also be used for service promotion. Questions to consider:

- How can you best use technology to promote your service?
- What information is available for young people — how can this be improved?
- How can you involve young people in creating or improving content?
- What creative methods can you use to involve young people in taking an active approach to promoting their own health?

4.3. *Youth Participation*

Technology can also enable youth participation in research, service delivery, and design. Via online modalities, young people can be actively involved in the development, implementation, review, and evaluation of services and programs in ways that create a sense of ownership, importance, and influence, as well as fostering mutual respect within the service or program.

Online surveys, online discussions in the form of focus groups, or using hand-held devices for recording information, all offer new ways of collecting data in research. The internet can be a good way to promote research opportunities, inform participants, gain consent, and conduct the research itself. Generally, information available in the public domain can be used in research, without consent, if it does not identify participants. On the internet it is not always clear which information is public or private. If information is potentially identifiable, consent from participants (and their parent or guardian) is usually needed (Chapter 6). Questions to consider include:

- What do you want to find out about your service?
- How can you use technology to gather that information?
- How can you use technology to engage young people to become more involved in shaping your service design and delivery?

5. Conclusion

Electronically communicating with young people brings many opportunities for increasing young people's health and well-being. Through the use of technology we can encourage young people to be engaged in their health care, adopt healthy lifestyles, and access appropriate services when required. This involves health professionals engaging with young people by using the communication media with which young people are most comfortable, as well as utilising innovative ways to promote young people's access to information and services.

References

Amon KL, Campbell A. (2008) Can children with AD/HD learn relaxation and breathing techniques through biofeedback video games? *Aust J Educ Dev Psychol* **8**: 72–84.

Andersson G, Cuijpers P. (2008) Pros and cons of online cognitive-behavioural therapy. *Br J Psychiatry* **193**(4): 270–271.

Barak A, Bloch N. (2006) Factors related to perceived helpfulness in supporting highly distressed individuals through an online support chat. *Cyberpsychol Behav* **9**(1): 60–68.

Beattie D, Cunningham S, Jones R, Zelenko O. (2006) I use online so the counsellors can't hear me crying: Creating design solutions for online counselling. *Media Int Aust, Incorporating Culture & Policy,* **118**: 43–52.

Burns J, Morey C, Lagelee A, Mackenzie A, Nicholas J. (2007) Reach out! Innovation in service delivery. *Med J Aust* **187**(7): S31–34.

Christensen H, Griffiths KM, Jorm AF. (2004) Delivering interventions for depression by using the internet: Randomised controlled trial. *BMJ* **328**(7434): 265.

Kato PM, Cole SW, Bradlyn AS, Pollock BH. (2008) A video game improves behavioral outcomes in adolescents and young adults with cancer: A randomized trial. *Pediatrics* **122**(2): e305–317.

Mcgorry, PDPR, Hickie, IB, Jorm, AF. (2007) Investing in youth mental health is a best buy. *Med J Aust* **187**(7): S5–S7.

Neal DM, Campbell AJ, Williams LY, Liu Y, Nussbaumer D. (2011) "I did not realize so many options are available": Cognitive authority, emerging adults, and e-mental health. *Libr Inf Sci Res* **33**(1): 25–33.

Newton NC, Andrews G, Teesson M, Vogl LE. (2009) Delivering prevention for alcohol and cannabis using the internet: A cluster randomised controlled trial. *Prev Med* **48**(6): 579–584.

Notley T. (2008) Online network use in schools: Social and educational opportunities. *Youth Studies Aust* **27**(3): 20–29.

Rickwood DJ. (2010) Promoting youth mental health through computer-mediated communication. *Int J Ment Health Promotion* **12**(3): 32–44.

Sethi S, Campbell AJ, Ellis LA. (2010) The use of computerized self-help packages to treat adolescent depression and anxiety. *J Technol Hum Serv* **28**(3), 144–160.

Woodruff SI, Conway TL, Edwards CC, Elliott SP, Crittenden J. (2007) Evaluation of an internet virtual world chat room for adolescent smoking cessation. *Addict Behav* **32**(9): 1769–1786.

Chapter 9

Education Issues

Margaret Allan

1. Introduction

Adolescents have a right to education. Schools can also promote healthy behaviours, sound nutrition, physical activity, and mental well-being. However, both acute and chronic illness can interfere with education. This disruption can be due to hospitalisation for prolonged periods, or as a result of cognitive or physical impairments due to illness, trauma, or medication. Schools for adolescents play a major role in integrating with the peer group and the development of social competency. These important roles should not be neglected while coping with an illness, and adolescents should be given every encouragement to engage in education in some way. Additionally chronic illness may interfere in more subtle ways with cognition.

2. The Hospital School

The aim of the hospital school is to support the student in their educational program whilst they are away from their 'home school'. Adolescents typically form 25% of the inpatient population of any paediatric hospital. These adolescents require educational support during their admission. Any adolescent who is well enough to attend the classroom can follow an educational program. Those adolescents who are not able to come to the classroom but well enough to receive schooling, may have access to bedside teaching.

Schooling aims to stimulate and support students through an enjoyable, positive educational experience, and to promote psychological well-being, whilst assisting and enhancing the recovery process. The hospital school provides a continuum of familiar educational activities, and for some students this may be the first positive experience of education that they have. Importantly, links are maintained with the student's 'home school'. The hospital school has to work in consultation with medical and nursing staff, other therapists, and allied health in order to adjust to changing needs of the young person.

In some cases, the exact program an adolescent was following at their 'home school' is not adhered to. Relevance and collaborative planning are key issues to ensure that the student is happy, positive, and continuing to learn. Learning needs to be relevant to the adolescent, particularly if there has been anxiety in the learning process. Collaboration with an adolescent team can bring about a range of styles, strategies, and processes for the adolescent. The older adolescent who is undertaking final school external exams can be helped to navigate educational rulings around illness and misadventure.

Key educational issues faced by adolescents with health conditions are mostly found in curriculum and welfare areas. Team approaches work best with the support of the student who moves between the school and hospital. The student, parent/carer, allied health, school personnel, and community members are integral to this process. Transition processes can be planned and programmed for the student and offer ongoing support through the high school years. Many educational jurisdictions offer formal links to mental health services or access to school nursing services, which may need to be involved in continuing care of the adolescent.

3. Adult Hospitals

Older adolescents in adult hospitals may not have access to school teachers. Here, the parents/carers may need to arrange ongoing education if the adolescents are capable of doing school work. Young adults in tertiary education can usually resolve education issues if they are provided with internet contact. They may however need supporting documents and certificates to assist with missed classes and assignment deadlines. Young people may not be aware that they can ask for these and clinicians should check this need before discharge.

4. Chronic Illness and Cognitive Ability

The effect of an acute illness or a temporary exacerbation of a chronic illness may have an impact on cognition and learning ability. Adolescents and young adults with a chronic illness may have experienced previous neurological assaults, including in infancy and early childhood. These assaults may have long term and often subtle effects on learning, both in school and university, and in learning about self-management in chronic illness.

4.1. *Metabolic Disturbances*

Severe hypoglycaemia in childhood, as defined by unconsciousness or convulsions, may result in lifelong cognitive impairment. The younger the age of the hypoglycaemic patient, the more likely is the impairment. Uncommon conditions which cause dehydration and electrolyte disturbance in the neonatal period may also result in long term learning difficulties. These conditions include nephrogenic diabetes insipidus and salt-wasting forms of congenital adrenal hyperplasia.

4.2. *Frontal Lobe Damage*

Examples of this damage include the hydrocephalus of spina bifida and post-cranial irradiation in early childhood. Executive functioning difficulties vary from patient to patient and impact on many areas of day-to-day use. These areas include planning and organising, problem solving, motivation and mental flexibility, all of which impact education. For young adults, these functional deficits may also be more obvious when dealing with novel situations, switching between tasks, setting personal goals, and altering behaviour to achieve these goals. These situations in turn create higher education challenges and re-evaluative psychometric testing may be needed to ensure that the young person is not placed in a learning situation in which he/she is likely to fail.

4.3. *Early Hypoxia*

Both cognitive and motor delays have been reported in complex congenital heart disease and its associated reparative surgery. Early intervention programs have been of assistance. Presently, there are inadequate data on outcomes in adolescents and young adults.

5. The Developmental Role for Schools

Learning and engagement in education in adolescence is critical to social and emotional development and well-being, and to enable successful participation in the workplace and community as an adult. Puberty has mostly been conceptualised as a stressful life event that can disrupt academic performance, and the age at which pubertal maturation occurs may influence academic performance. However, performance differences are not necessarily enduring. The influence of the pubertal hormone rise on motivation and engagement in education, particularly when compared with the well-identified effects of socio–economic status and mental health, is as yet unknown. In schools, where year levels are defined by age, rather than pubertal stage, such research information would assist school personnel to identify and deal with the wide developmental range in any given year group.

References

Asvold BO, Sand T, Hestad K, Bjorgaas MR. (2010) Cognitive function in type 1 diabetic adults with early exposure to severe hypoglycemia: A 16-year follow-up study. *Diabetes Care* **33**(9): 1945–1947.

Australian Health Promoting Schools Association Available online at: http://www.ahpsa.org.au/ (accessed 20 August 2011).

Dubas JS, Graber JA, Petersen AC. (1991) The effects of pubertal development on achievement during adolescence. *Am J Educ* **99**(4): 444–460.

Johannsen TH, Ripa CPL, Reinisch JM, Schwartz M, Mortensen EL, Main KM. (2006) Impaired cognitive function in women with congenital adrenal hyperplasia. *J Clin Endocrinol Metab* **91**(4): 1376–1381.

Nsw Public Schools *Supporting students, disability programs*. Available online at: http://www.schools.nsw.edu.au/studentsupport/programs/disabilitypgrms/dpre sources.php (accessed 20 August 2011).

Spence SH. (2003) Social skills training with children and young people: Theory, evidence and practice. *Child Adolesc Ment Health* **8**(2): 84–96.

The Hospital School & Westmead, C. S. H. A. *Useful links*. Available online at: http://www.chw.health.nsw.gov.au/kids/school/useful_links.htm (accessed 24 August 2011).

Chapter 10

Adolescents and Young Adults in Adult Hospitals

Gail Anderson, Tegan Sturrock and Patricia Kasengele

1. Introduction

Adolescents may not fit comfortably into either paediatric acute care or adult acute health care facilities. They present special challenges for paediatric staff who feel more comfortable with younger patients. In adult facilities, adolescents may feel out of place and isolated when mainstreamed into adult wards according to clinical specialty. Wherever possible, treatment should be provided in a dedicated adolescent ward with staff trained in the developmental stages and special needs of adolescents. This chapter addresses some of the generic issues for hospitalised adolescents and young adults, and discusses how to create a youth friendly ward and a positive hospitalisation experience.

2. Adolescents in Hospital: Opportunistic Health Assessments

The Australian Institute for Health and Welfare National Hospital Morbidity Database indicates that the main reason for hospitalisation in adolescents and young adults in Australia aged 15–24 years is pregnancy and childbirth for females, and injury and poisoning for males. The next most common reasons are diseases of the digestive system and mental health. Young people with chronic illness make up a lower percentage of admissions but are more likely to have repeated admissions.

Any admission of an adolescent or young person provides an opportunity to assess risk behaviours and mental health, the leading causes of morbidity in this age group. These may be related to the admission, for example, trauma after a road traffic accident when intoxicated or deliberate self-harm with suicidal ideation. There may also be a less obvious connection between risky behaviours or mental health issues and the admission, for example — a flare up of inflammatory bowel disease as a result of unacknowledged non-adherence to therapy or chronic anxiety which compromises nutritional status in cystic fibrosis. A risk factor may simply be incidental, such as heavy nicotine use disclosed during a pre-operative assessment for suspected appendicitis.

Hospitalisation provides an ideal opportunity for screening adolescents, both at the beginning of an admission when a youth specific care plan is devised, and throughout the admission. Paediatric care plans focus on childhood developmental health issues and the transfer of familiar home routines to the hospital. Adult care plans are more likely to address falls risk and drug interactions. For a youth specific care plan, the HEADSS assessment offers a good framework for identifying issues of concern in areas such as home life, education, substance use, sexuality, and mood disturbance (Chapter 5). Clinicians consistently identify substance use, sexuality, and mood disturbance as being difficult to initiate discussion around and specific training should be offered. The use of opportunistic screening must include access to defined referral pathways if high risk behaviours or mental health problems are identified.

Young people often present to emergency departments as a result of risk taking behaviour or mental health concerns. Anecdotally these presentations can be a negative experience for the young person if clinical staffs are not trained and skilled in engaging adolescents at the appropraite developmental level. Adolescent and young adult clinicians need to advocate strongly to enhance the skills of emergency department staff in areas of adolescent development, risk taking, and mental health.

3. Adolescent Wards

The concept of an adolescent ward was initially developed in paediatric hospitals. Adolescent Wards in paediatric services have a number of key features that contribute to their success:

- The age group for admission is defined and quarantined. The lower age limit is generally 12 years. The upper limit is dependent on local policies. As an example, some hospitals may have an upper age limit of 16 for acute presentations but 18 for patients with long standing chronic illness. For the latter group, it is important that they understand the implications of the upper age limit and when their admission will have to be transitioned to an adult facility (Section 5). Flexibility around upper age limit policy is useful in cases of developmental disability and for operative procedures where expertise resides solely in paediatric services. However, these situations should be infrequent and managed with clear institutional policies and with advocacy for appropriate services in adult health care facilities.

- Experienced ward staff are capable of dealing with regressive or acting out behaviours, which commonly occur in physically or emotionally stressed adolescents. Ward staff will also have the necessary skills to ensure that parents support their adolescents in an age appropriate manner. This includes allowing adolescents to actively participate in decision making, to learn to manage part of their hospital stay on their own, and to negotiate with ward staff around ward rules and permissions. Adolescent ward staff may also act as a hospital wide resource for adolescent health.

- A clinical mix of patients is maintained. This may require negotiation with medical and surgical specialty teams who argue that it is only possible to deliver specialist care on a specialist ward. Other examples which support a mix of patients are decisions around the maximum number of eating disorder patients and the maximum number of rehabilitation admissions for complex somatising disorders that are hospitalised at any one time.

- The promotion of developmentally appropriate care and environment, with support for schooling and school attendance. This promotion extends to the physical space, with room for young people to relax, prepare snacks, and the use of age appropriate colour schemes and decorations.

4. Adolescents and Young Adults in Adult Hospitals

Unfortunately there are fewer adolescent wards in adult hospitals than there are in paediatric hospitals. This is of particular concern, especially as survival rates for children with chronic illness have improved so significantly over recent years and the need for transitional care to adult health care settings has increased exponentially. Apart from a few specialist adolescent wards in adult facilities in Australia, the majority of adolescents and young adults who are in-patients in adult facilities will be scattered throughout the facility. The challenge then is to advocate for a multidisciplinary adolescent health team to locate these young people and help manage their special developmental needs in adult wards with variable patient mixes and therapeutic approaches. The role of this team would also include effective advocacy for the special needs of adolescent and young adult patients and the education of staff to be able to assess and manage these special needs of young people.

The effective management of adolescents and young adults in an adult facility without a specialist adolescent ward would be advanced by:

- Grouping adolescents together whenever possible.
- Appointing a multidisciplinary outreach team with expertise in adolescent and young adult developmental and health care needs. A potential model for hospitals without specialist adolescent medicine units is a 'service without walls' or liaison service which crosses all departments and specialities. Management problems that arise with this age group often relate to nonmedical, nonsurgical aspects of care. Adolescent health care staff can act as advocates and as trainers of other staff in the use of youth specific assessment processes and formulation of care plans so that bio–psychosocial aspects of care can be addressed from early on in the admission. It should be remembered that young people are unlikely to volunteer information unless

directly asked in a trusting and non-judgemental way. An age specific youth care plan may be useful in order to make sure developmentally appropriate information is obtained.

- Allowances will need to be made for first time hospitalisation of young people transitioning from paediatric facilities. Many staff in adult services do not appreciate the major physical and cultural differences that exist between paediatric and adult facilities. What is often a shock to the young person transitioning from paediatric hospital care is the lower staff:patient ratios that exist in adult-based hospitals and that interaction with staff is limited.
- Providing information on patient rights, responsibilities, and how the hospital works in youth-friendly language.
- Identifying ways to enhance peer contact, and providing dedicated space for young people to engage in developmentally appropriate diversional activities are important. This means identifying the young person's usual activity patterns and preferences, and incorporating these into the daily ward routine wherever possible, ideally involving an occupational therapist or leisure coordinator.

5. Hospitalisation as a Transition from Paediatric to Adult Care in Chronic Illness

For many adolescents with chronic illness, recurrent hospitalisation is a reality. Facilitating one or even several meetings with the new treating team in the adult based service prior to formal transition can provide opportunities for the young person to become familiar and confident with the new health care environment and personnel, **before** they experience their first hospitalisation in a new facility.

In some situations it may be possible to create a new patient record where transition information is kept prior to any physical visit to the new facility. In developmental delay, it is important to decide in advance which team will be responsible for the admission and to have clear instructions around the need for sedation with any procedure (including venepuncture and radiology). This can be detailed in a letter held by parents/carers as well as the hospital. The key person in transition can be any member of the health care team, and is often a specialist nurse or allied health worker who has the necessary knowledge, skills, and interest in this particular area of care. Transitional care coordinators are now being employed to work with young people, families, and clinicians. Where a designated specialist transitional coordinator does not exist, in-patient nursing staff may be ideally placed to take on a key leadership role in developing individual local transitional care plans.

It is preferable to avoid an acute hospitalisation as the first point of contact for a chronically ill adolescent with their new receiving adult service. This can happen in situations where a young person delays transition, such as with cystic fibrosis, or has an inherently unstable condition such as epilepsy (especially if associated with developmental delay) or has had a slow deterioration in control because of failure to engage in adult care. Diabetic ketoacidosis, acute exacerbation of inflammatory bowel disease on a background of malnutrition, and acute renal failure in spina bifida are all examples of the latter.

6. Creating a Youth-Friendly Hospitalisation

Surveys of young people admitted to hospital identify social interaction with friends and peers, education and work disruption, separation from family, and loss of freedom as aspects of life affected by hospitalisation. Making it easier for young people to stay in contact with family and friends and facilitating ongoing schooling are helpful strategies. Making sure that appropriate certificates and forms to cover absence are provided is another. Young people may not be aware that these are available and often spend significant time fretting about what will happen on discharge. While for some young people, hospitalisation can be a reminder of their own mortality, for others especially those with chronic debilitating conditions, it can be a positive experience due to enforced rest, feelings of getting better, and being taken care of.

Adolescents should not be co-located with severely ill or dying adult patients. Single rooms can be helpful in providing an opportunity for a parent or carer to stay overnight, especially when the young person has cognitive disabilities or some behavioural problems requiring close supervision. Adolescents and young adults should not be placed in mixed gender bays, for both developmental and safety concerns. This is an increasing problem, especially where mixed gender bays are a specific strategy for hospitals to deal with bed shortages. Ideally, hospitals should have a youth advisory committee to assist the hospital executive in the creation of youth friendly services.

Diversional activities and group therapy sessions are helpful for both peer contact and support, healthy expression of feelings and for meeting adolescent developmental needs; a recreation room should be made available for these reasons. A classroom-type facility and hospital-based school teachers assist adolescents to keep up their schooling.

Staff need to recognise and cater for special developmental needs of adolescents. They will need to be comfortable discussing intimate issues raised by young people in a sensitive and non-judgemental way and use age appropriate language to assist the young person in their understanding of their illness and treatment, which will promote their autonomy.

7. Summary

As young people develop and become more independent they generally and gradually begin to assume responsibility for their own health and start making their own life decisions. With this responsibility comes the opportunity to make choices that can have a positive or negative impact on their lives. Every presentation of an adolescent to a health care service, including hospitalisation, provides a window of opportunity to set the stage for establishing or reinforcing healthy and productive behaviours and reducing the likelihood of health related problems in the future.

Adolescents and young people can often feel overwhelmed in adult health care systems. Without particular attention paid to their biological, psychological, social, and developmental needs, young people new to the adult health care system may perceive it as unfriendly, uncaring, and irrelevant to their care. Communication difficulties can also occur between the young person and clinicians in adult health services when the young person is still struggling with the development of more adult skills such as decision making, problem solving, assertiveness, self-determination, and self-advocacy.

Adult health services need to develop specific policies around the care of adolescents and young people to ensure that their developmental needs as well as their health care needs are being met. To be most effective, clinicians need to have a genuine interest in, understanding of, and desire to work with this dynamic population.

References

Bernstein J, Heeren T, Edward E, Dorfman D, Bliss C, Winter M, Bernstein E.(2010) A brief motivational interview in a pediatric emergency department, plus 10-day telephone follow-up, increases attempts to quit drinking among youth and young adults who screen positive for problematic drinking. *Acad Emerg Med.* **17**(8): 890–902.

Blum RW, Hirsch D, Kastner TA, Quint RD, Sandler AD. (2002). A Consensus Statement on health care transitions for young people with special health care needs. *Pediatrics* **110**(6): 1304–1306.

Britto MT, DeVellis RF, Hornung RW, DeFriese GH, Atherton HD, Slap GB. (2004) Health care preferences and priorities of adolescents with chronic illnesses. *Pediatrics* **114**(5): 1272–1280.

Fisher M, Kaufman M. (1996) Adolescent inpatient units: A position statement of the society for adolescent medicine. *J Adolesc Health* **18**: 307–308.

Goldenring JM, Cohen E. (1988) Getting into Adolescents Heads. *Community Pediatrics* 75–90.

Kari J, Donovan C, Li J, Taylor B. (1999) Teenagers in hospital: What do they want? *Nurs Stand* **13**: 49–51.

Royal College of Nursing (2004). Adolescent transitional care: Guidance for nursing staff. Available from www.rcn.org.uk/__data/assets/pdf_file/0011/78617/002313.pdf

Sturrock T, Masterson L, Steinbeck KS. (2007) Adolescent Appropriate Care in an Adult Hospital; The use of a Youth Care Plan. *AJAN* **24**: 49–53.

Viner R. (2001) National Survey of use of hospital beds by adolescents aged 12 to 19 in the United Kingdom. *BMJ* **322**: 957–958.

Walton MA, Resko S, Whiteside L, Chermack ST, Zimmerman M, Cunningham RM. (2011) Sexual risk behaviors among teens at an urban emergency department: Relationship with violent behaviors and substance use. *J Adolesc Health* **48**(3): 303–305.

Watson AR. (2004). Hospital youth work and adolescent support. *Arch Dis Child* **89**: 440–442.

Chapter 11

Self-Management in Chronic Illness; Promoting Therapy Adherence

Michele Casey and Kate Steinbeck

1. Introduction

Self-management describes the decisions and actions that a young person takes to cope with and improve his/her health. It is a young person's ability to deal with all that a chronic illness entails. The management of chronic illness places significant demands on the young person with the illness, as well as the clinicians who look after the young person, and his/her family. The personal demands of self-management vary considerably depending on the type and severity of the chronic illness.

The broad theoretical framework underlying self-management is that improvement in self-management skills will build confidence and self-efficacy to perform three important tasks:

- Disease management.
- Role management.
- Emotional management.

2. The Requirements of Self-Management

2.1. *Knowledge*

Self-management requires knowledge, an understanding of the chronic illness which includes aetiology, and the effects (current and potential) on health and well-being. For many young people, this knowledge was provided to their parents in the past, but not to them.

2.2. *Plans*

The ability to manage care plans is essential. This includes the names of medication, doses, and reasons for each therapy, and what adverse or side effects exist for each medication. These plans need to be written somewhere as it is unrealistic to expect a young person to remember the details.

2.3. *What to do in an Emergency*

An emergency plan is required which includes what to do if there is a clinical deterioration. Many chronic illnesses also require a plan for what to do if the young person has an intercurrent illness which may affect chronic illness management. Examples are insulin treatment of Type 1 diabetes and where pharmacological doses of glucocorticoid which suppress the hypothalamic pituitary adrenal axis are being taken. Both require an increase in dose with an intercurrent infection, to cover increased insulin resistance and failure of the endogenous rise in adrenal steroid production respectively. Young people need to have the contact details of their health care professionals and to be able to manage day-to-day care when away from home, including sleepovers, camps, and holidays with friends. For the older adolescent and young adult, selected peers and their parents need to know what to do in an emergency.

2.4. *Local Health Care Knowledge*

An understanding of the processes around obtaining prescriptions, making appointments to see a primary care doctor, their specialist doctor and other health care professionals, and the costs of health care are all necessary for competent self-management. Discussions should include what to do if the young person runs out of medication and travel planning. Travel planning should cover insurance and access to medications and emergency health care. It may be prudent to provide an introductory letter and contact numbers for an overseas treatment team, especially if the young person plans to be away for more than a few weeks.

2.5. *Looking After Themselves*

This aspect is about understanding the physical, emotional, and social impact of the adolescent's chronic illness. For some young people this might be explaining to friends about what they can and cannot do or explaining absences from school, work, or social events. It might also be about a clear plan for energy conservation, as in 'Zest', a website publication of the Department of Adolescent and Transitional Medicine at Royal Prince Alfred, Sydney, Australia. Young people with a chronic illness need to adopt a lifestyle that generally promotes health. This includes knowing about the potential effects of tobacco, alcohol, and other drugs on their health, and having knowledge about contraception, fertility, and pregnancy (including the safety of their medication in pregnancy).

3. The Primary Goals for Self-Management

Optimal health and well-being for the young person is the ultimate goal. This means the achievement of the best possible balance between the intrusiveness of the day to day management and the requirements of illness control. A partnership between the young person and the health professionals involved in their care needs to be developed. Improvements in self-efficacy promote better levels of health and in turn allow the time spent with health professionals to be used more effectively.

4. Transitions to Self-Management

During adolescence, the goal is to gradually shift the responsibility of self-management from parents or carers to the young person. The assumption is that a young person who is educated about their illness and its management will improve their self-care. However, behaviour change does not automatically follow education and the attainment of new knowledge. Personal beliefs about the advantages of change, individual readiness to change, and the capacity to make change under their own personal circumstances are all important. A thorough HEADSS interview (Chapter 5) is essential.

The achievement of satisfactory self-management in adolescents with chronic illness has specific developmental aspects:

- At some time, self-management is passed from the parents to the young person, except if significant disability is present.
- The time when such knowledge transfer is expected to happen is when the young person is faced with a large number of developmental tasks, not related to the chronic illness, but which may be significantly affected by the chronic illness.
- The acquisition of self-management skills is essential to optimal transition to adult care in chronic illness. Clinicians will expect the older adolescent and young adult to take charge of their illness and its management and to make their own decisions about their illness. This can sometimes be perceived as uncaring by the young person.
- The consequences of failing to achieve illness management skills may result in drop out from care and a deterioration of physical condition, as the burden for the young person is too great to manage.

Case history:

Yasmin is 19 years old and has had Type 1 diabetes mellitus for six years. Yasmin has competing priorities, as she is juggling casual shift work, with medical appointments and study. She would like to move out of the family home, where there is considerable conflict which interferes with blood glucose control. She is unsure whether to disclose health issues to her employer, as she is afraid that she will lose her job. She has much less structure around medication regimens and time management since leaving the routine of school. She does not always take insulin because of concern about weight gain and because of her fear of having hypoglycaemia in front of others.

The intervention included goal setting according to Yasmin's changing routines which will need to change again as circumstances change. Making sure that she has a diabetes education nurse and specialist care closer to work, rather than home, has helped attendance at scheduled appointments considerably. Mild depression and incipient bulimia were addressed. New daily routines and management expectations were developed in consultation with Yasmin. Some compromises had to be made on both sides. Discussions about how to handle specific social and work scenarios took place so that she could solve the problem in advance.

5. Adolescent Development and Self Management

The most consistently challenging aspect of self-management in adolescence and in young adulthood is therapy adherence. The issues relevant to therapy adherence/self-management vary with developmental stage (Chapters 3 and 13).

5.1. *Early Adolescence*

Cognitive processes are concrete and the understanding of their illness is basic. 'I have something wrong with my heart and I take these tablets to keep me well and out of hospital.' Parents are generally responsible for reminding the young adolescent to take their medication and are the key coordinators around hospital visits, medication supplies, and negotiations with school. Young adolescents are immediately reactive to treatment if it is painful or if there are unwanted side effects and it may be hard to convince them to continue. They are starting to comprehend that not everyone their age has to do what they must do as part of a daily schedule.

5.2. *Middle Adolescence*

The process of achieving independence from parents has commenced. In parallel, the importance of the peer group has increased. Cognitive maturation progresses but adolescents in middle adolescence have a limited ability to conceptualise their future, including the future impacts of their chronic illness. If asked, they would acknowledge that it is impossible to imagine themselves as ever being thirty. The future is all about next weekend or next holidays.

However, the young person is able to comprehend that chronic means forever, and that they do not like. There is often an intense interest in potential cures. They are pushing the boundaries in many aspects of their life, chronic illness included. 'Taking insulin injections really sucks, and I do not believe that I will die if I miss one or two injections, even though that's what my parents and my doctor say.' The adolescent develops more privacy around their chronic illness and becomes more selective about whom they tell about their condition. If a young person suffers an exacerbation of their illness or if they have other psychosocial issues to deal with, their self-management skills may temporarily regress.

5.3. *Late Adolescence*

Cognition is maturing and in late adolescence the young person is able to understand their chronic illness in a more coherent fashion. There is a gradual attitudinal shift. 'I don't like it that the medication can make me feel sick on the stomach sometimes, but I also know that if I don't take it I may be in hospital for weeks or even die.' Young persons in their late teens will be less likely to accept their parents' views and instructions, and will often ask their clinician quite challenging and incisive questions about their condition. They are quick to detect if health professionals are not being straight with them. It becomes apparent that they need to intergrate their chronic illness into their life plans and aspirations.

6. Therapy Adherence

6.1. *Reasons*

Adolescents are not the only ones who have difficulties adhering to treatment regimens. A third of adults never fill the prescriptions that have been written for them. Parents may fail to deliver therapy to their children because of chaotic lives or mental illness. Adolescents and young adults with cancer demonstrate many of the issues associated with non-adherence. Adherence to therapeutic regimens, particularly oral chemotherapy, is more problematic in adolescents and young adults than in younger and older patients. Complex regimens, a need for substantial behavioural change, inconvenient or inefficient clinic systems, and inadequate supervision — as parents try to give the teenager the space they request — may coalesce to produce less than ideal management. Poor communication with health care providers, patient's health beliefs in favour of non-adherence (denial, invincibility, or fatalism), poor understanding of the illness, inadequate social support, concern over ineffectiveness, and fear of side effects can produce ambivalent or frankly avoidant feelings about adherence.

6.2. *Strategies*

Having identified adherence as a problem, several strategies should be employed. There needs to be clear acknowledgement of the reality of variable adherence, and engagement of the young person in problem-solving, rather than blaming. Appointment and medication reminders, mobile phone alarms and calendars, and transportable pill containers are useful. Especially for the younger adolescent, there should be a discussion to clarify whether the adolescent or their parent/carer is responsible for medication taking and other treatments in their schedule.

6.3. *What the Clinician Can Do*

Helping an adolescent or young adult adhere to a therapeutic regimen is possible with time, the development of a therapeutic alliance that is based on honesty, trust, and good will and with an understanding of their individual circumstances.

Initially:

- Ensure that the young person understands, using age and developmentally appropriate language, why they are being asked to adhere to a certain management programme. *Ask them to repeat back to you what you have said.*
- Keep the regimen as simple as possible — once or twice a day dosing avoids having to take medication at school or work.
- Understand the young person's schedule and commitments and how these might affect their ability to follow instructions.

- Where possible provide some flexibility within the regimen so that the young person has some choice and control.
- Identify a reminder system to help the young person remember schedules such as a mobile phone alarm or a link with a regular activity.
- Determine if there might be financial difficulties which may make adherence difficult.
- Discuss the expected results of therapy including the time frame in which the results might be expected to occur, in order to avoid cessation of therapy 'because it didn't work'. Young people might expect instantaneous results when in fact days or weeks may be needed to achieve a full response.
- Tell them about the known side effects and how these can be ameliorated.

Over a period of time:

- Ask carefully about side effects of new therapies.
- Ask the young person to contact you if they are worried that the therapy might be having adverse effects. It may be easier for a young person to text message or ask his/her parent to call.
- Ask the young person to contact you before stopping therapy.
- If a number of changes to treatment are needed, try to initiate one at a time.
- Praise the effort and look for concrete ways that the patient can demonstrate achievement.
- Enlist the help of others, but only if the young person agrees.

6.4 *What Parents/Carers Can Do*

While parents/carers acknowledge emerging autonomy, they will also be anxious about health outcomes if therapy regimens are ignored.

- Acknowledge that they ultimately have to hand over therapy control to their young person.
- Acknowledge their own anxiety and sometimes distress at handing over this responsibility.

- Allow their young person the same level of responsibility with medication that they have in other areas of their life, but when significant boundaries are crossed let them know.
- Avoid persistent nagging — it has never been shown to work.
- Be positive about their young person's ability to handle their medications and notice the effort.

Case history:

Jack is 18 years old and has had Crohn's disease since he was 12. Jack is not very good at discussing his condition with his doctors. His main priorities are completion of final school exams and sports. Illness induced lethargy is a significant problem and he is embarrassed by illness symptoms, especially frequent diarrhoea. His parents want full involvement with consultations and treatment decisions, while Jack's health care professionals are working on transition. Jack just feels that too much is happening all at once. It is important to identify current concerns and how these influence of illness control. Goal setting and prioritising was related to his own priorities. Jack was provided with some basic information on Crohn's disease and the website of a support group for his age. Simplified strategies (specific steps) for treatment regimens and increasing independence with illness management were negotiated and written down. This included the development of clear roles and boundaries for him, and his parents. His daily routines were reorganised to fit with both illness management and study demands. Jack found simple aids to stress management and relaxation techniques were useful, along with developing strategies for managing social situations, and an understanding of energy conservation.

References

Butow P, Palmer S, Pai A, Goodenough B, Luckett T, King M. (2010) Review of adherence-related issues in adolescents and young adults with cancer. *J Clin Oncol* **28**(32): 4800–4809.

Fredericks EM, Dore-Stites D. (2010) Adherence to immunosuppressants: How can it be improved in adolescent organ transplant recipients? *Curr Opin Organ Transplant* **15**(5): 614–620.

Kyngäs HA, Kroll T, Duffy ME. (2000) Compliance in adolescents with chronic diseases: A review. *J Adolesc Health* **26**(6): 379–388.

Osterberg L, Blaschke T. (2005) Drug therapy: Adherence to medication. *New England Journal of Medicine* **353**(5): 487–497.

Sawyer SM, Drew S, Yeo MS, Britto MT. Adolescents with a chronic condition: Challenges living, challenges treating. *The Lancet* **369**(9571): 1481–1489.

Zest Energy Conservation. Available online at: www.sswahs.nsw.gov.au/sswahs/youth/pdf/zest.pdf (accessed 1 May 2011).

Chapter 12

Complex Medicopsychosocial Conditions: Chronic and Functional Disorders

Susan J Towns and Helen E Bibby

1. Introduction

This chapter explores what Lipowski described as the *'borderland between psychiatry and medicine.'* Adolescents with physical symptoms which are medically unexplained such as somatoform disorders, with clinical syndromes where both psychological and psychosocial factors play a key role, such as post-viral fatigue, and with other chronic medical conditions all fit within this 'borderland'.

2. Definitions

A range of terms are used in the medical literature to describe complex medico–psychosocial presentations.

2.1. *Medically Unexplained Symptoms*

These are physical symptoms in the absence of an identifiable organic explanation, and may be seen as a continuum with minor aches and pains at one end, unexplained 'functional' symptoms in the middle, and diagnosable somatoform disorders at the other end.

115

2.2. *Functional Symptoms*

This term is sometimes used interchangeably with medically unexplained symptoms. 'Functional' may imply a problem with an organ or system's function, as distinct from its structure. It may be used to imply that the symptom serves some function in the patient's life or a secondary gain.

2.3. *Somatisation*

This term, coined by Lipowski, is often used to describe symptoms that are the manifestation of psychological difficulty or distress, but which the sufferer believes to be caused by a physical illness. More recently, Garralda's holistic view has been used which takes into account a range of interacting biological, psychological, and psychosocial factors.

2.4. *Somatoform Disorders*

A group of disorders where the main feature is one or more physical symptoms that cannot be completely explained by a medical condition, direct effects of a substance/medication, or a mental disorder. To receive the diagnosis of a somatoform disorder, the symptoms must cause significant distress and/or impairment. If any medical conditions are present, these are not sufficient to explain the nature/intensity of the symptoms and/or the associated impairment and preoccupation. This category of disorders is found in both ICD-10 and DSM-IV-TR (Table 1).

2.5. *Functional Clinical Syndromes*

These are diagnostic labels for specific sets of symptoms that are causing impairment, but which cannot be completely explained by biomedical processes and include irritable bowel syndrome, recurrent abdominal pain, fibromyalgia, and chronic fatigue syndrome.

2.6. *Abnormal Illness Behaviour*

This includes unhelpful perceptions, beliefs, and behaviours associated with a symptom or disease. The responses could be excessive, such as

Table 1: Common diagnostic classifications.

ICD-10	DSM-IV	Other
F45.0 Somatisation disorder.	300.81 Somatisation disorder.	
	300.11 Conversion disorder.	
F44.4–F44.7 Dissociative (conversion) disorders of movement and sensation.	300.82 Undifferentiated somatoform disorder.	
F45.1 Undifferentiated somatoform disorder.	300.7 Hypochondriasis.	
F45.2 Hypochondriacal disorder.	300.82 Somatoform disorder not otherwise specified.	
F45.3 Somatoform autonomic dysfunction.		
F45.8 Other somatoform disorder.		
F45.9 Somatoform disorder unspecified.		
F45.4 Persistent somatoform pain disorder.	307.80 Pain disorder associated with psychological factors.	
R52.1 Chronic intractable pain.	307.89 Pain disorder associated with both psychological factors and a general medical condition.	
R52.2 Other chronic pain.		
R52.9 Pain unspecified.		
F48.0 Neurasthenia.		Chronic fatigue syndrome:
G99.3 Post viral fatigue syndrome.		CDC criteria.
		Oxford criteria.
M79.7 Fibromyalgia.		Fibromyalgia: Smythe criteria.
G44.2 Tension headache.		
K58.0 Irritable bowel syndrome.		Recurrent abdominal pain: Rome criteria.
K59 Other functional intestinal disorders.		

(*Continued*)

Table 1:   (*Continued*)

ICD-10	DSM-IV	Other
F51 Nonorganic sleep disorders.	307.42 Primary insomnia. 307.44 Primary hypersomnia. 307.45 Circadian rhythm sleep disorder. 307.47 Dyssomnia not otherwise specified.	International classification of sleep disorders. Dyssomnias. Parasomnias. Sleep disorders associated with medical/psychiatric disorders. Proposed sleep disorders.
F54 Psychological and behavioural disorders associated with disorders listed elsewhere.	316 Psychological factor affecting medical condition.	

those seen in somatoform disorders and inadequate responses, such as denial of illness.

Symptoms associated with somatoform disorders and functional clinical syndromes are not under conscious control. These must be distinguished from the factitious and induced disorders, which are purposefully induced or feigned and which are rare in adolescence.

3. Epidemiology

Medically unexplained symptoms are common in children and adolescents. The incidence increases from childhood into adolescence, with adolescent girls reporting more symptoms than adolescent boys. Common complaints include headaches, abdominal pain/nausea, fatigue, myalgia, arthralgia, dizziness, breathlessness, and fainting, alone or in combination.

4. Diagnostic Considerations

There is a lack of consensus about the appropriate diagnostic labels to apply to adolescents presenting with complex medico–psychosocial conditions. Both ICD-10 and DSM-IV-TR list a number of relevant diagnoses, but there are some key differences in terms of the labels used, and the diagnostic criteria employed. Many of the diagnoses, which were developed for adults, have not been well validated with adolescents.

An excellent example of the diagnostic dilemmas facing clinicians is chronic fatigue syndrome. The syndrome is not mentioned in DSM-IV, while its closest approximation in ICD-10 is neurasthenia. Clinicians tend to use criteria that were originally developed for research purposes. The commonly used CDC criteria are:

- Unexplained fatigue of definite onset that has persisted for 6 months or more.
- The fatigue is not due to ongoing exertion, and is not substantially alleviated by rest.
- The additional presence of at least four of the following symptoms: sore throat, memory or concentration problems, muscle pain, joint pain, headache, tender lymph nodes, un-refreshing sleep, post-exertional malaise.

These criteria have been criticised for not being empirically based and it has been recommended that the six month criteria be dropped for adolescents to facilitate early intervention. There has also been considerable debate about the overlap between CFS and myalgic encephalomyelitis. We find the term 'post-viral fatigue syndrome' is often preferable to use with adolescents, to emphasise the fact that CFS has a better prognosis in teenagers compared to adults.

> *Practice Point*: A somatoform disorder or functional syndrome must always be a diagnosis of exclusion. Thus, a medical practitioner must rule out alternative physical and psychiatric explanations for the presenting concerns. Even if the onset of the symptom coincides with significant stressful life events, we cannot be sure that organic pathology is not present without a thorough medical assessment.

5. Aetiology

The aetiology of most complex medico–psychosocial conditions is unclear, and likely to differ between disorders and from patient to patient.

Many clinicians advocate taking a bio-psychosocial approach, which considers the interaction between physical, psychological, and social contributions to the condition. Therefore, we recommend developing a *case formulation* for each patient, which includes risk factors, triggers and maintaining factors. It is also helpful to consider the strengths of the adolescents and their families. The formulation should be based on a review of the relevant literature, and should be used to guide treatment.

5.1. *Examples of Risk Factors*

- Family history of chronic medical problems, complex medico–psychosocial conditions or psychological distress.
- Characteristic responses to physical symptoms, regarding them as medical or dangerous. Preoccupation with body sensations, or fear of illness.
- Family reinforcement of physical symptoms, for example with excessive attention or making special allowances.
- Avoidance/discouragement of expressions of negative emotions.
- History of high achievement or perfectionism. High parental expectations, or adolescent perception of high parental expectations.

5.2. *Examples of Triggers*

- Physical illness/injury, for example viral illness.
- Psychosocial stressors, for example bereavement, parental separation, bullying, transition to secondary school.
- A combination of several factors is very common.

5.3. *Examples of Maintaining Factors*

- Significant anxiety about the symptoms and hypervigilance to small changes in body sensations.
- Lack of symptom management skills.
- Excessive lifestyle changes in response to the symptoms.
- Secondary gain, for example, avoidance of stressful or unpleasant activities or extra attention/closeness from others.

- Family health beliefs; in particular, beliefs that a medical cause has been 'missed', that increasing activity levels will lead to exacerbation of the illness and that the only viable treatment is a medical intervention. A split between the family's understanding of the condition and that of their health professionals.

6. Presentation

The symptoms are typically longstanding and there is often a history of seeing multiple health professionals, with multiple investigations. Referrals are generally around:

- An atypical symptom pattern with disruption to normal activity in the presence of a stable or well controlled primary disease and/or
- Poor response to medication, especially analgesia.

7. Assessment

7.1. *A Detailed and Comprehensive History*

This is most important, including the assessment of the illness in the family context as well as an individual interview with the adolescent (see also Section 5.1–5.3). Key targets for assessment include the number of symptoms, site and duration of pain, triggers, relieving factors, response to treatments, number of consultations, previous investigations as well as musculoskeletal and sleep history. Diet and exercise history and use of media (in particular screen time) are useful. A detailed history may reveal previous episodes of unexplained symptoms, and recurrent soft tissue or joint problems. The family history could include multiple illnesses within family members.

7.2. *Psychosocial Assessment*

This focuses on exploring the likely risk and maintaining factors, as well as assessing current and pre-morbid functioning, the impact of the condition on family interactions, and the assessment of comorbid problems such as emotional, behavioural or learning difficulties. Self-report and parent-report questionnaires may also assist in screening for common comorbidities such as depression, anxiety, or family relationship problems. However, these should be introduced carefully. Introduce with the phrase 'I give this to all the adolescents I see,' as some families are very sensitive to any implication that the symptoms may be psychological in origin. The opinions and observations of siblings may also provide helpful insights.

Practice Point: Taking adolescents and their parents through a typical example of a time when the symptoms were particularly severe, or resulted in non-attendance at school, often reveals important beliefs and characteristic behaviour patterns that may be important for developing a case formulation.

7.3. *A Thorough Physical Examination*

This is necessary from a diagnostic point of view and also to reassure the adolescent and family. Include height and weight and BMI percentile.

- *For post viral fatigue syndrome*: Assess postural hypotension or tachycardia as orthostatic intolerance can be a feature. Joint hypermobility syndrome is also associated with pain and fatigue syndromes. Light sensitivity or hyperacusis may be noted.
- *For pain disorder:* Site of pain may be associated with hyperaesthesia, or abnormal responses to touch. Distribution of pain may be atypical, such as non-dermatomal.
- *For headache:* Normal CNS examination and normal affect despite high subjective pain score.
- *For gastro-intestinal symptoms:* Usually non-localising pain and stable weight. Asking about the location of pain or where nausea is felt may be helpful to clarify symptoms.

7.4. *Differential Diagnosis*

Conditions to exclude will depend on the presenting symptoms. Differential medical diagnoses may include hypothyroidism, inflammatory bowel disease, coeliac disease, autoimmune disorders, juvenile arthritis, complex regional pain syndrome and migraine. Differential psychiatric diagnoses may include anxiety disorders (separation anxiety, panic disorder, school phobia, and generalised anxiety disorder), depressive disorder, adjustment disorder, anorexia nervosa and psychosis.

7.5. *Investigations*

Obtaining the results of all previous investigations will help to reduce unnecessary tests. While it is not possible to provide an exhaustive list of the appropriate investigations for each symptom, Fig. 1

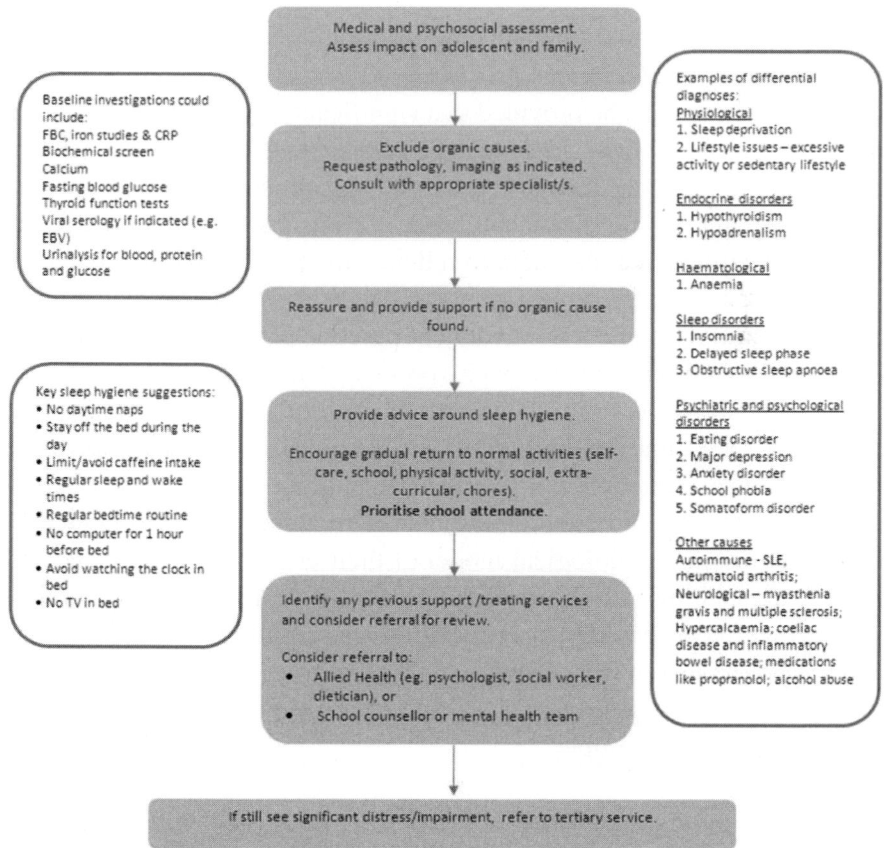

Fig. 1:   Fatigue in adolescents.

> *Practice Point*: Asking the adolescent to keep a symptom diary, such as for pain or sleep, may provide more detailed information around triggers, frequency, and context, and also reinforces that you are attending to their symptoms and seeking more information.

provides an example of guidelines we have developed for general practitioners/family physicians when assessing adolescents presenting with fatigue.

7.6. *Feed Back to the Family*

Once the assessment is complete, families should be provided with a clear explanation of the assessment process, test results, and examination findings. Reassurance can be provided that significant serious illness has been ruled out. However many adolescents and/or parents become increasingly concerned that 'no-one knows what is wrong'. In such cases, the provision of the appropriate diagnostic label, such as PVFS or pain disorder, with good explanation may help to relieve this distress. We also reassure patients and families that medical symptoms will continue to be assessed and monitored throughout the treatment process, particularly with changing or new symptoms.

The feedback session is also an opportunity to present the adolescents and their families with some of the information from the case formulation as a rationale for treatment. It is important not to overwhelm them, as part of the process of treatment is to help families to gradually move from a purely biological model of their condition to a more complex understanding of the processes involved. Abruptly confronting families with a psychological explanation may result in a loss of rapport, and continued searching for a biological diagnosis.

The use of demonstrations and analogies are a helpful way to introduce concepts, for example:

- Getting family members to focus their attention on a previously asymptomatic part of their body to demonstrate hypervigilance and the role of attention.

- Discussing how stress can impact on a range of chronic illnesses such as diabetes and asthma, to help normalise its role in the adolescent's condition.

8. Management

Regardless of the diagnostic label, the key goals of management generally include achieving more normal levels of function, and improving symptom management. A bio–psychosocial rehabilitation program is a multidisciplinary approach that is individualised based on the needs of the young person and their family. The emphasis is on normalising function and teaching symptom management techniques in order to achieve a progressive increase in physical activity, school attendance, and social interaction. The approach acknowledges both physical and psychological symptoms and aims to address these with the Three Ps:

- **P**harmacotherapy.
- **P**hysical therapy, including a graded exercise program, physiotherapy with stretching and strengthening exercises, TENS machine.
- **P**sychological therapy, including cognitive behavioural therapy, relaxation or mindfulness meditation, parent management training.

Adolescent and family health beliefs are also addressed throughout the course of treatment to support adherence. The young persons and their families are likely to need clear and repeated education about the rationale for this treatment approach, acknowledgement of the reality of their symptoms, and support to tolerate the uncertainty associated with the absence of a simple, biological diagnosis.

Treatment of comorbid problems may also be required, such as sleep disturbance, depression, anxiety, behavioural problems, or family relationship difficulties which may have been present already or may have developed as a result of long-standing physical symptoms and associated isolation and distress. Such difficulties should be addressed if these are thought to be exacerbating the presenting problem, interfering with treatment, or increasing the risk of relapse. Similarly, difficulties with identifying and expressing emotions, perfectionism, and parental anxiety may be appropriate targets of treatment.

8.1. *Inpatient Management*

A planned admission to hospital can provide adolescents with a much needed improvement in functioning, challenge family assumptions about the dangers of increasing activity levels, and provide the treatment team with an opportunity to observe the adolescent's behaviour when they are asked to engage in physical, educational, and social activities. However, there is also the risk that an admission may reinforce overvalued symptomatology and confirm the idea of organic illness. Therefore:

- It is generally undertaken only after failure of ambulatory management or for those from regional or remote areas where local services are not readily available.
- The rationale, goals and structure of the admission need to be considered and discussed in detail with the adolescent and family prior to its commencement.

Usually a two-week period is sufficient to facilitate progress, followed by discharge to practise the new routine that has been developed. The initial 24–48 hours in hospital comprises medical review with appropriate investigations. Thereafter a structured timetable of activities is developed reflecting the hours required for a normal school day; rise at 7 am, breakfast, attend school and groupwork program with daily physiotherapy, occupational therapy, and psychological counselling. Weekly family meetings to report on progress and plan a post-discharge timetable are the key.

An adolescent ward and nursing staff trained in adolescent nursing are integral to the success of the admission and the rehabilitation program. The nursing staff can support and encourage emerging independence and self-management, improve adherence to treatment and facilitate transition to adult care when appropriate. A dedicated adolescent ward provides a supportive and nurturing environment with clear expectations around behaviour, maintaining routine, and encouraging supportive peer interaction.

8.2. *Ambulatory Management*

Patients are initially seen quite frequently (1–2 times per week) to establish a good therapeutic relationship and reinforce the graded structured home program. This allows the adolescent and parents to understand the condition more fully and become motivated to participate in all aspects of therapy. An important role for the treating team is coordination of care, particularly among the other subspecialty teams, community or local services, and the adolescent's school. This will involve case conferencing (including telephone or video) and a school visit if possible.

Practice Point: The goals of a school visit include discussion of support around a flexible and graded return to full-time education and to negotiate other arrangements such as regular rest-breaks, support for symptom management plans and special provisions for assessments. Such a visit is therapeutic in itself for families as they see the health professionals as experts advocating for their needs. It also provides an opportunity to clarify any misconceptions held by teaching staff.

Encouraging participation in creative and peer-related activities can also be helpful for young people with complex psychosocial illness to support the development of healthy self-esteem, promote social well-being, and enable peer support.

8.3. *Pharmacological Management*

Drug therapy is trialled in the context of psychological and physical therapies to provide additional relief of symptoms; however, pain disorders are often relatively refractory to medication. The addition of a non-steroidal anti-inflammatory agent may be helpful alternating with paracetamol or alone. With chronic pain, longer term options may include gabapentin or similar to avoid opiate use. Tricyclic anti-depressant medications can also be beneficial for pain management. SSRIs may be indicated if comorbid depression or anxiety are present.

8.4. *Management Challenges*

Complex medico–psychosocial disorders tend to be associated with disproportionate disability when compared with chronic illnesses. Some of the challenges to successful management include:

- Significant, and often unacknowledged, mental health problems in the adolescent or parents which may predate or complicate ongoing physical symptoms.
- Adolescents in rural and remote areas may experience delays in diagnosis and treatment and a lack of coordinated resources for ongoing care.
- Adolescents of indigenous or culturally and linguistically diverse backgrounds, for whom cultural perceptions of health and well-being may make management more difficult. It is important to use qualified interpreters whenever they are required.
- Resistance to treatment, where some families are highly defended against any non-biological explanation or treatment for the adolescent's symptoms. It is important to both validate the subjective reality of the adolescent's symptoms, and to provide a model for understanding these that acknowledge a role for both physical and psychological factors.

9. Prognosis

Adolescents with somatoform disorders and PVFS may have a better prognosis than adults, particularly if intervention commences before disability has become too entrenched. During treatment, the adolescent's symptom levels typically fluctuate, and do not generally improve at the same pace as functional abilities. Treatment progress should be judged according to day-to-day functioning, with reassurance provided that symptomatic improvement will follow.

The attitudes of parents are crucial. As parents become increasingly open to the role of non-medical contributions to symptoms, and less hypervigilant to changes in symptom intensity, their adolescents can progress to more normal function. Parental care and support is often a better prognostic indicator, even if the adolescent does not acknowledge or understand the psychosocial aspects of their illness.

10. Common Challenges in Complex Chronic Illness

Patients with chronic illnesses such as asthma, inflammatory bowel disease, and diabetes are also influenced by a complex interplay of medical, psychological, and systemic factors, which in some cases include a functional component. Consideration needs to be given to physical triggers of an exacerbation as well as acknowledging the role of psychological or stress-related factors such as anxiety or mood disorders. In adolescence, developmental changes often conflict with the demands of living with a chronic condition. This is a time when participating in peer group activities and 'fitting in' is of paramount importance. The label and/or management demands of a chronic illness may interfere with the adolescent's efforts to 'be normal'. Adolescents are particularly sensitive about their physical appearance, with changes in weight or in the pace of puberty of particular concern. It is important to consider developmental factors, and to explore areas at home, at school, and with peers that may be affecting therapy and producing new symptomatology.

References

Calvert P, Jureidini J. (2003) Restrained rehabilitation: An approach to children and adolescents with unexplained signs and symptoms. *Arch Dis Child* **88**(5): 399–402.

Campo JV, Fritz G. (2001) A management model for pediatric somatization. *Psychosomatics* **42**(6): 467–476.

Chambers D, Bagnall A-M, Hempel S, Forbes C. (2006) Interventions for the treatment, management and rehabilitation of patients with chronic fatigue syndrome/myalgic encephalomyelitis: An updated systematic review. *J R Soc Med* **99**(10): 506–520.

Deary V, Chalder T, Sharpe M. (2007) The cognitive behavioural model of medically unexplained symptoms: A theoretical and empirical review. *Clin Psychol Rev* **27**(7): 781–97.

Garralda ME. (1999) Practitioner review: Assessment and management of somatisation in childhood and adolescence: A practical perspective. *J Child Psychol Psychiatry* **40**(8): 1159–1167.

Kirmayer LJ, Looper KJ. (2006) Abnormal illness behaviour: Physiological, psychological and social dimensions of coping with distress. *Curr Opin Psychiatry* **19**(1): 54–60.

Kreipe RE. (2006) The biopsychosocial approach to adolescents with somatoform disorders. *Adolesc Med Clin* **17**(1): 1–24.

Lipowski ZJ. (1988) Somatization: The concept and its clinical application. *Am J Psychiatry* **145**(11): 1358–1368.

Rangel L, Garralda ME, Jeffs J, Rose G. (2005) Family health and characteristics in chronic fatigue syndrome, juvenile rheumatoid arthritis, and emotional disorders of childhood. *J Am Acad Child Adolesc Psychiatry* **44**(2): 150–158.

Sperber AD, Drossman DA. (2010) Functional abdominal pain syndrome: Constant or frequently recurring abdominal pain. *Am J Gastroenterol* **105**(4): 770–774.

Stone L. (2011) Explaining the unexplainable: Crafting explanatory frameworks for medically unexplained symptoms. *Aust Fam Physician* **40**(6): 440–444.

Taylor S, Garralda E. (2003) The management of somatoform disorder in childhood. *Curr Opin Psychiatry* **16**(2): 227–231.

Chapter 13

Transition from Paediatric to Adult Care in Chronic Illness

Sandra Whitehouse, Lynne Brodie and Susan Towns

1. Introduction

In developed countries, young people with chronic illnesses arising in childhood are now surviving into adulthood in numbers that were unanticipated twenty years ago. Over 90% of children born today with chronic or disabling conditions will survive beyond their 20th birthday. For example, 85% of individuals born with spina bifida survive into adulthood, while 35 years ago less than one third survived to 20 years of age. Similar increases in survival rates are seen for conditions such as cystic fibrosis, haemophilia, chronic renal failure, and many types of cancer, whilst other illnesses such as diabetes and inflammatory bowel disease have increased in prevalence. Many such young people are enrolled in tertiary education, entering the workforce, marrying, having children, and living independently. However, a significant number with complex chronic illnesses and disabilities continue to rely on ageing parents and carers for even basic care. Irrespective of their level of independence, all young people with a chronic illness or disability will need to transition from paediatric to adult health services.

2. Prevalence of Chronic Illness

The prevalence of chronic illnesses arising in childhood in the population of developed countries is estimated between 10%–20%, depending on the definition used. In Australia, approximately 300,000 individuals aged 12–24 years live with a chronic illness or disability.

3. The Definition of Transition

Transition is described by Blum as *'the purposeful, planned movement of adolescents and young adults with chronic physical and medical conditions from child-centred to an adult oriented health care system.'* Transition takes time and is a process, not an event. Adult health services and support organisations worldwide are often under-resourced to meet the needs of these young people, and the young people and their families may be inadequately prepared to leave paediatric services. Transition has been described as a time when young people's complex health needs become superimposed on an adult health system with fragmented services.

Engaging young people to take increased responsibility for their health care, as part of transition planning, presents many challenges as health transition is only one of many important transitions that occur in late adolescence. The transition period can therefore be a difficult, confusing, and frustrating experience for all involved — young people, their parents or carers, and health professionals. The potential for loss of continuity of appropriate care and support has been well documented.

4. Principles of Transition

Recognition of the need to address transition processes has evolved slowly over the last two decades. An increasing number of generic and condition specific guidelines and position statements have been published internationally and within Australia. The overarching transition message is that healthcare should be continuous, comprehensive, and coordinated, as well as flexible and individualised to meet the diverse needs of young people. The best practice to facilitate successful transition is summarised in the following sections.

4.1. *Transition Planning*

4.1.1. *The process*

* Focuses on developmentally appropriate care that enhances autonomy and facilitates self-reliance while addressing common concerns of adolescents such as sexuality, mental health, and the impact on lifestyle and relationships.
* Occurs over time, beginning in early adolescence with gradually increasing personal responsibility. A written health care transition plan should be developed by the age of 14 years.
* Requires an identified health care professional to take responsibility for facilitating the transition process. These professionals should have core knowledge and skills in transition requirements.

4.1.2. *Culminates in transfer and follow up*

* There should be formal systems in place that enable young people to leave the children's hospital and move to adult care with all the information both they and their health care providers require. This includes an up-to-date medical summary that is portable and accessible.
* Young adults should receive youth friendly, developmentally and culturally appropriate care in adult facilities.

4.1.3. *Effective transition from a young person's perspective should*

* Offer quality developmentally appropriate health care that is flexible and responsive.
* Promote the development of communication and decision making skills in order to maintain assertiveness and self-advocacy.
* Ensure a sense of control and independence in health care and personal life.
* Maximise lifelong functioning and potential.

4.2. *Developmental Issues Related to Health Care Transition*

For all teenagers, coming to terms with the physical changes of puberty, becoming more independent and making decisions around further education and employment can be challenging. The demands of living with a chronic illness can conflict with the normal developmental tasks of adolescence, which can be divided into early, middle, and late (Chapter 2):

- Early adolescence (11–14 yrs). The early years of puberty are characterised by rapid physical change and young people can become preoccupied with being 'normal'. This may result in considerable anxiety if there is either early or delayed puberty — the latter more common in chronic illnesses.
- Middle adolescence (14–16 yrs). The middle years are a time of establishing a sense of self-identity and the peer group becomes very important. Chronic illness can result in frequent hospitalisations with social isolation and persistent reliance on family members for medical management, which in turn affects the normal developmental changes of increasing independence and decision-making. Conversely as young people challenge the status quo, adherence to treatment plans may become increasingly problematic.
- Late adolescence (16–18 yrs). Future considerations such as work, lifestyle, and relationships become central. However, young people with special health care needs may not be able to plan their future with certainty. They may have to deal with issues of grief and loss associated with complications of their condition. These may include diminished fertility, the genetic implications of their illness, limited vocational opportunities, and reduced life expectancy.

Early 11-14 yrs	Middle 14-16 yrs	Late 16-18 yrs
Distortion of body image.	Enforced dependency.	Reduced vocational options.
Isolation from peers.	Less acceptance by peers.	Concerns about relationships and fertility.

Fig. 1:   Impact of chronic illness on development according to developmental stage.

4.3. *Preparation, Planning, and Communication*

Preparation of the young persons, their families, and the paediatric and adult teams is essential but frequently inadequate (Table 1). Discussions with the young persons and their families about the expectations of transition should commence early, shortly after diagnosis. In the older child

Table 1:   What do I have to do? Clinician planning made easy.

Preparation Phase (Up to 16 yrs)	Discuss transition.
Focuses on	Check out the internet for information
• Education regarding the condition.	about transition planning.
• Developmentally appropriate care.	Give out transition information.
	Discuss self management checklist and
	initiate transition plan.
• Enhancing self management skills.	Address issues raised in self management
	(Chapter 11).
	Assign case manager if needed.
Active Phase (16–18 yrs)	
Involves	
• Developing individual transition plan.	Make sure all care teams are aware of transition plans.
• Engaging a primary care doctor for ongoing coordination of management.	Complete an individual transition plan and prepare a comprehensive summary of care for the adult team.
• Arranging the first appointment with adult services.	Arrange a visit to adult clinic if possible to assist decision making process.
	Copy all relevant documents to the young person and primary care doctor.
	Ensure the young person has an emergency plan and contact details for adult clinicians.
Post Transition Phase (Late teens and young adulthood)	
Requires	
• Feedback from adult services regarding engagement and subsequent attendance at clinic visits.	Ensure adult clinic attended. Evaluation of transition process.

and adolescent, the promotion of self-care, in conjunction with the parents can:

- Increase awareness of the need for self-management.
- Allow the adolescent to understand why each therapy is prescribed.
- Enhance the development of independence by,
    - o making appointments,
    - o negotiating changes in treatment,
    - o increased communication with the clinicians. The regular use of electronic transition planning tools and/or self-management checklists can facilitate this communication.

4.4. *Communication Between Health Care Teams*

Communication between paediatric and adult health care teams is an opportunity to provide and receive feedback about transition care and may include:

- Joint planning and the development of agreed transition policies.
- Ensuring continuity of care by encouraging clinicians in both paediatric and adult clinics to discuss and plan for adult issues such as employment (including tertiary studies and work choices), fertility, and sexual health advice. Research has demonstrated that adolescents with chronic illness and their parents expect their clinicians to be raising these issues and to provide guidance around appropriate assessment and management.
- Acknowledging the importance of 'moving on' with a Graduation Ceremony for those young people and families with long-term and/or intense association with paediatric care.
- Aiming for an initial adult appointment with minimal gap in regular care. In some situations a period of overlap between paediatric and adult teams may be needed. Problems can arise due to acute illness prior to the first appointment and with transfer of information. These situations are more likely to occur when there is a prolonged period before the first ambulatory care visit at the adult centre.

- Discussing education for the adult team on adolescent and young adult health care.
- Identifying transition 'champions' in adult health care.

4.5. *Practical Advice, Resources, and Support*

Parental support of the transition process is integral to its success. Regular information forums for parents and young people providing up-to-date knowledge of clinical care, challenges, and realistic expectations following transition to adult care can reduce associated anxiety.

Practical steps include providing parents and young people with:

- Details on the location of the clinic and/or hospital, parking arrangements, expected duration of the visit, and details of whom they may meet at their first appointment.
- A preliminary visit to the adult centres whilst still attending the paediatric clinic can alleviate some of the associated transition anxiety.
- Written information about the adult services with subsequent discussion.
- Information regarding differences in policy and practice for infection control, intravenous therapy, or other specific services.

Young people consider the most important factors for successful transition to be:

- The opportunity for a joint meeting with the paediatric and adult services.
- A preliminary visit to the adult service prior to transition.
- Having their first appointment made for them.

4.6. *Transferring Medical Information*

For the adult health service, receiving comprehensive referral information from the paediatric centre to help the adult team understand the extent of complications (such as prior drug allergies and toxicities, venous access challenges, changes in clinical status in recent years, and the emotional well-being of the young person) will improve continuity of care subsequent to patient transfer. It is most important that paediatric health care providers provide a written summary of health status at the time of anticipated transition including:

- A comprehensive discussion of the diagnosis (and copies of relevant results) and associated clinical issues.
- Current clinical findings and latest results of investigations.
- Medications, management plan, and current level of adherence.
- Paediatric and other adult care providers' names, contact information, and services.
- The primary care doctor's name and contact information and their level of involvement.
- An assessment of significant psychosocial, family and individual issues that may affect overall well-being and transition to adult care.

This should be provided well before the first appointment to allow the adult team to be prepared for the young person and their family.

Patients themselves should carry a personally held, portable, accessible, up-to-date summary of care. The Hospital for Sick Children in Toronto, for example, provides transitioning adolescents with both a condition specific paper health record summary that fits inside a wallet and an electronic version that can be emailed (www.myhealthpassport.ca). A carefully planned transitional care process should result in a seamless movement from paediatric care to adult care with an engaged young person who is responsible for day-to-day care, supported by his/her family.

5. Challenges to the Transition Process

5.1. *Multiple Stakeholders: Health Care Services, Providers, Parents, and Young People*

During the transition process, the relationship between the young person, the family, the paediatric health care provider and the health care service shifts when a new health care relationship begins with an adult health care provider. The goal is to maintain continuity of care through attendance at adult clinics and avoid use of emergency services. Transfer of care is likely to be more successful if the young person and his/her family are well prepared for differences in health care provision with appropriate transition planning around integration into the available adult care service and health care resources.

5.2. *Paediatric and Adult Care Systems: Bridging the Divide*

When adolescent patients are transferred from a paediatric sub-specialty team to an adult health care provider, they are shifting between two systems of care that serve distinctively different populations with divergent health care needs. The differences are evident in the type and level of support from health care providers, decision-making and consent processes, and the amount of family involvement (Table 2).

5.3. *Transition Challenges for the Adolescent Patient*

While many adolescents are highly motivated to move on to adult care and enjoy a more adult therapeutic relationship, some may be ambivalent with concerns including:

- Leaving a familiar environment and having to develop a new relationship of trust with unfamiliar health professionals in an unknown setting.
- Lacking the confidence to contact the adult health professional to whom they have been referred.
- Resisting the changes in relationship with their parents who are expected to be less responsible for health care and check-ups.
- Increasing expectations of their understanding of the patho-physiology of their condition.
- Leaving school, moving on to further education or finding employment or psychosocial issues such as depression and risk taking behaviour may take priority, interfering with the transition process.

Young adults have suggested a number of strategies that facilitate effective transition. These include connecting with mentors and peer support groups where possible, and having a health care professional oversee the transfer phase who has knowledge and personal understanding of

Table 2: Differences between paediatric and adult health care systems.

Paediatric care systems	Adult care systems
Care provided in a multidisciplinary clinic by a range of health care providers.	Care provided by adult specialist with referrals to other health care providers as needed. Limited time and resources available for teaching and counselling.
Increased access to some medications and treatment.	Variable insurance services and payment requirements.
Adolescent clinics with peer support and youth friendly care.	Few young adult clinics.
Family is active partner in health care team.	Physician visits encouraged to be independent of family/carers.
Child/adolescent visit the physician together with their parents.	
*Parent or guardian understands the condition, ensures adherence and has a strong advocacy role.	Patient is assumed knowledgeable about their condition and plans their own care.
*Parent or guardian gives consent.	Patient responsible for consent.
*Parent or guardian takes responsibility for treatment and daily care needs.	Patient expected to self manage personal care and decision- making.
Specialist knowledge with rare paediatric conditions.	Lack of experience with rare paediatric conditions.
Focus on developmental perspective.	Focus on risks of long term complications.

*This situation evolves and changes as the adolescent develops skills in self-management.

their condition. Cohesive and communicative family support has also been shown to be beneficial during transition.

5.4. *Transition Challenges for Parents: Role of the Family*

Parents and guardians may find difficulty in 'letting go' to enable the young person to take on the skills and behavioural changes necessary for independent decision-making and self-management. It is important that the young person has the opportunity to confidentially address social, developmental, and lifestyle issues such as sexual health or alcohol use during their consultation.

Parents or guardians can:

- Encourage their adolescent to make their own appointments and to ask their own questions during a consultation.
- Allow their adolescent time with the health care provider alone.
- Offer opportunities for the young person to participate in home responsibilities such as chores and seek outside part-time employment where appropriate.
- Engage in a gradual process of offering support without being over-protective, thereby encouraging self care and management.

Parents and care-givers may also benefit from networking through condition-specific associations or parent support groups.

5.5. *Role of Paediatric Sub-Speciality Providers*

During transition, clinicians focus on teaching and consulting with the young person, while role modelling and providing support and anticipatory guidance to the parent. Effective communication is essential and strategies include:

- Using accessible language.
- Taking a comprehensive approach rather than exclusively focusing on the condition.
- Ensuring the young person of confidentiality and privacy during the consultation.
- Demonstrating respectful communication that can contribute to the development of self esteem and self confidence.
- Facilitating the development of self management whilst simultaneously respecting the family's role.

5.6. *Adult Health Care Providers*

One of the major emerging transition issues is that adult health care services are under resourced to manage the large numbers of young people transitioning to adult care.

Adult health care providers need the *opportunity to acquire the clinical knowledge and skills* to treat and care for adolescents and young adults with chronic health conditions, including:

- Understanding the process of adolescent development.
- Using a non-intrusive, non-judgemental, supportive, and positive approach to foster an environment of acceptance.
- Maintaining a collaborative attitude to help young adults build confidence in their new setting.
- Assessing and managing the psychosocial needs of the patient and family unit.
- Being aware of new financial burdens that may emerge as paediatric benefits are discontinued and that families need support to adapt.

One of the particularly challenging areas for adult service clinicians is to manage new patients who are facing end of life issues. Adult physicians in some areas such as cystic fibrosis are providing leadership and expertise in palliative care and post-transplantation management as these issues previously faced in the paediatric clinics are now delayed to adulthood.

5.7. *Primary Care Doctor*

The primary care doctor has a unique opportunity to address primary health care needs, facilitate the transition process and provide continuity of care. All young people with chronic health problems need to have a primary care doctor who is able to provide support and ongoing management in collaboration with specialist clinicians. At this stage in life, other transitions including changes in school, education, employment, and insurance may impact the young person's ability to retain the same primary care doctor. On the other hand, young people may wish to choose a new primary care doctor who is different from the one they have seen during childhood and adolescence, a health professional who they can get to know on their own terms.

6. Emerging Adulthood

Emerging adulthood, the period from 18–30 years, is distinct from both adolescence and adulthood, and coincides with extended periods of educational training, postponed marriage, and reduced family obligations. The concept of adolescent/young adult clinics for some sub-specialty areas in adult hospitals is helpful as this acknowledges the unique requirements of the age group; allowing appropriate peer interaction, parental/carer involvement and continued promotion of self management skills. Many such clinics run on an 'assertive case management' model where the clinical coordinator will keep in regular phone contact, providing reminders and contacting to reschedule nonattenders. With cognitive and emotional maturity usually developing by the mid-twenties most young adults are then ready to confidently move on to an adult clinic.

Young adulthood is associated with other transitions and instability, making management of chronic conditions even more challenging. For example, young adults with diabetes attending university find self-management challenging as it requires attention to alcohol, sexual health, and sick day diabetes management plans. Barriers to optimal self-care include time constraints, erratic schedules, limited available food choices, concerns about hypoglycaemia, and absence of social support. A high level of family support is the strongest predictor of adherence to the diabetes regimen, implying that connectedness and family engagement remain critical in this unstable period.

7. Models of Care

Transition planning is not straightforward and requires both a global and local understanding in order to determine best practice service delivery models. It is apparent both from the literature and from discussions with local clinicians that there is no 'best fit' model of care for young people with chronic illnesses as each health condition has particular requirements. The model may describe the level of health care required such as primary, secondary, or tertiary care or a combination, along with the type of service

Table 3: Models of care.

Adult models of care	Appropriate patient populations
Single specialist working in an ambulatory setting.	Diabetes, rheumatology, inflammatory bowel disease.
Multidisciplinary team working in an ambulatory setting.	Spina bifida.
Complex multidisciplinary specialist care with a large inpatient component.	Cystic fibrosis, muscular dystrophy.

Key questions to consider when deciding on appropriate models of transition care:

1. How many young people need the service? Is the disease incidence increasing? What is the age distribution?
2. Are they a homogenous group or might they need different service models?
3. What sort of service is needed and are there any factors that need to be taken into consideration, such as cohorting patients if possible?

   - specialist tertiary care for all aspects of management (inpatient and ambulatory).
   - tertiary care for regular review and assessment +/− tertiary inpatient care.
   - local hospital management.
   - general practitioner/family doctor.

4. How many services are needed?
5. Where should these be located?
6. What professionals constitute the adult team?
7. How should young people be prepared to transition from paediatric to adult services according to the model of care used?
8. Who should coordinate care?
9. How should services be funded?
10. How do young people pay for services and ensure access to medications and equipment?

required such as multidisciplinary teams versus a single clinician on an ambulatory or inpatient basis.

In the state of New South Wales in Australia, a State-wide Transition Network has been established to coordinate and support transition services at all levels of care. Each sub-specialty area needs to decide which model of care is most applicable to their area. The questions above (Table 3) provide a framework to determine which type of model suits each specific practice.

8. Conclusion

With good preparation and planning, young people with chronic illness can be equipped to move on to the adult health care system. However we must endeavour to not only recognise but address the cultural and system challenges that can lead to adolescents falling through the gaps in our health systems. By recognising the developmental challenges for adolescents and their families, appropriately resourcing adult services to increase their capacity, providing equity of access and facilitating transfer of complex patient information, smooth transition to adult care should ensure optimal health outcomes for the increasing numbers of young adults requiring ongoing, lifelong health care.

References

Arnett JJ. (2001) Conceptions of the transition to adulthood: Perspectives from adolescence through midlife. *J Adult Dev* **8**(2): 69–79.

Beresford B, Sloper P. (2003) Chronically ill adolescents' experiences of communicating with doctors: A qualitative study. *J Adolesc Health* **33**: 172–179.

Holmes-Walker J, Llewellyn AC, Farrell KA. (2007) A transition care programme which improves diabetes control and reduces hospital admission rates in young adults with type 1 diabetes aged 15–25 years. *Diabet Med* **24**: 764–769.

Kennedy A, Sawyer S. (2008) Transition from pediatric to adult services: Are we getting it right? *Curr Opin Pediatrics* **20**(4): 403–409.

Lotstein DS, McPherson M, Strickland B, Newacheck PW. (2005) Transition planning for youth with special health care needs: Results from the National Survey of Children with special health care needs *Pediatrics* **115**: 1562–1568.

Manjo D, Yader A, Williams J, Moli P, Kelly D, Petchey R, Carter YH. (2009) Transition to adult services for children and young people with palliative care needs: A systematic review. *Arch Dis Child* **96**: 78–84.

Peter NG, Forke CM, Ginsburg K, Schwarz DF. (2009) Transition from pediatric to adult care: Internists' perspectives. *Pediatics* **123**: 417–423.

Reiss JG, Gibson RW, Walker LR. (2005) Health care transition: Youth, family, and provider perspectives. *Pediatrics* **115**(1): 112–120.

Scal P, Ireland M. (2005) Addressing transition to adult health care for adolescents with special health care needs. *Pediatrics* **115**(60): 1607–1612.

Steinbeck K, Brodie L, Towns S. (2007) Transition care for young people with chronic illness. *Int J Adolesc Med Health* **19**(3): 295–303.

Resources available at NSW Government, Dept of Health, Agency for Clinical Innovation: http://www.aci.health.nsw.gov.au/networks/transition-care (accessed 5 June 2012).

The Children's Hospital at Westmead http://www.chw.edu.au/prof/ (accessed 5 June 2012).

Chapter 14

Resilience

Emily Klineberg

Why is it that when faced with the same adversity, some people will fare better than others? Is there a reason why some individuals have the capability to beat the odds, and overcome problems more easily than others? What is it that makes a person able to bounce back better psychologically or physically? One explanation lies in the concept of resilience; the capacity to cope with and overcome adversity.

1. What Is Resilience?

The definitions of resilience may vary between disciplines, however the core concept of successfully weathering adversity is shared across different fields. Resilience implies the presence of strength and resources that have a buffering effect. These may be within the individual, or drawn upon from external sources. Resilience may be a *process of adaptation* when overcoming a challenge, or may be an *outcome*, being able to maintain functioning and competence despite the challenge being faced. Different components of resilience may counteract a risk factor, or may reduce the effects of a risk factor. Resilience may vary with time, age, context, and when facing different adversities. It may also be accumulated, with development of resilience reflecting life experience over time.

Resilience at an individual level involves cognitive or emotional resources and self-esteem. It includes individual traits, but is not a single definable trait. Resilience also involves the capacity to draw upon social support, and wider strengths in terms of identity, environment, culture, and community. In this chapter, individual and contextual components of resilience will be discussed, followed by an outline of the role of adversity, and then how this concept of resilience may be useful in practice.

1.1. *Components of Resilience*

1.1.1. *Individual components of resilience*

The various components of resilience are listed below. This is not an exhaustive list, however, it provides a selection of features to consider when looking for an individual's strengths to work with in practice:

- Cognitive style, fluidity in thinking, which would improve chances of flexibility in adaptive responses.
- Personality, including regulation of affect, flexibility, humour, capacity to adapt.
- An easy, positive temperament may resonate across different aspects of a young person's life, regulate emotional reactivity to stress and promote resilience.
- Interpersonal skills such as sociability, capacity to see things from another's perspective, the ability to relate to, and communicate with others.
- Positive attachments, showing the ability to form attachments with others, or having had some positive attachment experience.
- Self-esteem and self-reliance, having confidence and belief in oneself, and a positive self-view.
- Self-regulation, planning, organising and goal-directed behaviour, executive functioning, and self-management.
- Internal locus of control, the perception of being able to alter situations, rather than attributing everything to external circumstances or fate.
- Intelligence in decision-making, success of planning and ensuing consequences.
- An ability to attend to tasks, capacity to focus, and prioritise appropriately.

- Coping style, taking a flexible, pragmatic or problem-solving approach rather than an emotional focus which might increase anxiety and depression.
- Having a sense of meaning and purpose.
- Aspirations for the future, having a vision of what must be overcome, or an aim to strive towards.
- Showing perseverance, persistence, and capacity to keep going.
- Capacity to maintain motivation and focus, without becoming demoralised by the challenge.
- Health literacy, knowledge about self-care, and help-seeking.

1.1.2. *External components of resilience*

A key part of resilience is each individual's social and environmental context. This context may be the source of the adversity being faced, but it may also be a place from where resources could be drawn. Buffering from adversity may stem from social, psychological, interpersonal, financial, or environmental influences, all of which may contribute to resilience. External aspects of resilience rely upon the existence of positive influences and the young person's capacity to draw upon those influences.

Features of resilience stemming from a young person's context may demonstrate multiple sources of support and more general social capital able to be utilised in relation to their health and well-being. For example, social and family relationships both reduce exposure to risk and provide stability, through support, connectedness, encouragement, and acceptance. A positive parent–child attachment and a warm parental style may increase resilience, as do other positive role models. The absolute minimum to enhance resilience appears to be having one adult in whom the young person can trust, and talk to when in need of support. Different sources of support can have variable impacts on the psychological well-being of young people. As an example, the impact of social support from family may differ from peer emotional support during adolescence. Family and friends may influence attitudes to health and health behaviours by modelling behaviours, or providing information to the young person about service use and sources of help.

Access to healthcare is a society-level factor for promoting resilience in health and responding to adversity of illness. Additionally, identification with a group and utilisation of a group identity may function as a buffer, adding to resilience in marginalised youth. In the wider community, resilience may be built through cultural influences, values, and spirituality. A school may present opportunities for support and connectedness through structured communications with adults, peer relationships, sports, and group activities in the classroom. Connectedness and involvement within the community may also foster resilience.

1.1.3. *Adversity required for demonstration of resilience*

Risk or adversity needs to be present in order for resilience to be shown. Akin to a quality such as bravery, resilience may only become apparent when there is a need for it to be tested. For example, if a young person was bullied, being able to access support, and learning socially constructive responses to such an experience may function to promote more adaptive responses to future social adversity. As such, coping skills, perseverance, and resourcefulness may be tested and developed in response to a crisis. The adversity may relate to challenges at an individual level, an interpersonal level, or a wider social, cultural, or community level.

Low levels of exposure to risk factors may function to promote learning about how to overcome adverse events, and thus increase resilience. This introduces the idea that low levels of adversity may benefit young people's resilience, promoting experience in utilising resources and showing them their own coping skills.

In research on risk and resilience, risk factors such as experience of abuse may be clearly identifiable, whereas protective factors, such as social support or social capital are more challenging to define, assess, and compare. Thus there is a greater history of research on risk than resilience. With different types of adversity, different aspects of resilience may be more or less useful. In practice, it is important to consider which resources may need to be drawn upon to assist an adolescent's capacity to deal with the circumstances that they face.

Adversity may relate to individual experiences, or stem from a combination of individual experiences, within the community or social context of that individual. For example, adversity such as chronic illness may stem from individual factors, while also being influenced by the environment. Resilience may be shown at an individual level, in the way that a young person responds to severe illness or injury both physically and psychologically. The adversity of an illness experience may vary with the symptom severity, nature of the diagnosis, prognosis, how the family responds and what community resources exist for the support, and management of ill health.

Adversity may be the experience of abuse or neglect. The resilience fostered may be psychological or behavioural defences adopted to deal with such traumas, being able to seek and accept help, as well as identifying potential ways to prevent repetition of such experiences. It is also feasible to view adolescent adversity as occurring with a lack of protective factors. Adversity leading to marginalisation could relate to social or socio–economic deprivation, unstable housing, and disengagement from education.

Social and cultural differences within society may lead to complex challenges for young people. This type of social adversity may be more apparent in adolescents in minority ethnic groups, indigenous adolescents, young refugees, or those who are marginalised through deprivation or social exclusion. Changes in lifestyle and exposure to different socio–cultural influences may emerge through relocation or changes in family structure.

Adversity may stem from adaptation to change, which is inherent in adolescence. Adolescents face a multitude of changes in terms of physical development, identity development, social interactions, and schooling. Adversity may take the form of health risk behaviours. For example, opportunities to experiment and adopt adverse health behaviours such as alcohol or substance use may be present throughout adolescence, along with different manifestations of psychological distress and an increased likelihood of adopting maladaptive ways to deal with emotional distress, such as self-harm. Changes such as coming to terms with sexuality, gender identity or negotiating conflicts with cultural norms may function as a source of distress. Resilience plays a role when an individual is able to function and move on, despite such adversity or distress being faced.

On a larger scale, adolescents may experience adversity affecting the entire community such as natural disasters, which could be stressful in themselves, as well as disrupting potential sources of support.

2. Why Is Resilience Important when Working with Adolescents?

Utilising resilience in practice means working with the strengths that an adolescent demonstrates. It involves adapting practice to emphasise how their interests, beliefs, relationships, and environment can contribute to a positive or adaptive response to the situations that they face. Working with a young person's strengths to foster engagement and concordance with treatment may be used implicitly in practice. It involves being aware of 'what is working' for him/her at the moment, what are the motivations for current behaviour, and how professional input could enhance that capacity to bounce back.

Adolescence is a period of transition. When roles, social relationships, and contexts change, so might an individual's capacity to respond to challenges. An adolescent's sense of resilience may vary with their perceptions about themselves, their developing sense of identity, and independence. Adolescence is also a time when young people may test boundaries and take risks. Clinicians need to consider how adolescents perceive adversity, and the proportionality in their response to stress. This could function to emphasise or minimise the adversity being faced. For example, a peer conflict or rejection may be particularly sensitive and emphasised, while other issues may be concealed or played down, with a sense of bravado. Adolescents experiment with different personas, and thus in a health situation, they may wish to present as being more resilient than they actually are.

It is important to note that resilience can be shown when young people survive early life adversity; however, this implied resilience does not guarantee that they will continue their lives free from psychological distress.

3. How Do You Assess Resilience?

Resilience is difficult to assess clinically, as it is dependent on the type of adversity being faced and how resilience is conceptualised. A number of scales have been developed and used in both research and practice. The *Resiliency Scale* is based on the theory of stress, appraisal, and coping. It has three sub-scales to assess skills that are employed by resilient people: future orientation, active skill acquisition, and independence/risk taking. A second scale is *The Resilience Scale* which assesses constructs including perseverance, equanimity, meaningfulness, self-reliance, and existential aloneness.

4. Interventions Relating to Resilience

Instruction on how to build and stimulate resilience in a clinical setting remains challenging and diffuse. Interventions may relate to preventative actions, or as responses to crises. There is scope for components of resilience to cascade and influence other components, for example, an increase in confidence may lead to an increase in the likelihood of feeling worthy of seeking social support.

As a clinician working with adolescents, it is important to consider resilience as both a process and an outcome. That is, maintaining an awareness of any potentially modifiable factors which could be identified and used to enhance resilience, to build capacity and influence a young person's developmental trajectory. Such modifiable factors may include:

- Attitudes and beliefs.
- Self-esteem.
- Assistance in identifying strengths.
- Competence in negotiating and minimising known risks.
- Interpretations and appraisal of stressors.
- Social and school engagement.
- Perceived resources the young person can draw upon.
- Encouragement to use available resources.

One function of professional input relating to resilience would be to foster coping outside of health service input. That is, working with the young person within his/her own context and social networks, amongst peers, family, and other accessible sources of support in the community. It is an ongoing challenge to propose theories for this complex, changeable idea which could be tested and validated to practice. Two models proposed for use in practice with adolescents are presented below: The Resilience Doughnut and the Resourceful Adolescent Project.

4.1. *A Model of Resilience for Use in Practice: The Resilience Doughnut*

This model presents a doughnut; where the hole in the middle represents the individual. The 'doughnut' is comprised of seven segments surrounding the individual, and each segment represents an external factor which interacts with the person in the middle and which has scope to foster resilience. The seven segments are: the parent factor, the skill factor, the family factor, the education factor, the peer group factor, the community factor, and the money factor. This model was developed from strength-based approaches to provide an accessible structure for thinking about and working on resilience. At different phases in life, the different segments of the doughnut may seem more robust, showing where a young person draws their strength at that time, and also which areas may benefit from input from services, their family or wider community.

4.2. *Program for Building Adolescent Resilience: RAP — Resourceful Adolescent Project*

This project was designed to foster resilience and mental well-being in adolescents, informed by cognitive behavioural therapy. The Resourceful Adolescent Project is comprised of three programs with a preventative focus; targeting the young person, parents, and teachers. This program can be implemented in schools. It also contains an adaptation of the parent program developed for working with Indigenous families. The RAP emphasises self-esteem, problem solving, keeping calm, and personal strength in young people. It promotes skills for dealing with conflict, understanding others, self-regulation, and creating and utilising support networks. The parent program has a focus on promoting strong parental attachment, warmth, management of negative over-reactions, and promoting a harmonious family environment to engender self-esteem and resilience in adolescents. RAP has been evaluated over 10 years, and has been adopted across Australia and internationally.

5. Summary

Resilience is a multifactorial concept, with many inter-related components. The different aspects of resilience may have greater or lesser salience, depending on the individual, his/her context and the adversity being faced. The promotion of resilience in young people involves considering different aspects of the concept, gauging and working with the young person's strengths and resources to enhance their capacity to overcome the challenge being faced.

References

Blum LM, Blum RWM. (2009) Resilience in adolescence. In: Diclemente RJ, Santelli JS, Crosby RA (eds.), *Adolescent Health: Understanding and Preventing Risk Behaviours*, pp. 51–76. Jossey-Bass, San Francisco, CA.

Fergus S, Zimmerman MA. (2005) Adolescent resilience: A framework for understanding healthy development in the face of risk. *Annu Rev Public Health* **26**: 399–419.

Hearn SP. (2010) *Adolescent health in an indigenous context — the potential role for resilience.* University of Sydney.

Jew CL, Green KE, Kroger J. (1999) Development and validation of a measure of resiliency. *Meas Eval Couns Dev* **32**(2): 75–89.

Klineberg E, Clark C, Bhui KS, Haines MM, Viner RM, Head J, Woodley-Jones D Stansfeld SA. (2006) Social support, ethnicity and mental health in adolescents. *Soc Psychiatry Psychiatr Epidemiol*, **41**(9): 755–760.

Olsson CA, Bond L, Burns JM, Vella-Brodrick DA, Sawyer SM. (2003) Adolescent resilience: A concept analysis. *J Adolesc* **26**(1): 1–11.

Robards F. (2009) *Increasing the Resilience of Young People at Risk: A Literature Review.* Available online at: http://www.caah.chw.edu.au/policy/CAAH_policy_literature_report.pdf).

Rutter M. (2007) Resilience, competence, and coping. *Child Abuse Negl* **31**(3): 205–209.

Shochet I, Hoge R, Wurfl A. (2009) Building resilience in adolescents: The resourceful adolescent program (RAP). In: K. Geldard (ed.), *Practical interventions for young people.* Sage Publications Ltd.

Wagnild G. (2009) A review of the resilience scale. *J Nurs Meas* **17**(2): 105–113.

Wexler LM, Difluvio G, Burke TK. (2009) Resilience and marginalized youth: Making a case for personal and collective meaning-making as part of resilience research in public health. *Soc Sci Med* **69**(4): 565–570.

Worsley L. (2006) *The resilience doughnut.* Wild & Woolley, Sydney, Australia.

Chapter 15

Alcohol and Other Drugs

Bronwyn Milne, Yvonne Bonomo and Gilbert Whitton

1. Introduction to Substance Abuse in Young People

Drug and alcohol use during the teenage years is often seen as a normal part of the risk taking and experimentation of adolescent development. Although it may be seen as a rite of passage with little harm, some young people come to significant harm as a consequence of alcohol and/or other drug use. It is important for health professionals to be competent in identifying young people at risk and to be able to offer brief interventions and ongoing management for drug and alcohol issues.

Almost 90% of 14 year olds have drunk alcohol. Over 20% of those who have drunk alcohol identify as weekly drinkers, half of whom binge drink at harmful levels. More than half of all secondary school students report having tried illicit drugs at least once in their lifetime, with around 15% reporting recent use. Cannabis is the most common illicit substance used by teenagers. The use of other illicit substances such as ecstasy, amphetamines, LSD, and cocaine are less common in adolescence, but increase in prevalence in the older age group and into young adulthood.

Young people traditionally use substances that are easily accessible and low cost. Young teens are more likely to use inhalants and over the counter medications, while older teenagers are more likely to use alcohol, cannabis, and party drugs. An adolescent's use of heroin and methamphetamine closely reflects drug availability. Drug patterns vary widely from location to location and are influenced by policy, customs, policing, and supply and demand.

1.1. *Spectrum of Drug Use*

There is a broad spectrum of substance use in adolescence, from experimentation, substance abuse and misuse to substance dependence. Progression from one stage to the next is generally related to the age of initiation, frequency, and quantity of the substance used.

1.1.1. *Substance use*

Experimentation with substances by young people is much more common than progression to regular use. There are many reasons young people experiment with alcohol or other drugs including simply just to 'try it', peer pressure, social context, assistance with sleep, or desire to self-medicate for emotional difficulties.

1.1.2. *Substance abuse*

Substance abuse refers to drug or alcohol use that is causing recurrent problems. These may include relationship difficulties, deterioration in school performance, financial difficulties, or trouble with the law. Harm associated with adolescent substance abuse includes violent behaviour and injury, drunk-driving and motor vehicle accidents, mental health issues such as anxiety, depression and suicide attempts, engaging in risky sexual behaviour and being victims of sexual abuse.

1.1.3. *Substance dependence*

Substance dependence is a maladaptive pattern of substance use leading to clinically significant impairment or distress. According to the

Diagnostic and Statistical Manual of Mental Disorders IV criteria it is manifested by three or more of the following occurring at any time in the same 12 month period:

- A great deal of time is spent in drug related activities.
- Social, occupational or recreational withdrawal.
- The substance use is continued despite knowledge of having a persistent or recurrent physical or psychological problem.
- Tolerance develops so greater or more frequent amount required.
- Withdrawal symptoms occur.
- The substance is taken in larger amounts or over longer periods of time than initially intended.
- Persistent or unsuccessful efforts to cut down or control substance use.

It is important to note that the DSM criteria were developed with adults in mind and an accurate history needs to be taken from the young person to determine whether they are dependent on a given substance.

Neuroadaption is used to describe the changes inferred from observing tolerance to and withdrawal from a substance. It assumes adaptive changes in the central nervous system as a result of exposure to the substance.

2. Risk and Protective Factors

Usually a complex interplay of several risk factors and a paucity of protective factors in a young person's life leads to drug use and its associated high risk behaviours.

3. Assessment

3.1. *Screening*

CRAFFT is an acronym of six screening questions (Table 1). This tool has been recommended by the American Academy of Pediatrics Committee on Substance Abuse. If a young person answers yes to two or

Table 1:　CRAFFT screening tool.

C	Have you ever ridden in a CAR driven by someone (including yourself) who was 'high' on alcohol or drugs?
R	Do you ever use alcohol or drugs to RELAX, feel better about yourself or 'fit in'?
A	Do you ever use alcohol/drugs while you are by yourself, ALONE?
F	Do you ever FORGET things you did while using alcohol or drugs?
F	Do your family or FRIENDS ever tell you that you should cut down on your drinking or drug use?
T	Have you gotten into TROUBLE while you were using alcohol or drugs?

Source: Ref: Knight *et al.* 2002.

more questions, a high risk substance abuse is identified, and then a more thorough drug and alcohol assessment is required.

3.2. *History Taking*

Polysubstance use is common. Ask about each substance group individually. Start at the most commonly used substances by young people such as tobacco, alcohol, and cannabis, and then progress to substances with less prevalent use such as amphetamines (speed, base, ice, and ecstasy), opiates, benzodiazepines, inhalants, and hallucinogens such as LSD and ketamine. Ascertain the age of onset, age of regular use, pattern (weekend use versus daily use), approximate date the substance was last used and an estimate of the amounts, and cost. It is also important to ask about problems related to drug and alcohol use, and previous treatments (for example 'detox', counselling, pharmacotherapy).

3.3. *Clinical Assessment*

The revised HEADSS framework for taking a broad psychosocial history about drug and alcohol use is helpful.

Assessment should include the following six items:

1.　Presenting problem and motivation for treatment.
2.　Drug use history and severity of dependence.
3.　Medical and psychiatric history.

4. Psychosocial history.
5. Examination.
6. Formulation and development of an initial treatment plan.

3.4. *Risk Assessment*

There are many risks associated with substance abuse and dependence. A thorough drug and alcohol assessment includes assessing the following:

- Medical complications of the substance used.
- Nutritional status.
- Blood-borne viruses associated with intravenous drug use including hepatitis B and C and HIV.
- Immunisation status.
- Adverse effects of IVDU including thrombophlebitis, skin abscesses, septicaemia, and infective endocarditis.
- Sexual health.
- Mental health including screening for anxiety, depression, suicidal ideation, and psychosis.
- Family situation.
- Educational attainment and presence of ADHD and specific learning difficulties.
- Forensic review and current legal issues.
- Unwanted harms associated with alcohol and drug use including sexual assault, motor vehicle accidents, trauma, violence or aggression.

4. Drug and Alcohol Treatment Principles

Effective approaches to prevention and intervention should be 'strengths-based', aiming to increase protective factors, reduce risk factors, and build resilience in young people. This approach can result in positive outcomes across a range of health and social domains including reduction in drug use and criminal activity, and improvement in mental health.

4.1. *Primary Intervention*

This is the prevention of, or delay, in the onset of drug use. Early intervention can take place in schools, and during consultations with general practitioners, hospital clinicians, and other professionals who work with young people.

4.2. *Secondary Intervention*

This refers to reducing problems early in the drug use spectrum, including preventing further use or progression to drug dependence.

4.2.1. *Brief intervention*

This is the provision of information and advice aimed at reducing risky alcohol or other substance use. It is usually opportunistic and offered by general practitioners, paediatricians, youth workers, family therapists, and addiction specialists who encounter young people who use alcohol or other drugs. Brief intervention is generally most appropriate early in the substance use spectrum, but may also be used in the context of harm reduction for individuals who are at the more severe end of the substance use spectrum. Brief intervention may include motivational interviewing techniques or counselling according to the stage of change with which the young person identifies. An example of brief intervention is the 5As as used for smoking cessation (Chapter 34).

4.2.2. *Stages of change*

A significant part of drug and alcohol assessment and intervention is understanding both the stages of change model and where the adolescent 'sits' with regard to their drug use. The stages of change are as follows.

Precontemplation — these young people do not recognise their alcohol or drug use as a problem and are not ready to change. They usually focus on the positive aspects of their drug use.

Contemplation — these young people are ambivalent or unsure about their alcohol or drug use and are thinking about making some changes. This group is particularly amenable to motivational interviewing.

Action — This group is ready to change. They may have already taken some action to change their behaviours.

Maintenance — This group of young people has ceased their alcohol or drug use and are maintaining the change.

Relapse — This group of young people has returned to alcohol or drug use. It is important to treat this as a part of the process of change rather than a failure. Relapse is common in the natural history of substance abuse.

4.2.3. *Motivational Counselling*

The goals of motivational counselling are to identify where the young person is in the stages of change and to help him/her progress to become ready for change or maintain that change. There are five general principles of motivational interviewing:

1. Express empathy.
2. Develop and explore discrepancy.
3. Avoid argumentation.
4. Roll with resistance.
5. Support self-efficacy.

4.3. *Tertiary Intervention*

Here, strategies are aimed at achieving abstinence and/or reducing harm in those young people at the severe end of the substance use spectrum who are not able to achieve abstinence. This more intensive intervention is usually performed by youth-specific drug and alcohol services and using an assertive case management approach.

4.3.1. *Harm minimisation*

Harm minimisation considers the actual harms associated with the use of a particular drug (rather than just the drug use itself), and how these harms can be minimised or reduced. The harm minimisation approach includes abstinence but does not insist on abstinence as the objective of treatment or community prevention initiatives. Some examples of harm reduction include educating young people on strategies to reduce potential harms from alcohol consumption, party safe campaigns and needle exchange programs for intravenous drug users aimed at decreasing the risk of blood-borne viruses such as hepatitis B, C, and HIV.

4.3.2. *Individual cognitive behaviour therapy*

CBT is a commonly used, evidence-based treatment for young people who abuse substances. The research mostly relates to cannabis and amphetamine use. CBT can be of assistance in the following ways:

- To teach relaxation techniques.
- To provide anxiety management.
- To manage cravings.
- To promote relapse prevention.
- As counselling.
- To substitute substance use with healthier options.
- To address spiritual fulfilment.

4.3.3. *Pharmacotherapy*

This approach refers to the use of medications in substance abuse treatment. An example includes opioid replacement therapy, such as methadone or buprenorphine for young people who are opioid dependent. Medications are also sometimes used for the short term alleviation of withdrawal symptoms, and to manage comorbid mental health disorders such as anxiety, depression or psychosis.

4.3.4. *Family therapy*

Family therapy has proven efficacy for many adolescents with substance use problems, assisting parents and the family unit. The involvement of parents in treatment indirectly assists the adolescent by addressing parental concerns, influencing parenting style and capacity, and breaking unhealthy patterns of communication and interaction between parent and teenager. Intervention can involve meeting with the parents alone, with the parents and the substance using teenager, or with the whole family. The goals of intervention are to assist parents to take a strong, containing, protecting, and nurturing stance, to promote respectful communication, conflict resolution, and to incorporate an understanding of the views of all family members.

4.3.5. *Residential drug and alcohol rehabilitation*

This is a treatment option for young people who are substance dependent. Programs are specifically geared to assist with breaking the cycle of drug use, to re-engage the young person in school, education or employment, and to promote healthy family and social supports. Effective treatment ideally includes an extensive aftercare program.

5. Common Substances of Abuse

5.1. *Alcohol*

Alcohol is the most commonly used recreational drug in Australia and many other countries. The current NHMRC guidelines for reducing the risks of alcohol related harm in young people include the following:

- Parents and carers should be advised that children under 15 years of age are at the greatest risk of harm from drinking and that for this age group, not drinking alcohol is especially important.
- For young people aged 15–17 years, the safest option is to delay the initiation of drinking for as long as possible.
- For women who are pregnant or planning a pregnancy or breast feeding, not drinking is the safest option.

5.1.1. *Effects of alcohol*

The short term effects of alcohol include relaxation, slower reflexes, dis-inhibited behaviour and slurred speech, confusion, nausea, vomiting and blackouts.

There are many long term effects of alcohol that are common in adults after years of heavy drinking including alcoholic liver disease and pancreatitis and neurological damage. In young people however, there is emerging evidence that frequent episodes of binge drinking affect short and long term memory and concentration.

5.1.2. *Pattern of alcohol use in young people*

The majority of alcohol related harms in young people are caused by drinking to intoxication or 'binge' drinking. Young people are rarely aware of what volume comprises a standard drink, or of the alcohol content of their beverage. Surveys suggest that some young people consume extremely large amounts, 10–20+ standard drinks, on any given drinking occasion.

5.1.3. *Risks associated with adolescent alcohol use*

The most commonly described risks associated with excessive alcohol consumption are detailed in Section 3.4. It is increasingly understood that adolescence is a critical time for brain development and that alcohol abuse can affect cognitive abilities, including learning and memory.

Alcohol affects adolescents differently from adults in the following ways:

- Adolescents appear less sensitive to the impairment of coordination and to the sedative effects of alcohol.
- Adolescents appear to be more sensitive to the learning and memory impairments associated with heavy alcohol use.
- Early initiation of alcohol use increases the risk of alcohol dependence in adulthood up to four fold.
- Research suggests that it is not only repeated alcohol exposure but also withdrawal (hangover) that may be damaging to the developing adolescent brain.

5.1.4. *Management of acute alcohol intoxication*

The management of acute alcohol intoxication is often required when young people present with medical complications from binge drinking. The mainstay of treatment is supportive therapy and includes the following:

1. Airway management: a patient with a Glasgow Coma Scale of less than or equal to eight should be electively intubated and ventilated.
2. Treatment of agitation: 2.5 mg IV diazepam boluses, administered at five minute intervals until the patient is no longer agitated to a maximum of 20 mg. There is a risk of further respiratory depression and monitoring is essential.
3. Intravenous fluid and glucose: all adolescents should be on maintenance IV dextrose/saline. Hypoglycemia should be treated with a bolus of 5 mL/kg of 10% dextrose. Thiamine should be added to intravenous therapy if there is a history of prolonged, heavy drinking.
4. Management of hypothermia using appropriate warming techniques.
5. Monitor with GCS: consider investigation for head injury if there is fluctuation in consciousness.
6. Referral to drug and alcohol services or mental health services.
7. Consider urine drug screen: polysubstance use is common.
8. Collect blood alcohol level if required: it is a legal requirement in Australia to collect blood alcohol levels in adults and adolescents 15 years and over involved in motor vehicle accidents.

5.1.5. *Alcohol dependence*

Initiation of alcohol consumption at an early age has been associated with increased frequency and quantity of alcohol intake in adolescence and increased risk of abuse and alcohol dependence. People who start drinking alcohol before the age of 15 are four times more likely to develop alcohol dependence than someone who starts drinking at 21 years.

5.1.6. *Alcohol withdrawal syndrome*

The syndrome occurs uncommonly in young people. It commences between 6–24 hours after the last drink and may last up to 14 days. Features include sweating, tachycardia, hypertension, insomnia, tremor, fever, nausea, vomiting, anorexia, abdominal cramps, diarrhoea, craving, insomnia, headache, seizures, confusion, perceptual distortions, disorientation, and hallucinations. Diazepam is the current treatment of choice for alcohol withdrawal and may be given as a loading dose in an inpatient setting or as a tapered dose in an outpatient setting. Prevention of dehydration is important. Parenteral administration of thiamine to avoid Wernicke's encephalopathy is essential.

5.1.7. *Longer term treatment of alcohol dependence*

Medications commonly used for long-term treatment of adults with alcohol dependence include naltrexone, acamprosate, and disulfiram. These are sometimes also used in the management of young people with alcohol dependence, although the focus is on psychosocial interventions. Management of concurrent mental health disorders is an important aspect of treatment.

5.2. *Cannabis*

Cannabis is derived from the hemp plant *Cannabis sativa.* Marijuana is the dried leaves and flowers of the plant. The resin contains about 60 cannabinoids, the most abundant being delta tetra hydrocannabinol. Cannabis is commonly smoked as cones or bongs and usually mixed with tobacco.

5.2.1. *Effects of cannabis*

The effect lasts for 2–3 hours in which the user describes being stoned, 'high' or 'bent'. This includes relaxation, loss of inhibition and impaired concentration, judgement, memory, and cognition. The physical effects include tachycardia, hypotension, increased appetite or 'munchies', conjunctival injection, anxiety, panic attacks, restlessness, excitement, altered perception, de-realisation, irritability, paranoia, hallucinations, and risk of psychosis.

5.2.2. *Pattern of cannabis use in young people*

Many young people will try cannabis and experience no apparent harm. However a minority experience harmful outcomes, particularly those with recurrent use or daily use. These include depression, anxiety, and acute psychosis.

5.2.3. *Cannabis dependence*

About 90% of daily users meet criteria for dependence.

5.2.4. *Cannabis withdrawal syndrome*

The severity of withdrawal increases with heavier use, earlier age of first use, and comorbid mental illness. Figure 1 details the timeline of withdrawal symptoms. Less common symptoms include chills, depressed mood, abdominal pain or physical discomfort, tremulousness, sweating, and acute psychosis.

No specific medications have been shown to be effective in the management of cannabis withdrawal. Benzodiazepines may alleviate aggression and agitation. An anti-depressant such as mirtazapine which has a sedative effect can be helpful for withdrawal related insomnia and mood disorder. Mental health assessment and follow up is important in these young people as they are often at risk of developing more complex mental health issues.

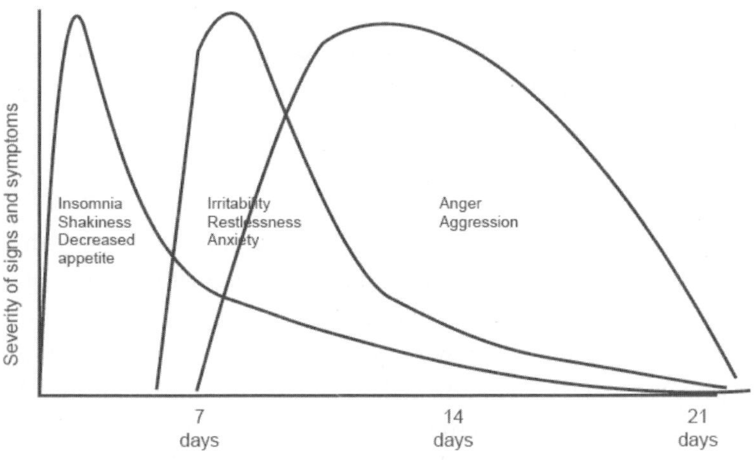

Fig.1: Course of cannabis withdrawal.

5.3. *Psychostimulants*

Psychostimulants include the amphetamine group (speed, base, ice), ecstasy, and cocaine. Speed is a powder form of methamphetamine. Base is a brown, viscous mixture. 'Ice' is a street name for crystal-methamphetamine hydrochloride, which is the most potent form of amphetamine. Other street names for ice include 'meth', 'crystal', 'shabu', 'batu', 'tina', and 'glass'. Amphetamines may be ingested, injected, smoked, snorted, or inserted anally.

5.3.1. *Effects of amphetamines*

The immediate effects are of increased alertness, talkativeness, increased confidence and euphoria. These effects are accompanied by decreased appetite, insomnia, dry mouth, nausea and vomiting, diarrhoea, jaw clenching, sweating and hot and cold flushes. Common physical signs include tachycardia and hypertension, tachypnea, and pupillary dilatation.

The effects of higher doses include dizziness, restlessness, anxiety and panic attacks, depression, confusion, hallucinations, and acute psychosis. Cardiac arrhythmias may be present.

The longer term effects of stimulants are many and include cardiomyopathy and congestive cardiac failure, stroke and its sequelae, movement disorders, chronic lung disease, and chronic skin infections.

Ecstasy 3,4-methylenedioxymethamphetamine, is a common 'party drug'. It is usually sold as a coloured pill and may contain a variety of amphetamine-related substances and other impurities. The effects of ecstasy are felt approximately 20–40 minutes after use and the 'high' usually lasts from 4–6 hours.

In addition to the general effects of amphetamines, ecstasy produces feelings of euphoria, increased self-confidence, lack of inhibition, feelings of relaxation, self-exploration and emotional openness, and increased energy. Caution must be taken when prescribing SSRI medication to young people who use ecstasy due to the risk of acute serotonin syndrome. Ecstasy has been associated with hyperthermia, particularly when used during raves or dance parties. Excessive water consumption whilst intoxicated with ecstasy increases the risk of hyponatraemia, cerebral oedema, and death.

Cocaine is derived from the leaves of the coca plant. This plant is processed in different ways to make different types of cocaine. *Cocaine hydrochloride* is the white powder type of cocaine most common in Australia. In this form it is sniffed through the nose. *Freebase cocaine* can be smoked and this makes the user feel 'high' quickly. *Crack cocaine* is a type of freebase cocaine sold in the form of small crystals or rocks. It is usually smoked.

Cocaine is often mixed or cut with other substances to make the drug go further. Some mixed-in substances can have unpleasant or harmful effects.

In addition to the harms associated with amphetamine use, cocaine users are at risk of nosebleeds, sinusitis, and damage to the nasal septum. Intravenous drug use increases the risk of blood-borne viruses, septicaemia, thrombophlebitis, and infective endocarditis. There is increased risk of sexual promiscuity and sex working in young people who frequently use cocaine or other amphetamines.

5.3.2. *Amphetamine use in young people*

The incidence and prevalence of amphetamine use increases in late adolescence and the early twenties. Amphetamine withdrawal syndrome is well described in those with amphetamine dependence. It typically follows the pattern below:

Day 1–3: 'The Crash'; exhaustion, hypersomnia, depressed affect.
Day 2–10: cravings, mood swings, irritability and anxiety, headaches, myalgia, paranoia.
Day 7–28: most symptoms settle but cravings, mood swings, insomnia, and irritability may persist.
Months 1–3: mood and sleep start to return to normal.

5.3.3. *Specific treatment of amphetamine use*

Treatment of young people who use amphetamines depends on the frequency of use, associated harms, risk of dependence, and comorbidities. General drug and alcohol treatment principles apply. There is growing evidence to support CBT as an effective treatment to maintain abstinence, including managing withdrawal and relapse prevention. There is no specific pharmacotherapy for amphetamine dependence, however diazepam may be used short term to assist with anxiety. Anti-psychotic medication may be used for drug induced psychosis. Rarely an inpatient admission its required to assist with attaining abstinence, particularly in the case of poor social support networks and prior to admission to a residential rehabilitation, if there is inappropriate housing or if the young person is homeless.

5.4. *Opioids*

Opiates are compounds extracted from the juices of the poppy *Papaver somniferum*, such as morphine and heroin. Opioids include both opiates and synthetic compounds such as methadone and pethidine that bind to the opiate receptor. Heroin is a potent 'mu' receptor agonist, a subclass of opiate receptors known as morphine receptors. It is commonly used intravenously, giving its effect within minutes. It can also be smoked or used by inhaling fumes from heating heroin but cannot be taken orally due to high first pass metabolism in the liver.

5.4.1. *Effects of opioids*

Mu opiate receptor agonist drugs have the following pharmacological actions: analgesia, euphoria, sedation, CNS depression including respiratory depression, pupillary constriction, hypotension and bradycardia. Opioid intoxication is indicated by drowsiness, drawling speech, pinpoint pupils, decreased respiratory rate, deceased heart rate and hypotension.

5.4.2. *Pattern of opioid use in young people*

Young people who smoke heroin often are in denial about their dependence on the substance and delay seeking treatment. Those who inject are at high risk of blood-borne viruses and other risks associated with IVDU. Another population of opioid using young people that is recognised are those who use over the counter medications including combinations of codeine, paracetamol, and/or ibuprofen. Young people can become opioid dependent from abuse of codeine. Due to the combination pills, they also may suffer complications of either paracetamol or ibuprofen abuse.

5.4.3. *Opioid withdrawal syndrome*

The onset and duration of withdrawal from opioids depend on the half life of the drug being taken. For heroin, the onset of subjective symptoms of withdrawal is usually 8–24 hours after the last dose, reaches a peak at 24–48 hours, and resolves after 5–7 days. For methadone, onset is usually 24–48 hours after the last dose. The peak severity of withdrawal from methadone tends to be considerably lower than for heroin withdrawal, but withdrawal is more prolonged, with a debilitating low-grade withdrawal lasting for 3–6 weeks.

Opioid withdrawal syndrome symptoms include anorexia and nausea, abdominal cramps, diarrhoea, bone, joint and muscle pain, rhinorrhoea, hot and cold flushes, increased lacrimation, yawning, agitation and insomnia. Piloerection and dilated pupils are common physical signs. Cravings, anxiety, insomnia and/or anhedonia may persist for weeks or months.

5.4.4. *Treatments for opioid dependence*

Symptomatic treatment for withdrawal may include the following: Clonidine 75 mcg every 6 hours for sweating, hypertension and agitation, buscopan 20 mg every 6 hours as needed for abdominal cramps, and paracetamol 500–1000 mg as required (maximum 4000 mg in 24 hours) or ibuprofen 400 mg every 6 hours as needed (if no history of peptic ulcer or gastritis) are commonly used for general pain or discomfort. Metoclopramide 10 mg, 4–6 hourly, prochlorperazine 5 mg, every 4–6 hours or ondansetron 4–8 mg, every 12 hours for nausea or vomiting are used. Diphenoxylate/atropine 5 mg, 4–6 hourly is used for diarrhoea.

Buprenorphine is increasingly used as the principal treatment to relieve withdrawal symptoms, so that other symptomatic medication is not usually required. Buprenorphine is a partial mu receptor agonist and may precipitate withdrawal in someone who has used heroin in the previous 6–12 hours or methadone in the previous 24–48 hours. Buprenorphine may also be used as an opioid replacement maintenance therapy.

5.4.5 *Opioid replacement therapy*

Longer term opioid replacement therapy can be offered with either methadone or buprenorphine. The goals of treatment are to reduce the need for heroin use with opiate substitution, to reduce injecting drug use and to facilitate social functioning of opioid using individuals. These medications are usually prescribed and dispensed daily in either a public hospital drug and alcohol clinic, or community pharmacy. Caution is required when undertaking this form of intervention in young people. Firstly, it is necessary to ascertain opioid dependence. A urine drug screen to confirm presence of opioid in the system before commencing opioid replacement therapy is also mandatory.

Methadone is a useful substitution treatment for opioid dependent individuals because of its long half life and its opioid effects. The half life of methadone is approximately 24 hours. Methadone should be started at low dose, and increased slowly as steady state equilibrium with methadone is not achieved until approximately 4–5 days. A starting dose of 10–20 mg is appropriate for someone who has a low or uncertain level of neuroadaptation or who is engaging in high risk polysubstance use. A higher starting dose of 20–30 mg is recommended for individuals with a greater level of neuroadaptation. Individuals commenced on methadone should be reviewed once or twice per week until the dose is stabilised and monthly thereafter. High risk individuals require more frequent review.

Buprenorphine maintenance is usually in the form combined with naloxone and is administered sublingually. Buprenorphine is a mixed opioid agonist/antagonist with high affinity for mu opioid receptors. Buprenorphine/naloxone is particularly favoured for young people because of its safety profile and limited abuse liability. Principles of buprenorphine/naloxone maintenance are to give a low first dose (4–6 mg sublingually) in case precipitated withdrawal occurs. Thereafter, the dose can be increased reasonably rapidly. Maximum daily dose varies between individuals. However, a plateau effect for both efficacy and toxicity is likely beyond 32 mg daily.

5.5. *Lysergic Acid Diethylamide, Hallucinogens and Others*

Hallucinogens are a group of drugs that affect the senses and cause hallucinations. *LSD* is a hallucinogen, also known as a 'psychedelic drug' or 'acid' and usually comes in the form of a liquid, tablet, capsule, or square of gelatine or blotting paper. *Ketamine* also known as 'Special K' is a powerful anaesthetic used in surgery. It is a dissociative drug, producing the sensations that the mind seems to 'leave' the body. Ketamine comes as a liquid (for injecting), pill, powder, and a formulation for smoking. *Gamma-hydroxybutyrate* comes as a colourless, odourless liquid or as a crystal powder. GHB is a powerful, rapidly acting central nervous system depressant and is often used in 'date rape'. Its effects last for 3–6 hours.

5.5.1. *Effects of hallucinogens*

The effects of hallucinogens begin within half an hour of taking the drug, peak at 3–5 hours and may last up to 12 hours. These effects include distorted perceptions, intense sensory experiences, mixing of the senses (hearing colours or seeing sounds), changed sense of time, strange bodily sensations, and changed and intense thoughts and emotional swings. Physical effects include muscle fasciculation, weakness, paresthesia, pupil dilatation, tremor, nausea, vomiting, tachycardia, hypertension and lack of coordination. There are few known long-term effects from hallucinogens. However, 'flashbacks' can happen days, weeks, or even years after taking the drug. These visual hallucinations may be triggered by other drugs, stress or fatigue, and may be very disturbing.

5.5.2. *Hallucinogen use in young people*

Hallucinogens are more likely to be used by older adolescents either experimentally or occasionally. Less frequently they are used on a regular basis. There is little evidence that physical dependence or withdrawal syndromes exist for hallucinogens. It is possible however to become psychologically dependent. General principles of drug and alcohol treatment as outlined in Section 4.0 are used.

5.6. *Inhalants*

Inhalants contain volatile substances that are self-administered as gases or vapours to induce a psycho-active effect. These are available in legal, relatively inexpensive, and common household products. Young people sniff glue, felt-tipped pens, butane gas for lighters or barbecues, aerosol sprays, nail polish removers, paint thinners, correction fluids and chrome-based paint. Petrol sniffing, particularly by Indigenous young people has been a particular concern in some remote areas in Australia.

5.6.1. *Effects of inhalants*

Inhalants have many short-term effects: rapid intoxication, euphoria, hallucinations, loss of muscular coordination, slurred speech and blurred vision, confusion and incoherence, aggression, increased risk-taking behaviours, and vomiting.

Most studies on long term effects that have been conducted have examined inhalant use by industrial workers. Some work in Indigenous communities has shown that inhalant abuse results in significant cognitive impairment which, in the early stage only, is still reversible. Peripheral neuropathy, liver and renal impairment and bone marrow suppression have also been described.

Other harms from chronic use include recurrent nose bleeds with oral and nasal ulceration, sinusitis, indigestion, conjunctivitis, chronic cough, tinnitus, chest pain, depression, and anxiety.

5.6.2. *Pattern of inhalant use in young people*

As with other drug use by young people, patterns of inhalant use can be classified into four types: experimental, regular, chronic, and situational. Inhalant dependence disorders have the same diagnostic criteria sets as other substance use disorders, except that a characteristic withdrawal syndrome is not included. Habitual use can lead to tolerance and at least psychological dependence, plus weight loss, and malnutrition.

Inhalants are the only drug class where use tends to decline with age through the adolescent years and into young adulthood. Treatment is mostly psychosocial with a harm minimisation approach, acknowledging that young people who use inhalants are likely to grow out of this behaviour.

5.7. *Benzodiazepines*

Benzodiazepines are depressant drugs, prescribed to reduce anxiety and sleeplessness. Young people with anxiety sometimes self-medicate with benzodiazepines. More commonly young people abuse benzodiazepines on a sporadic basis, placing themselves at risk of disinhibited behaviour, injury, and overdose. Self-medication with benzodiazepines can cause tolerance and dependence through regular use. Benzodiazepine withdrawal can occur with therapeutic doses when given for two months or more. The onset is typically 1–2 days after the last dose for short-acting benzodiazepines and 2–4 days after the last dose for long-acting benzodiazepines. The peak symptoms occur at 5–7 days, but symptoms may last for several weeks.

Withdrawal symptoms include anxiety and panic attacks, poor concentration, insomnia and bizarre dreams, depersonalisation, headaches, tremulousness, sweating, nausea, vomiting, and abdominal pains, and heightened senses of sight, touch, and hearing. More severe withdrawal can occur with short-acting benzodiazepines that have been used for longer duration at very high doses. Abrupt cessation is particularly hazardous and may cause seizures, hallucinations, or delirium.

Slow tapering of the daily dose is recommended to treat dependence. This is best done in a controlled environment with daily pick up of benzodiazepine dose, communication with all health professionals involved in the young person's care regarding the management plan and regular urine drug screens. Doctor shopping for benzodiazepine prescriptions must be prevented.

6. Common Comorbidities of Substance Abuse

6.1. *Attention Deficit Hyperactivity Disorder*

There is a 1.5 increased risk of substance abuse in young people with ADHD. Comorbid oppositional defiant disorder, conduct disorder, and major depression are significant predictors of substance use disorder. Continued monitoring of stimulant treatment and receiving additional help at school are protective factors against substance abuse for young people with ADHD. This approach in turn may increase retention in education and subsequent employment, thus decreasing further risks for the young person.

6.2. *Mental Health*

6.2.1. *Anxiety and depression*

Young people may use alcohol and other drugs as self-medication for depression and/or anxiety. Daily cannabis users report high levels of anxiety, depression and fatigue, and low motivation. Early onset weekly cannabis use in adolescence predicts a twofold increase in rates of depression and anxiety among young women, with daily use increasing the risk fourfold. Within the Australian Indigenous population, heavy cannabis use increases the risk of depression four fold.

6.2.2. *Risk of psychosis*

The relationship between cannabis and psychosis is bidirectional. Regular cannabis use doubles the risk for schizophrenia and psychosis, with an even greater risk in youth who have early onset and more frequent use. Among those with psychosis, chronic cannabis use impacts negatively on both illness course and treatment outcome and is associated with poor medication compliance, more severe psychotic symptoms and earlier and more frequent psychotic relapses.

Drug induced psychosis is often due to psychostimulant drugs such as cannabis, cocaine, LSD, amphetamines, and occasionally alcohol. Symptoms may resolve after cessation of substance use or may take months to improve. Differentiation between diagnoses is difficult on first presentation of early psychosis. Treatment services for young people with early psychosis work closely with youth drug and alcohol workers to decrease substance abuse and reduce the risk for recurrence of psychotic symptoms.

6.3. *Young People In Out of Home Care*

Young people in out of home care are a complex, high needs group. They often have a background of neglect, abuse, parental substance abuse, school disruption, conduct and behavioural issues, and complex mental health concerns. They are at increased risk of substance use, abuse, and dependence. Treatment of this group is often challenging, requiring engagement to build trust, and a comprehensive management plan to address all the issues the young person is facing.

6.4. *Young Offenders*

Young people in custody and others who come into contact with the criminal justice systems are at greater risk than most of developing alcohol and other drug problems. Young offenders are more likely to have had parents who have been in prison and had drug and alcohol problems themselves. A history of childhood abuse and a sense of being abandoned by their parents is common, as is school dropout.

7. Transition

Youth drug and alcohol clinicians may work within a number of settings. These include youth health clinics, adolescent medical services, child and adolescent mental health services, or adult drug and alcohol services. Many of these services work within a developmental framework and offer treatment for young people to their mid twenties. Older adolescents with complex substance abuse and dependence will require transition to adult drug and alcohol services for ongoing management. Principles are the same as for other areas of adolescent medicine (Chapter 13).

References

Bertolin-Guillen J, Lopez-Arquero F, Martinez-Franco L. (2008) Cannabis-induced mania? *J Subst Use* **13**(2): 139–141.

Bonomo Y, Proimos J. (2005) Substance misuse: Alcohol, tobacco, inhalants, and other drugs. *BMJ* **330**(7494): 777–780.

Czucta D, Ryan K. (1999) *First Episode Psychosis: A Guide for People with Psychosis and their Families.* Available online at: http://www.camh.net/About_Addiction_Mental_Health/Mental_Health_Information/First_Episode_Psychosis/fep_guide.pdf. (accessed 13 Jan 2012).

Degenhardt L, Coffey C, Carlin JB, Swift W, Moore E, Patton GC. (2010) Outcomes of occasional cannabis use in adolescence: 10-year follow-up study in Victoria, Australia. *Br J Psychiatry* **196**: 290–295.

Hall W, Degenhardt L. (2000) Cannabis use and psychosis: A review of clinical and epidemiological evidence. *Aust NZJ Psychiatry* **34**(1): 26–34.

Hides L, Dawe S, Kavanagh DJ, Young RM. (2006) Psychotic symptom and cannabis relapse in recent-onset psychosis. Prospective study. *Br J Psychiatry* **189**: 137–143.

Hill DJ, White VM, Williams RM, Gardner GJ. (1993) Tobacco and alcohol use among Australian secondary school students in 1990. *Med J Aust* **158**(4): 228–234.

Knight JR, Sherritt L, Shrier LA, Harris SK, Chang G. (2002) Validity of the crafft substance abuse screening test among adolescent clinic patients. *Arch Pediatrics Adolesc Med* **156**(6): 607–614.

Moore THM, Zammit S, Lingford-Hughes A, Barnes TRE, Jones PB, Burke M, Lewis G. (2007) Cannabis use and risk of psychotic or affective mental health outcomes: A systematic review. *Lancet* **370**(9584): 319–328.

Patton GC, Coffey C, Carlin JB, Degenhardt L, Lynskey M, Hall W. (2002) Cannabis use and mental health in young people: Cohort study. *BMJ* **325**(7374): 1195–1198.

Shrier LA, Harris SK, Kurland M, Knight JR. (2003) Substance use problems and associated psychiatric symptoms among adolescents in primary care. *Pediatrics* **111**(61): e699–670

Wilens TE, Martelon M, Joshi G, Bateman C, Fried R, Petty C, Biederman J. (2011) Does ADHD predict substance-use disorders? A 10-year follow-up study of young adults with ADHD. *J Am Acad Child Adolesc Psychiatry* **50**(6): 543–553.

Chapter 16

Unintentional Injuries Among Adolescents and Young Adults

Richard E Bélanger and Joan-Carles Suris

1. Introduction

Over the last century, causes of mortality and their prevalence have seen dramatic changes in developed countries. In ageing populations, most deaths are now the result of cancers and chronic conditions as threats related to infectious diseases have largely been controlled. The picture is however quite different for individuals aged 10–24. Injuries are by far the leading cause of deaths and long term disabilities among adolescents and young adults living in North America, Europe, and Australia.

Previously referred to as accidents, injuries have long been considered solely the result of misfortune. As a result, authorities have for years considered injuries a lesser public health priority. We now know that injuries are both predictable and preventable events that can directly, and even indirectly, result in harm.

In the first place, injuries are classified according to their premeditated intent. Unintentional ones are of particular interest to adolescent and young adult health: more youths from developed countries die each year in such circumstances than from all other causes combined. This disproportion is even more extreme for young adults alone (Table 1).

In 2005, unintentional injuries resulted in the loss of more than 15,000 individuals aged 15–24 in the US, 1,022 in Canada, and 922 in Australia.

Table 1:   Five leading causes of death (and number) by age group, United States (2005).

Rank	Age 10–14	Age 15–19	Age 20–24
1	Unintentional injuries 1,343	Unintentional injuries 6,616	Unintentional injuries 9,137
2	Malignant neoplasms 515	Homicide 2,076	Homicide 3,390
3	Suicide 270	Suicide 1,613	Suicide 2,599
4	Homicide 220	Malignant neoplasms 731	Malignant neoplasms 986
5	Congenital anomalies 200	Heart disease 389	Heart disease 730

This is only part of the picture in these countries, as many more adolescents
and young adults attended an emergency department or were hospitalised
because of unintentional harms. For every youth death in the US, there are
nearly 12 hospitalisations and more than 600 emergency visits. Roughly,
one-third of all emergency consultations are directly related to injury.
However, many injured adolescents and young adults do not reach the hospital, as they are treated in the office or at home. In 2002, 28% of individuals
aged 16–20 years living in Switzerland reported at least one accident needing medical care in the previous 12 months. Worldwide, it is estimated that
10–30 million children and adolescents are affected by non-fatal injuries
every year. These non-fatal injuries can result in long-lasting disabilities that
may hinder adolescents reaching their full potential. Moreover, the social
and psychological impacts of unintentional injuries in the youth population
are well recognised but still need to be thoroughly studied.

1.1. *Risk and Protective Factors*

Adolescents and young adults' increased risk for unintentional injuries is
partly explained by the vast range of activities to which they are exposed.
Their appetite for exploratory behaviours certainly explains part of this
risk as well. Managing risk and distinguishing between safe and unsafe
behaviour are important developmental skills for protection and survival.
The prolonged time needed to reach full cognitive potential of adulthood

provides much of the explanation for the apparently poor judgment of adolescents and the taking of unacceptable risks.

Other factors influence the incidence of youth's unintentional injuries. Globally, injuries among adolescents seem to decrease with age, while fatal ones increase up to age 24. Males are almost twice as likely as females to experience unintentional injury, in part because activities to which they are exposed are more hazardous. Previous psychological difficulties and behavioural problems are additional identified risk factors, with aggressive and anti-social behaviour being more consistently reported than ADHD. Social factors cannot be overemphasised as potent determinants of unintentional injuries. Poverty and remoteness from health facilities are associated with an increased likelihood of injuries and other unfavourable consequences among the vulnerable population that youths represent.

Substance use is one of the greatest contributors to unintentional injury. Alcohol is the preferred substance and binge drinking the common pattern (Chapter 15). Alcohol impairs cognitive abilities such as attention and judgment, and decreases fine motor functions and balance, a perfect mix for being injured. Alcohol is associated with over one third of fatalities in adolescents aged 15–20. It is a predominant factor in more than 30% of drowning deaths, 34% of pedestrian deaths, 40% of deaths in house fires, and 51% of adolescent traumatic brain injuries. Alcohol unsurprisingly contributes to motor vehicle injuries. While some data report that adolescents drink and drive less frequently than do adults, their crash risks are much higher when they do. One in 10 of 9–12th-graders in the US reports driving after drinking. More than a quarter admitted to riding with drivers who were intoxicated. Cannabis seems to impair driving performance as well. Similarly to alcohol, its influence is greater with higher intakes, and more in novice than in experienced drivers. Concomitant use of both substances increases driving risks.

1.2. *Causes of Unintentional Injuries*

Commonly, unintentional injuries are grouped by their origin, either from acute exposure to energy (kinetic, thermal, chemical, electrical energy, and radiation), or from the absence of an essential one (oxygen or heat). Injuries can also be classified by their general mechanism, as for example, being

Table 2: Leading causes of lethal unintentional injuries. (Number and percentages) by age group, United States (2005).

	Age 10–14	Age 15–19	Age 20–24
Transportation	893 (66.5%)	5114 (77.3%)	6124 (67.0%)
Poisoning	34 (2.5%)	637 (9.6%)	1847 (20.2%)
Drowning	132 (9.8%)	310 (4.7%)	339 (3.7%)
Burns/fire/flames	166 (12.4%)	116 (1.8%)	199 (2.2%)
Other	118 (8.8%)	439 (6.6%)	62 (8.9%)

struck by or hitting an object, or being cut. We rather prefer a description based on the underlying circumstance as it enables health professionals to highlight some particularities and possible preventive strategies (Table 2).

1.2.1. *Transportation*

1.2.1.1. Motor-vehicle

Annually, 450,000 US teenagers are injured due to motor-vehicle crashes. As in other parts of the world, road-traffic crashes are the leading cause of mortality and morbidity for youths in the US. Cars rather than motorcycles are usually involved. Despite this fact, being on four wheels appears to be safer than being on two. For every mile travelled, motorcyclists are at much greater risk than car occupants to die or to be injured in a motor-vehicle accident. Motor-vehicle deaths usually result from single vehicle crashes, leaving the road due to driving error and/or speed.

Most pedestrian and biking deaths also involve motor-vehicles. Among the 900 adolescents and young adult pedestrians dying each year in the US, four out of five are hit by a motor-vehicle. Similarly, even if non-fatal injuries account for the vast proportion of emergency visits related to bicycle riding, 90% are attributed to collisions with motor-vehicles, with severe head injuries explaining most of these. Overall, of the 2.6 million deaths having occurred worldwide in 2004 among people aged 10–24, more than a third were due to traffic injuries.

Despite adolescents driving less than older age-groups, they are disproportionately involved in motor-vehicle crashes. For each mile driven in the US by an adolescent aged 16–19, there are four times more crashes than for older drivers, and crash rates are the highest at age 16, nine times greater than among the general driver population. Adolescents may therefore be willing to accept a higher level of risk, or to be pressured into it by their peers while driving. Yet, more non-fatal injuries result from inexperience, rather than from speeding or obvious risky behaviour. The attention capacity of adolescents can also be altered by many factors. First, crashes happen mostly at night in all age groups. An adolescent's focus can simply be diverted to other activities while driving, such as cell phone use and text messaging. A recent Australian study reported that the amount of time young drivers spend not looking at the road when texting is up to four times greater than when not involved in this dangerous activity.

1.2.2. *Poisoning*

Any adverse health consequence related to the absorption (mainly ingestion) of chemical products (man-made or natural) is labelled as poisoning. From the 2,479,355 human exposure cases reported by the American Association of Poison Control Center's National Poison Data System for 2009, two thirds involved the under twenties, among which 163,615 (6.6%) involved adolescents aged 13–19. In comparison with children, for which unintentional toxic exposure is the rule, the number of accidental and intentional events among adolescents is roughly equal.

From emergency department records, consultations for poisoning among adolescents mostly involve alcohol, followed by illicit substances, non-prescription drugs, and prescribed ones. Corrosives and caustics, as well as gases and vapours, are uncommonly reported. Even if most exposures do not result in major problems or toxicity, adolescents are proportionally the largest group requiring hospitalisation. For this latter group, pharmaceutical agents are the main cause. Fortunately, a decrease in hospitalisation rates has been seen over the last few decades.

1.2.3. *Drowning*

Drowning is when an individual experiences respiratory impairment from submersion or immersion in a liquid. Adolescent drowning deaths rank second after those of children aged 0–4 years old. For non-fatal submersions, severe long-term adverse outcomes can result. This is largely explained by length of immersion, prolonged resuscitation efforts and lack of early resuscitation by bystanders.

While drowning can occur in diverse settings, most events take place in natural waters and mostly during the warmer seasons. A study carried out in the Pacific coast of the US reported that between 1980 and 1995, 76% of drowning among 15–19 years old had been witnessed by a friend or others.

Swimming ability and judgment about the safety of water are two important skills that everyone should acquire early in life. Medical conditions may play a part in the risk of some adolescents drowning. As an example, individuals with epilepsy have a 15–19 fold increase in risk of death by drowning compared to the general population.

1.2.4. *Burns, fire, and flames*

House fires account for 93% of all fire and burn-related deaths in the US. While most residential fires are related to cooking and heating equipments, cigarette smoking is the commonest underlying cause of death.

For most house fires, suffocation rather than burning causes the fatality. For that reason, smoke detectors are of crucial importance. Working smoke alarms in residential fires can reduce the risk of death of its inhabitants by nearly 50%. In the US, more than 90% of households have at least one smoke alarm. Unfortunately, one quarter of these are not working because batteries are not replaced properly each year, or are simply removed. Fire brigade figures from New South Wales in Australia show that in the decade to 1999–2000, 88% of fire deaths occurred in dwellings with no smoke alarms.

1.2.5. *Sports*

Despite its well-known positive effects on health, sports participation accounts for an impressive percentage of non-lethal injuries among adolescents and young adults. Sports related injuries are the most frequent reason for which adolescents seek medical care, representing up to 40% of injuries in some surveys. In Edinburgh, Scotland, a quarter of all fractures in adolescents aged 10–19 were caused by sport activities. Among these, nearly 85% involved upper limb compared to 16% in the lower limb, with football (soccer), rugby, and skiing causing the majority. Such statistics however represent sports preferences, and population and country specific data are essential.

Concussion is a concerning injury in any sport due to its long-term associated developmental and cognitive problems. From 2001 to 2005, among the 502,000 estimated emergency visits for concussion among 8–19 year old youths in the US, half were sports-related. Organised team sports such as football and ice hockey seem, among others, particularly risky.

In contrast, overuse injuries resulting from small but repetitive stress to the musculoskeletal system without sufficient recovery time may seem minor compared to other trauma. Yet, these now represent up to 50% of all injuries seen in paediatric sports medicine consultations.

1.3. *Prevention*

Moving from the term accident to injury has enabled significant advances in the prevention of harm related to regrettable, yet predictable events.

Prevention advice has long been integrated in consultation agendas in the paediatric and adolescent medicine fields. For example, the HEADSS mnemonic has integrated a section where discussion around safety can be included during a visit (Chapter 5). As several safety issues might be relevant, practitioners should tailor their advice according to both risk assessment and evidence-based effective interventions. Recommendations can now be found in up-to-date review documents produced by scientific groups around the world. As an example, the Greig Health Report from the Canadian Paediatric Society strongly advocates for bicycle helmet safety discussion for adolescents aged 10–17. This is based on research clearly showing that wearing a helmet while riding a bicycle saves lives. From a limited-scale prospective cohort, riding with a helmet provides an 85% reduction in the risk of head injury and an 88% reduction in the risk of brain injury. Unfortunately, in the US, for example, 85% of high school students rarely or never use bicycle helmets.

Since not all youths have access to comprehensive health care services and proper counselling, population based safety interventions are an essential public health approach. Such interventions are based on three strategic pillars: educational, environment, and legislation.

1.3.1. *Educational interventions*

Educational interventions should start early, with parents modelling the desired intervention for their children who will be more likely to continue the desired behaviour during adolescence. School-based programs can be carried out from kindergarten to college when relevant. We know that educational programs directed to adolescents are more likely to provide results if these are heard, viewed, and discussed in multiple settings. Media campaigns are usually of significant importance for these reasons. Peer education is also of great interest, as it is based on adolescents' own perceptions and motives.

1.3.2. *Environmental interventions*

Environmental factors are probably the most powerful way to reduce unintentional injuries among adolescents and young adults. In comparison to educational interventions, which need active efforts from the individual, environmental measures, also known as structural interventions, act passively, and are directed at the source of potential threats. As an example, households where handguns or rifles are present have an increased risk of injuries related to firearms. This is particularly true in the US where 7,000 individuals aged 10–24 die every year from firearms, with nearly 200 of these events due to unintentional causes. The four practices of keeping a gun locked, unloaded, storing ammunition locked, and in a separate location are each associated with a protective effect regarding related injuries. Similarly, keeping as few medications as possible at home, keeping them in safe places, and safely disposing of unwanted medications are environmental measures that should reduce the risks of poisoning.

1.3.3. *Legislation*

Legislation is a powerful instrument for prevention. Like environmental measures, these interventions act passively but necessitate the active participation of authorities to translate these measures into practice.

Therefore, creating a regulation is one step, implementation is another, and enforcement yet another. To work effectively, a law needs to be supported by the public, as well as being consistently enforced by local institutions.

Automobile-related injuries are perhaps the setting in which legislation and regulations have mostly had an effect. Three key elements are part of this success in the decreased mortality of adolescents from the late seventies to the present. First, consistent use of seatbelts (both shoulder and lap types) can prevent up to 60% of motor-vehicle crash fatalities. Secondly, laws on alcohol drinking and car driving have also been implemented. Thirdly, a graduated licensing approach has also been shown to be effective in decreasing fatal crash injuries among adolescents. Licensing programs include constraints on adolescents starting to drive, curfews, limiting the number of passengers in the vehicle and driving with individuals who have a legal license. Under the most comprehensive graduated driver licensing, fatal crashes for 16 year-old drivers can be decreased by more than one-third.

1.4. *Conclusions*

In summary, because of both frequency and related morbidity and mortality, unintentional injuries are not only a problem for public health authorities, but also for all health professionals caring for adolescents and young adults. Adolescents seem particularly at risk for unintentional injuries as they increase their physical capacity for activities, but remain more likely to accept risk. Transportation injuries, mostly those related to motor-vehicles, are of primary interest as these are the leading cause of mortality among adolescents and young adults in developed countries. Substance use, mostly alcohol, and the paradox surrounding sports are two of the important issues that also require the attention of society. Finally, prevention of unintentional injuries among adolescents and young adults starts in the family, continues in the health professional's office and ends through large scale educational, environmental, and legislative interventions.

References

American Academy of Pediatrics Committee on Injury, Violence and Poison Prevention. (2010) Prevention of drowning. *Pediatrics* **126**(1): 178–185.

Australian Institute of Health and Welfare, Henley, G. & Harrison, J. E. (2009) *Injury deaths, Australia* 2004–05. Injury research and statistics series no 51. Report for (Adelaide, http://www.nisu.flinders.edu.au/pubs/reports/2009/injcat127.pdf).

Bell GS, Gaitatzis A, Bell CL, Johnson AL, Sander JW. (2008) Drowning in people with epilepsy: How great is the risk? *Neurology* **71**(8): 578–582.

Bronstein AC, Spyker DA, Cantilena LR Jr, Green JL, Rumack BH, Giffin SL. (2010) 2009 annual report of the American association of poison control center's national poison data system (npds): 27th annual report. *Clin Toxicol (Phila)* **48**(10): 979–1178.

The Greig health record (2010). Canadian Paediatric Society. Available online at: http://www.cps.ca/english/statements/cp/preventivecare.htm (accessed February 5, 2011).

Web-based injury statistics and query and reporting system (wisqars) (2011). Centers for Disease Control and Prevention & National Center for Injury Prevention and Control. Available online at: http://www.cdc.gov/injury/wisqars/. (accessed February 5, 2011).

Grossman DC, Mueller BA, Riedy C, Dowd MD, Villaveces A, Prodzinski J, Nakagawara J, Howard J, Thiersch N, Harruff R. (2005) Gun storage practices and risk of youth suicide and unintentional firearm injuries. *JAMA,***293**(6): 707–714.

Hosking SG, Young KL, Regan MA. (2009) The effects of text messaging on young drivers. *Hum Factors* **51**(4): 582–592.

Fatality facts 2008: Teenagers. Insurance Institute for Highway Safety & Highway Loss Data Institute. Available online at: http://www.iihs.org/ research/fatality_facts_2008/teenagers.html. (accessed February 5, 2011).

Lenne MG, Dietze PM, Triggs TJ, Walmsley S, Murphy B, Redman JR. (2010) The effects of cannabis and alcohol on simulated arterial driving: Influences of driving experience and task demand. *Accid Anal Prev* **42**(3): 859–866.

Mytton J, Towner E, Brussoni M, Gray S. (2009) Unintentional injuries in school-aged children and adolescents: Lessons from a systematic review of cohort studies. *Inj Prev* **15**(2): 111–124.

Sleet DA, Ballesteros MF, Borse NN. (2010) A review of unintentional injuries in adolescents. *Annu Rev Public Health* **31**:195–212.

Weiss JC. (2006) The teen driver. *Pediatrics* **118**(6): 2570–2581.

Child and adolescent injury prevention: A global call to action (2005). World Health Organization. Available online at: http://whqlibdoc.who.int/publications/2005/9241593415_eng.pdf).

Zador PL, Krawchuk SA, Voas RB. (2000) Alcohol-related relative risk of driver fatalities and driver involvement in fatal crashes in relation to driver age and gender: An update using 1996 data. *J Stud Alcohol* **61**(3): 387–395.

Chapter 17

Rural and Remote Australian Adolescent Health Issues

Catherine Hawke

1. Introduction

Rural inequalities in health are experienced in many countries. The greater the distance from urban areas, the greater the burden of disease in the population as there are fewer services, and more dispersed populations, a higher price of goods along with lower income, education, literacy, and employment opportunities. Australia is an urbanised society with about 70% of the population living in capital or major cities. In 2005, 873,546 (32%) of 15–24 year olds lived outside major cities, 25,909 (0.9%) lived in very remote areas and over 50% of these were Indigenous young people. Thirty-nine percent of those living in remote areas have low socio–economic status compared to 24% of those in regional areas and 17% of those in major cities.

This chapter describes issues in Australian adolescent rural and remote health and some of the major determinants and inequalities of health experienced by adolescents living outside metropolitan areas. While country specific, many of the health issues described are similar to those in other countries which have large tracts of under-populated and physically inhospitable space.

In Australia, remote populations include a high proportion of Indigenous people whose burden of disease is greater than the non-Indigenous

193

population. There is also great diversity between rural communities; some rural populations have similar health outcomes to national standards while others fall well below, and the contribution of socio-economic and other health determinants in Australia to rural health outcomes often remains unclear. When clinicians see young people from rural and remote areas, knowledge of context and corroboration of that context is essential.

2. Individual Experiences — Growing Up in the Country

For primary school aged children, the country often provides more freedom and more opportunities to be physically active and play team sports. There are stronger community connections and many community members may be involved in the child's upbringing. Unlike much of urban life, a rural childhood may provide opportunities for greater vertical connectivity with adults of all ages. A situation with a balance in favour of advantage may shift rapidly to disadvantage during adolescence. The young person may have very limited privacy and is unable to blend into a larger crowd. Risk taking behaviour becomes public property. Young people are not exposed to cultural diversity as they would be in urban areas, and neither do they have access to youth sub-cultural experiences. Young people who are same sex attracted or who develop ideological views dissimilar to their families are at high risk of having no support to come to terms with their apparent difference.

3. The Importance of Climate Change

There is evidence that globally the number of weather related disasters has doubled over the last two decades. Adolescents and young people around the world nominate climate change and its effects as a major personal concern for their future. In Australia, a country with a highly variable climate, prolonged droughts, devastating bushfires, and destructive floods and cyclones are the weather events which impact most on rural populations. These natural disasters have long term financial, psychosocial, mental health, and community impacts. In an individual, prior disaster experience, including evacuation experiences and threat to the life of or separation from parents, and chronic anxiety may all increase the impact. These impacts can be worsened by the stereotyping of rural Australians as resilient and stoical.

4. Inequalities in the Determinants of Rural Adolescent Health

Adolescence in Australia is among the physically healthiest times of life, but in rural areas young people are more at risk of death, and the development of behaviours that put their future health at risk than their urban counterparts. This risk is even greater if the young person is Indigenous. The obstacles to health and well-being faced by many rural adolescents are different from those in urban areas. They face a unique combination of factors that create disparities in health outcomes: socio–economic factors, cultural and social differences, educational shortcomings, lack of youth-specific services, and gaps in services, the impact of natural disasters, poor access to transport (other than the car), and lack of anonymity, compounded by the isolation of living in some rural areas may all affect the adolescent's transition to healthy adult life.

4.1. *Education*

Learning and engagement in education is vital for the social and emotional development and well-being of adolescents and for their success at work and in the community as adults. Young people, especially boys living in rural and remote areas, are less likely to finish school than those in the cities. In Australia in 2008, final school year completion rates were 68% in metropolitan areas, 60% in rural areas, and just 51% in remote areas. Fewer students in remote areas met national benchmarks for reading, writing, and numeracy. Young people in rural and remote areas may think that education is less relevant to their life and careers than those in major cities and are less likely to know adults or other young people who have gone on to higher education. Many young people have to leave remote farms for secondary and tertiary education. They worry about the costs of their education, and the need for them to succeed in another career (particularly if the family's most successful business asset — the farm — may no longer be viable with climate change or other world economic conditions). Young people also worry about their parents' mental health, made worse by separation and the concern that their parents may be putting on a brave face. When they come home for holidays they may need to work physically hard and confront towns that are dying, so that vacations are no longer rejuvenating.

4.2. *Social Support*

Young people in remote areas may find it harder to build and maintain social networks, and young people in outer regional and very remote areas are less likely to have weekly contact with family and friends than those in major cities. Leaving home to continue their education may compound the situation. At a time when young people need to increase peer group interaction they may lose friendships both in the country and the city because they are never in one place for a long enough period of time.

4.3. *Transport*

Transport is a critical issue for young people in rural and remote areas. Non-existent public transport in all but medium sized towns make them dependent on lifts for any event other than school attendance until they are old enough to drive and/or able to afford a car. Their after-school activities, socialising, work experience, part time work, college attendance, and access to health care and hospitals are all affected by their lack of mobility.

4.4. *Health Services*

Rural and remote Australia has suffered from health professional workforce shortages for a long time. Provision varies across States and there has been some improvement in the number of doctors due to a lifting of restrictions of overseas trained doctors working in rural and remote areas. Forty-one percent of all doctors in rural and remote Australia are overseas trained. There is concern that these doctors are neither well supported professionally nor trained about Australian culture. Other concerns related to the rural health workforce are:

- The workforce is ageing, with newer graduates preferring to practise in better supported urban and regional areas.
- Limited choice of health professionals.

For a young person this may mean that they cannot choose a primary care doctor who is different to their own family doctor. This situation may discourage the disclosure or discussion of significant health concerns because of worry about confidentiality. Young people may choose not to seek help for mental health problems because of lack of privacy and the stigma of attendance when there is only one counsellor in town.

4.5. *Nutrition*

Young people in rural and remote areas and their family may have difficulty in eating a healthy diet because of the limited availability and high cost of fresh food items. Young people living in rural and regional areas are less likely to consume the recommended number of daily servings of fruit and vegetables than those in cities. The likelihood of inadequate fruit and vegetable intake increases with remoteness, as does the prevalence of overweight and obesity.

4.6. *Smoking, Alcohol and Other Drugs*

Smoking prevalence in Australia is inversely related to socio-economic status and to remoteness in young people over the age of 14 years. Twenty-five percent of young people in remote and very remote areas smoke, compared with 18% in metropolitan areas. Rates are even higher for Indigenous Australians. Alcohol and other drug use in adolescence increases the likelihood for reduced educational attainment, comorbid mental health disorders, substance abuse and dependence, criminality, and psychiatric disorders in adulthood. Risky and high risk drinking among 12–24 year olds increases with remoteness from 30% in major cities, to 37% in remote and very remote areas. Long term harm increases from 11% in major cities to 15% in remote and very remote areas. Alcohol use in rural youth is increasing at a higher rate than in the metropolitan areas and rural youth experience disproportionate harm because of their alcohol intake. The reasons behind this are unclear, as is knowledge about effective interventions to reduce this harm.

5. Other Inequalities in Rural Adolescents

5.1. *Life Expectancy*

Life expectancy of adolescents in Australia varies by geographical remoteness from urban areas. A 15 year old male living in remote or very remote areas has a life expectancy that is 3.7 years less than a 15 year old male from a highly accessible area. For females the difference is 2.5 years.

5.2. *Mortality Rates*

Mortality rates for young Australians aged between 15 and 25 years increase substantially with remoteness, with the rate for very remote areas almost five times that for major cities: 199 per 100,000 compared to 42 per 100,000. Mortality rates between young people living in major cities and very remote areas has widened in this age group over the last decade. The difference in the rates is due both to a decline in the death rate in major cities and an increase in very remote areas. Much of this health disadvantage is due to higher death rates of Indigenous young people. Factors that contribute to higher death rates outside of major cities include limited access to health services, occupational hazards, and the dangers associated with driving outside of major cities.

5.3. *Self Reported Health*

The more remotely a young person lives from urban areas the less likely they are to rate their health as very good or excellent compared with those in major cities or inner regional areas. Indigenous young people are likely to rate their health less well than non-Indigenous young people.

5.4. *Injury and Accidents*

5.4.1. *Injury*

Injury is the leading cause of death and a major cause of hospitalisation in Australian adolescents. Death rates and hospital separations increase with remoteness. Adolescents who live in very remote areas have an injury death rate greater than five times that of those who live in metropolitan areas: 145 per 100,000 versus 28 per 100,000. Injury mortality is about three times as high among Indigenous Australians, compared to the remainder of the population, even when controlling for remoteness.

5.4.2. *Traffic accidents*

Almost two-thirds of recorded road traffic fatalities are related to crashes on country roads. The majority of these crashes are on roads between country towns. In remote and very remote areas, the death rate from motor vehicle crash injuries is 1.7 times higher in Indigenous than non-Indigenous young people. However, the death rate in non-Indigenous young people in these areas is still twice that in major cities. The young driver fatality rate over the last decade has actually decreased significantly in urban areas. Factors related to death in rural traffic accidents are driver inexperience and risk-taking behaviours, such as speed and failure to use seat belts. The majority of deaths are male and there are often multiple young passengers in the same vehicle. While these scenarios are not unique to rural youth, high posted speed limits, long distances promoting fatigue and drink driving in areas where policing is limited make driving in rural regions potentially more hazardous.

5.4.3. *Violence and assault*

The health consequences that result from violence and assaults have higher rates outside the metropolitan area. Hospital separation rates for injuries due to assault among 15–24 year olds increase significantly with remoteness: 210 per 100,000 in major cities, 240 per 100,000 in regional areas, 706 per 100,000 in remote regions and 1,771 per 100,000 in very remote Australia. Similarly those living in regional and remote areas are more likely to report being the victim of physical or threatened violence than young people living in the city. Indigenous youth are over-represented in the juvenile justice system to a degree that is far greater than non-Indigenous youth for similar degrees of violence.

5.4.4. *Poisoning*

Hospitalisation from venom poisoning (spider, snake, and insects) is, not unexpectedly, higher in rural areas where there is greater exposure to risk. Less explicable is that hospitalisation rates for psychotropic drug poisoning are consistently greater in rural areas for both males and females. There is no reported variation of hospitalisation rates for poisoning from chemicals and analgesics between urban and other areas.

5.4.5. *Farm accidents*

Motor bicycles, particularly 'all terrain', other vehicles and dams pose the greatest risk of death on farms for rural adolescents. Males aged 15–19 years are the most at risk of serious injury on farms. Motorbike and horse riding are also the most common cause of serious farm injuries in younger adolescents aged between 10–14 years. Males are most likely to be injured on motorbikes, while the majority of those injured in horse riding are female. The rate of hospitalisation after farm injury increases with remoteness across both genders and age groups.

5.5. *Chronic Illness and Disability*

At least 15% of adolescents in Australia have a chronic physical illness or disability. There is little information on the prevalence of disability in rural young people, but they are disadvantaged by lack of services in rural areas. Services are dispersed and lack consistency as these often depend on short term funding which aggravates the problem of retaining staff. Urban paediatric services often provide multidisciplinary outreach clinics for rural adolescents. These terminate at school leaving age, and often there is no equivalent adult service available. This means that transition from paediatric to adult care is unsatisfactory and may result in deterioration in health status. Type 1 diabetes mellitus is a good example of this deficiency, where inadequate routine specialist care in youth results in the use of acute services for crisis management, and deterioration in diabetes control. Alternate methods of health care delivery such as teleconference and e-communication may have a role to play but will not take away the need for regular specialist consultation.

5.6. *Mental Illness*

Mental illness is the most prevalent burden of disease in young people. There is little known about the prevalence of mental illness among rural Australian adolescents. Depression and anxiety are the most prevalent disorders in adolescents and a number of aspects of rural life might be expected to increase this prevalence of mental health problems. The challenge is to provide appropriate services and support to meet the mental health needs of young people, particularly for early intervention in rural areas where the culture and characteristics of the communities may reduce willingness to access services. A culture of stoicism, issues around confidentiality and anonymity in rural areas where specialist services are limited, and potentially the social stigma of mental illness compound the problems of geographical distances and the lack of service provision.

Suicide is raised as a major health concern almost exclusively by rural adolescents when comparing health concerns between urban and rural young people. Suicide rates increase with remoteness, and 15–24 year old males in the country are nearly twice as likely to commit suicide when compared with those in the cities. The incidence of suicide may be up to six times higher in remote areas compared to urban rates. These figures may be underestimates; accidental deaths are high in rural areas and some of these may indeed have been intentional but not reported as such because of stigma and the lack of identification in Indigenous deaths. Mental health literacy is improving, especially in young rural males, but the impact of this on mental health outcomes is yet to be seen.

5.7. *Teenage Pregnancy*

Teenage births are more common among Indigenous Australians, and among mothers from remote areas. Limited access to family planning information and services may contribute to relatively high numbers of teenage births in rural communities. The Indigenous teenage birth rate in Australia is five times the non-Indigenous rate. The teenage birth rate increases with increasing remoteness, with teenage girls in remote and very remote areas being five times as likely to give birth as their peers in major cities (63 per 1,000 compared with 13 per 1,000). There is no significant difference in birth rates between those in the lowest and highest socio–economic status areas. Teenage pregnancy rates do not appear to be in decline, as these are in more accessible areas. Pregnant teenagers in remote areas smoke more cigarettes, and have worse birth outcomes and higher Caesarean rates than urban teenagers.

6. Conclusion

Inequalities and the deficits in rural and remote health are well described. Inequalities in the health of rural Australian adolescents are less researched and more information is required, not only to understand their needs but also to provide baseline data to monitor interventions. Health service providers must not only be able respond and communicate effectively with adolescents but also have an understanding of the complexity of rural practice. Improvement in health may not progress without a multidisciplinary approach and a comprehensive understanding not only of health but also the geographic, socio–economic, political, psychological, and environmental factors that lead to poor health in rural and remote adolescents.

References

Australian Institute of Health and Welfare. (2006) Rural, regional and remote health-mortality trends 1992–2003. AIHW cat. No. Phe 71(Rural Health series no. 7). Report for AIHW (Canberra).

Currie G, Gammie F, Waingold C, Paterson D, Vandersar D. (2005) Rural and regional young people and transport. Report for National Youth Affairs Research Scheme.

Dean JG, Stain HJ. (2010) Mental health impact for adolescents living with prolonged drought. *Aust J Rural Health* **18**(1): 32–37.

Liaw S-T, Kilpatrick S. (eds.) (2008) *A Textbook of Australian Rural Health,* Australian Rural Health Education Network Canberra.

Mathews RRS, Hall WD, Vos T, Patton GC, Degenhardt L. (2011) What are the major drivers of prevalent disability burden in young Australians? *Med J Aust* **194**(5): 232–235.

Morrissey SA, Reser JP. (2007) Natural disasters, climate change and mental health considerations for rural Australia. *Aust J Rural Health* **15**(2): 120–125.

Perry L, Steinbeck KS, Dunbabin JS, Lowe JM. (2010) Lost in transition? Access to and uptake of adult health services and outcomes for young people with Type 1 diabetes in regional New South Wales. *Med J Aust* **193**(8): 444–449.

Quine S, Bernard D, Booth M, Kang M, Usherwood T, Alperstein G, Bennett D. (2003) Health and access issues among Australian adolescents: A rural-urban comparison. Rural and Remote Health 3 (online) 245.

Roufeil L, Lipzker A. (2007) Psychology services in rural and remote Australia. In Psych: The Bulletin of the Australian Psychological Society Ltd [online], **29**(5): 8–11.

Smith KB, Humphreys JS, Wilson MGA. (2008) Addressing the health disadvantage of rural populations: How does epidemiological evidence inform rural health policies and research? *Aust J Rural Health* **16**(2): 56–66.

Chapter 18

Important Medical and Mental Health Issues for Incarcerated and Homeless Youth

Stephen Stathis, Lee Hudson and Andrew Kennedy

1. Introduction

There is a broad overlap in the medical and mental health needs of these most marginalised and disadvantaged young people, and similar challenges in providing health care and services for them. Incarcerated and homeless young people suffer from higher rates of medical and mental health problems. Both groups are characterised by complex needs requiring multidisciplinary input from a number of government and non-government services. These young people are frequently transient or itinerant and some fail to see their health needs as a priority. Continuity of care is challenging. Despite their significant needs, incarcerated and homeless youth are often not viewed as a high priority at governmental level. There are also divergent community views on the management of homeless and incarcerated youth, including the role of youth detention. *Addressing these young people's health needs or problems can seem futile as these sometimes appear insurmountable, but small changes can and often do make considerable differences in their lives.*

2. Incarcerated Youth

2.1. *Background*

In Australia, children younger than 10 years cannot be convicted of an offence. Generally, once a young person reaches 18 years, they enter the adult justice system. However in some states there is provision to keep 18 year olds in the youth justice system in certain circumstances. Similar age delineations exist internationally.

2.2. *International and National Guidelines*

The juvenile justice system should be seen to uphold the rights of young people and promote the physical and mental well-being of juveniles within its care. The quality of services provided to young people in custody is fundamental to realising this objective. There are a number of international treaties and consensus statements that promote the rights of young people in general, and incarcerated youths in particular. These include the Convention on the Rights of the Child, the United Nations Rules for the Protection of Juveniles Deprived of their Liberty, the United Nations Standard Minimum Rules for the Administration of Juvenile Justice (Beijing Rules) and the WHO Promoting the Health of Young People in Custody. The Australasian Juvenile Justice Administrators Standards for Juvenile Custodial Facilities have developed criteria that need to be met for the accreditation of youth detention centres. All these documents should form the cornerstone in developing evidence-based programs focused on the specific health needs of these young people.

2.3. *Demographics*

2.3.1. *Epidemiology and psychosocial adversity*

Adolescents held in youth detention rank amongst the most disadvantaged in the community, and share a number of vulnerabilities including chronic social, family or educational adversity, and a history of traumatic life events. High levels of overcrowded accommodation, poverty, unemployment, and violence are common. The majority suffer from mental health problems and substance abuse. Almost half have an IQ ≤79, 60% have experienced childhood abuse and/or trauma and 45% have a parent currently or previously in custody. The average age for leaving school is 14.4 years. Of those in detention, 79% have previously been in custody, with 50% having been incarcerated five or more times.

2.3.2. *High turnover*

Over one third of young people are detained in custody for less than a month and almost two thirds less than three months. High rates of short-term incarcerations are often counter-productive, as neither custodial nor community services can effectively manage a young person's medical or psychological needs as they repeatedly move between court, custodial centres, and the community.

2.3.2. *Recidivism*

Several factors contribute to recidivism, including a history of previous offences, substance abuse, social adversity, poverty, and abuse. The transition from adolescence to adulthood for marginalised youth in the justice system is extremely complex and often contributes to a repetitive cycle of crisis and crime. Toxic peer influences, dysfunctional environments, and lack of pro-social supports all contribute to re-offence and return to custody, and thus the cycle is repeated. Unfortunately, many young people entering the youth justice system subsequently enter the adult correctional system. Children of prisoners are more likely than children in the general community to commit offences that result in their own incarceration.

2.3.3. *Indigenous youth*

In many countries, including Australia, indigenous youth are over-represented in juvenile detention centres. Less than 5% of Australians aged 10–17 years identify as Indigenous, but Indigenous young people are 14 times more likely to be under supervision than their non-Indigenous peers.

2.4. *Health Needs*

Young people in the youth justice system suffer from high rates of medical, mental health and substance abuse problems, but many fail to take advantage of available health care in the community prior to their admission into detention. As a result, their health and substance misuse problems remain undiagnosed or inadequately treated. A custodial sentence is a limited window of opportunity if high quality youth health care services are available. However, complex medical and psychological histories, high turnover, limited collateral history, and difficulties establishing trust and rapport restrict the time available to complete a comprehensive medical, psychological, and substance use assessment or treatment plan. Traditional health screening and service provision both in detention and when back in the community simply may not work. A trans-disciplinary approach, which links health care between custodial and community services to education, employment, housing, and other related issues needs to be coordinated across government and non-government sectors. Given their high rates of reoffending, there should also be links with health and other services in the adult prison system.

2.4.1. *Health*

It is common for young people to rate their own health well and this is seen even in groups where it is known their health status is relatively poor, such as those in custody. Asthma, poor dental care, ear infections and hearing deficits, poor sleep hygiene, overweight and obesity, and injuries, particularly head injuries, are common.

2.4.2. *Mental health*

The majority of young people in youth detention suffer from some form of mental illness (community prevalence about 20%). Over 50% suffer from three or more mental disorders (excluding conduct disorder), which include depression, anxiety, ADHD, and symptoms of post-traumatic stress, and which reflect the long standing stresses of abuse and neglect.

2.4.3. *Abuse*

Young people in custody report high levels of past trauma, abuse, and neglect. Violent abuse is most frequently reported (36%) followed by emotional abuse (27%) and neglect (18%). When combined, almost half of young people (46%) report experiencing at least one of these types of abuse in their lifetime.

2.4.4. *Consequences of conduct disorder*

Childhood conduct disorder is strongly correlated to increased rates of criminal behaviour, medical problems and mental health disorders, suicide attempts, and substance abuse in both males and females. Prevention and early intervention programs have been demonstrated to reduce rates of conduct disordered behaviour in adolescents, but there is limited evidence that these programs can effectively be implemented for young people in custody.

2.4.5. *Substance use*

The link between substance abuse and offending behaviour is complex. Up to 90% of young people in custody report using substances at dangerous levels or having a substance dependency. Youth in detention begin using alcohol and drugs at an earlier age and more frequently than young people in the community, and up to 70% of juveniles state that they were under the influence of drugs at the time of their offence.

2.4.6. *Sexual health*

Detained youth have a high level of sexual activity (>90%), coupled with low age of sexual debut, low levels of contraception use and relatively high rates of chlamydia infection, especially in females, and of blood borne viruses such as hepatitis B and C. Screening for these infections must be part of the initial health assessment and treatment provided together with education around sexual health offered to all.

2.5. *Recommendations for Achieving 'Best Practice'*
for Health Care Needs

System of care: This should be integrated, comprehensive, and uniform.

Health professionals: health professionals who work in detention centres need to understand adolescent development and common health issues in the age group particularly in such a high-risk population.

Indigenous youth: there is emerging evidence that indigenous health workers contribute to the health care needs of indigenous young people by reducing barriers to accessing mental health and substance abuse services, by the engagement and maintainence of youth in treatment services, and acting as a 'cultural broker'.

Health assessment and referral pathways: general and mental health screening should be offered to all new detainees as soon as possible after admission into custody. Attendance at mental health and substance abuse services should be voluntary. Detention centres should have access to paediatric/adolescent medical and psychiatric services as well as on-call back up. There should be clear pathways linking these services to youth justice and health care services in the community.

Assessment of suicide: young people in custody have a number of factors that put them at an increased risk for suicide. Detention centres require processes to rapidly identify youth who are at an acute risk of self-harming or suicidal behaviours in order to develop strategies to ensure their safety.

Substance abuse: psycho-education about drug and alcohol use should be offered to all youth in detention. Those young people who abuse substances should be offered individual and group counselling while in detention. Detention centre staff should be educated about symptoms of drug withdrawal (Chapter 15).

Opportunistic intervention: the immunisation status of individuals can usually be tracked via state or national databases and catch up and/or routine immunisations must be offered to all detainees. Oral hygiene is often poor. Commonly detainees, who regard some aspects of their health as unimportant, worry about their teeth and are keen for dental care when in custody. The majority of youth in detention who abuse substances are pre-contemplative about changing their substance use. However, time in detention does provide an opportunity to impart psycho-education to young people about the risks of substance use.

Potential role for screening: validated screening tools not only give a measured indicator for the level of unmet need, but also reduce the risk of under-diagnosing mental disorders in a setting where distress is to some degree omnipresent. The Massachusetts Youth Screening Instrument Version 2 (MAYSI-2) is commonly used in the United States. Given the very high levels of mental health and substance abuse disorders in this population, screening tools that identify resilient and protective factors might be of more practical use.

Follow-up on release: an expectation of sustainable change is unreasonable unless the real gaps in community services for marginalised adolescents are addressed. It is important that young people are not lost to follow-up on release back into the community. Attention needs to be given to barriers in the community, such as the lack of suitable services and the limited availability of other community facilities that hamper young people from engaging with community interventions and supports.

The need for an adolescent forensic evidence base: there now exists a strong evidence base for the treatment of those adolescent mental health problems commonly suffered by young people in youth detention. However, this evidence base is almost exclusively obtained from community samples and incarcerated young people are the very ones that are excluded from the majority of studies. A separate evidence base, specific to adolescent forensic mental health, is therefore needed to assist the clinician working within the youth justice context.

3. Homeless Youth

3.1. *Definition and Demographics*

Defining homelessness is complex, but it can be broadly defined as an absence of a permanent residential abode which adequately meets an individual's basic social and health needs. Homelessness is much more than the popular image of sleeping roughly on the streets (primary homelessness) and includes those living transiently in temporary locations such as hostels (secondary homelessness), as well as those living in make-shift or shanty accommodation. There also exist acute and chronic states of homelessness.

The size of the problem of homelessness is always underestimated, because of difficulties reaching this section of the community. The 2006 Australian Bureau of Statistics Census reported that 21,940 young people aged from 12–18 were homeless, representing approximately 20% of all homeless individuals in Australia. In the US, around 1.6 million people are believed to use sheltered accommodation or transitional housing per year, 20% of them being under 18 years. Prevalence of homelessness is higher in the developing world, but reliable statistics are lacking and definitions vary from country to country.

3.2. *Health Needs*

The health needs of young people who are homeless are thought to be substantial although accurate research is limited in this difficult to reach group who are less likely to seek healthcare. Transience is common making follow-up difficult. The limited data available reveal a similar health burden as for youth in custody with the main issues being general health and nutrition, high levels of mental illness, substance use, and sexual and reproductive health issues.

3.3. *Seeing Young People in Context: Barriers to Health Care for Young People with Homelessness*

Unfortunately, a number of popular misconceptions about people who are homeless exist, including the idea that people with homelessness have made an active decision to 'drop-out' from regular society or refuse to work. In reality, factors leading to homelessness are many and varied.

These factors include a background of child abuse and neglect, mental illness and learning difficulties with low levels of educational attainment, chronic illness, lack of social capital and affordable housing, and personal debt, relationship failure, and unemployment.

Misconceptions increase the barrier between young people who are homeless and the health care services that exist to help them, especially when those providing such services share those popular misconceptions. By the time they seek health care, young people with homelessness may well have had more than one negative experience with people older than they, leading to understandable fear and suspicion of those in authority and those providing health care. Coexisting mental health problems or learning difficulties can also compound difficulties in accessing health care.

Where health care services generally require an upfront financial payment for care, patient access will be severely curtailed for young people with homelessness. Measures to provide free services for such patient groups can help alleviate this problem, but are in turn vulnerable to times of national economic hardship.

3.4. *Type of Health Care Interaction*

Health care interaction with a homeless young person can include encounters within hospital emergency departments, sexual health clinics, and specific clinics for homeless people. Thus training regarding particular issues required in caring for young people and adults with homelessness is important for all health care providers. While the provision of services within inner cities is more likely to provide for a greater number of young people, a large number of young people with homelessness live in rural areas and provision of services in these areas is important. Mobile health services are effective ways to reach a large number of young people and may be seen by young people as better services to visit compared to static, sometimes stigmatised public locations. Mobile services often provide only a basic and infrequent level of care due to limited resources.

The nature of health care interactions also varies, with most being once only due to the transient and chaotic lifestyle of many young people with homelessness. These young people are more likely to seek health care during crisis periods, viewing health as less of a priority during less critical times. With efforts from health care staff, it may be possible to facilitate more frequent interactions allowing approaches aimed at more regular treatment of chronic illnesses such as asthma and mental health problems. To maximise the chances that this will occur, some core and generic principles must be applied.

3.5. *Core Principles for Health Care Providers Caring for Homeless Young People*

The young person's circumstances and background are likely to be quite alien to the health care provider. Training in caring for young people with homelessness is often limited, and experience lacking. However, health care providers frequently possess a number of generic skills which can be applied to this patient group, and the principles are really no different from those relevant to caring for any young person. Working with such patient groups, with patience and persistence, is very rewarding. *The following seven core principles are central to effective care for young people with homelessness.*

Listen: at a first visit or interaction, the health care provider may be surprised by the absence of an obvious presenting medical complaint. Young people who are homeless do not often encounter people who will listen to them or care about their health, and so they may wish to spend a significant amount of time just talking. This in itself is of therapeutic value, leads to the establishment of rapport, and with time to revelations regarding health and social problems. It also increases the likelihood of re-attendance.

Avoid becoming frustrated: not being able to solve all of the young person's issues can be uncomfortable and frustrating. Dealing with what may seem to the health care provider as a small, relatively insignificant issue may in fact be huge to the young person, especially if they themselves have brought it up or acknowledged it as a problem.

Be non-judgemental: as with any adolescent patient, this is an important attitude which increases rapport, engagement, and re-attendance.

Apply opportunistic health care: opportunism is not simple and requires considerable thought and thorough consideration of the multiple problems within the young person's life. Such approaches can also reduce the burden on other members of the community, for example sexual health screening for chlamydia, and providing hepatitis B vaccinations.

Encourage re-attendance: application of the above principles will go a long way to achieve this, and will broaden the health care service from opportunistic screening alone. This may just be returning to review results performed at the first encounter, but will preferably be more regular and include regular provision of medications for chronic illness.

Rethink follow-up and after care: pragmatic approaches in assisting young people to continue to engage are important in this population group. Holding onto medications for young people and providing them as they are needed is one example. Attendance with a young person to a hospital appointment is another way. Communication between individuals involved is essential.

Think laterally: if the young person attends with a medical problem, is there an underlying psychosocial problem also at play? A laceration may be easily fixed with suturing, but did it happen in the first place because the young person is a victim of abuse, or is the young person self-harming? Assisting engagement with other services is another key example of lateral thinking for this age group.

3.6. *The Initial Assessment*

3.6.1. *History*

First, identify the young person's agenda and then spend time engaging and interacting on general topics. The HEADSS assessment (Chapter 5) may be useful. This will help identify where the young person has been living, and what are their social needs. Be aware that their expectations may be very low. This will include questions about their involvement with social services, and other supporting agencies. Specifically enquire about fever, cough and smoking, and nutrition and body weight. Determine if there has been recent trauma, particularly a head injury. Ask about drug and alcohol use, sexual encounters and protection, and symptoms of sexually transmitted infection. Pregnancy should be considered and a vaccination history sought where possible.

3.6.2. *Examination*

This should be focused, especially at the first visit. Measure height and weight and determine body mass index, and check for signs of malnutrition and poor dentition. Look for signs of head injury or other trauma. If there are signs of head trauma or if faints or fits have been revealed in the history, check for any neurological deficit. Skin infections are common and pay particular attention to digits and peri-orbital skin. A respiratory examination for pneumonia or tuberculosis is essential, as is palpation for enlarged lymph nodes which may indicate an infective site.

3.6.3. *Investigations*

These must all be appropriately consented. Testing may include hepatitis B and C serology (and HIV serology if appropriate), iron studies if poor nutrition (especially in young women), pregnancy testing, urine for chlamydia PCR, and a chest X-ray in those with chronic chest symptoms, especially if associated with weight loss.

3.7. *Specific Health Care Problems*

3.7.1. *Skin infections and infestations*

Skin complaints such as pruritus, infection and infestations, and trauma are the most common reasons for homeless young people to seek health care. Special consideration should be given to the causative agent of infection in homeless populations. Infections such as MRSA and Bartonella Quintana, less common in the general community, are more prevalent in the homeless. These may be suggested by failure to respond to initial antibiotic therapy. Swabs of lesions and nasal swabs are useful in identifying causative lesions, but are unhelpful at the time of presentation when empirical treatment decisions must be made. Knowledge of local bacterial sensitivities can be helpful in making initial antibacterial decisions. Adherence with antibiotics, especially completion of entire courses, can be problematic. Storing dispensed antibiotics for young people at centres supporting them and allowing daily visits for medications can be useful and also allows for regular review. Alternatively, for young people where transience is most likely to be an issue, intramuscular administration may be preferential, such as benzylpenicillin. Homeless young people, especially those with malnutrition, are more likely to suffer from pressure sores, as well as systemic illness and septicaemia. Consideration of hospital admission is important, particularly if adherence is likely to be an issue. In all cases, clear discussion with the young person about their understanding and requirements is essential. As well as treating infections, attention and support should be made where possible to attend to hygiene. Provision of showers and soap can be important preventative measures, as well as assisting the recovery of acute infections. In the case of infestations, efforts must be made to liaise and treat those in shared accommodation who may contract the infestation too — this needs to be handled with much sensitivity to avoid stigmatisation of the young person, including unfortunately, by those managing accommodation.

3.7.2. *Trauma*

Presentations with trauma can range from physical and sexual assault, accidental injury and self harm, and present as burns, fractures, and lacerations. Special consideration should be given to pain relief and prevention of infection, including ensuring recent tetanus vaccination. Management of young people with significant head injuries, such as large haematomas or history of loss of consciousness or seizure, can be difficult, especially if there is a need to rely on a prompt return for medical review if their condition deteriorates. A low threshold for CT imaging should be applied, with regular check-ups if possible. Referral to local specialist services such as emergency departments is important and most health care staff working in emergency departments will be well accustomed to treating young people with such injuries. Considering safeguarding or coexisting mental health problems is important, as it is for any young person presenting with an injury. When departments and staff are busy there is a temptation for these aspects of care to be overlooked. An attendance at an emergency department by a young person may be one of a few opportunities to identify social and mental health needs.

3.7.3. *Nutrition*

Poor nutrition and food insecurity are common problems, as are under-weight and overweight. Overweight results from cheap, high fat food on the streets, as well as reduced exercise and the use of anti-psychotics. Micronutrient deficiency can occur, especially iron deficiency in menstruating young women. Measuring iron levels and providing regular iron replacement should be considered. Direction to local services providing food support is an important role that health professionals can play.

3.7.4. *Dental*

Poor dentition can be a major cause of pain and infection affecting quality of life. Dental abscesses can provide a focus for spread of infection. Poor opportunity for self care, reduced access to dental professionals and poor nutrition all contribute to this problem. Ideally, local services dealing with homeless young people can involve a local dentist to help with dental care, as well as providing education, hygiene advice and dental care products.

3.7.5. *Mental health*

The interaction of mental health and homelessness is complex, both contributing to each other. Young people with mental health problems will have higher morbidity and mortality. The range of mental health problems can be huge, from depression to psychosis as well as personality disordered behaviour. The risk of young people to themselves and others is a key consideration when formulating appropriate management and referral and where the normal requirements for a place of safety and supervision are often lacking. Involvement of a mental health professional is essential for complex cases.

3.7.6. *Alcohol and other drugs*

Like mental health, drug and alcohol problems and homelessness have a complex interaction upon each other. Drug and alcohol problems contribute to poor financial situations, involvement in crime, personal neglect and trauma, as well as mental health problems. Harm minimisation strategies can also be discussed and needle exchange centres can be offered. Testing for blood borne viruses may also be appropriate.

3.7.7. *Respiratory health*

Asthma is common in all young people, and living from place to place, especially on the streets can be key triggers for exacerbations from the cold, pollutants, and infection. Respiratory infections are also problematic, with a higher incidence of infection with respiratory viruses, and vaccination is important in this patient group, as is a low threshold for referral to secondary care and hospital admission to monitor deterioration. Tuberculosis is also more common in this patient group and symptoms should be actively sought with referral to a specialist mandatory, both for the young person themselves and from a public health perspective. Smoking may exacerbate respiratory illness and efforts to help young people cut-down on or quit smoking can have significant impacts on general and respiratory health.

3.7.8. *Sexual health and pregnancy*

Health professionals working with homeless young people can have a significant impact on the sexual health and behaviours of young people, but it requires appropriate training. There should be no assumptions made about sexual identity and orientation. Sensitivity, confidentiality, and a non-judgemental approach are essential. Screen for and treat chlamydia. Screen for and vaccinate for hepatitis B. Early referral to specialist care for treatment of hepatitis improves morbidity and mortality. The provision of free contraception to both sexes and the identification of a local sexual health clinic, family planning clinic, or general practitioner who can accept referrals is required. The provision of emergency contraception and early diagnosis of pregnancy are also important, as is the identification and support of those who have been raped. Pregnancy care requires obstetric staff with an interest and experience in this patient group. Standard pre- and early-pregnancy screening, provision of vitamin supplementation (including folate), the monitoring of foetal health, education about alcohol and other drug use and finding an appropriate place to deliver are all necessary.

3.7.9. *Safeguarding and child protection*

This is one of the most complex aspects of caring for young people with homelessness, not least because of a number of areas of safeguarding: mental health, non-intentional injury, and sexual abuse, can all lead to homelessness. A professional's mandatory responsibility of notification to safeguard the young person should over-ride any other considerations. Professional support in this area is essential, and the health professional who discovers areas of potential safe-guarding should discuss and consult widely amongst colleagues, with careful and thorough documentation.

References

Abram KM, Teplin LA, Charles DR, Longworth SL, Mcclelland GM, Dulcan MK. (2004) Posttraumatic stress disorder and trauma in youth in juvenile detention. *Arch Gen Psychiatry* **61**(4): 403–410.

Standards for juvenile justice facilities, Australia (1999). Australasian Juvenile Justice Administrators. Available online at: http://www.djj.nsw.gov.au/pdf_htm/publications/general/Finalstandards.pdf 2011.

Cantor C, Neulinger K. (2000) The epidemiology of suicide and attempted suicide among young Australians. *Aust N Z J Psychiatry* **34**(3): 370–387.

Carlson JL, Sugano E, Millstein SG, Auerswald CL. (2006) Service utilization and the life cycle of youth homelessness. *J Adolesc Health* **38**(5): 624–627.

Golzari M, Hunt SJ, Anoshiravani A. (2006) The health status of youth in juvenile detention facilities. *J Adolesc Health* **38**(6): 776–782.

Hyde J. (2005) From home to street: Understanding young people's transitions into homelessness. *J Adolesc* **28**(2): 171–183.

Littell JH, Campbell M, Green S, Toews B. (1996) Multisystemic therapy for social, emotional, and behavioral problems in youth aged 10–17. *Cochrane Database of Syst Rev*. CD004797, John Wiley & Sons Ltd.

Putnin AL. (2005) Assessing recidivism risk among young offenders. *Aust N Z J Criminol* **38**(3): 324–339.

Raoult D, Foucault C, Brouqui P. (2001) Infections in the homeless. *Lancet Infect Dis* **1**(2): 77–84.

Sawyer MG, Guidolin M, Schulz KL, Mcginnes B, Zubrick SR, Baghurst PA. (2010) The mental health and wellbeing of adolescents on remand in Australia. *Aust N Z J Psychiatry* **44**(6): 551–559.

Tarasuk V, Dachner N, Li J. (2005) Homeless youth in Toronto are nutritionally vulnerable. *J Nutr* **135**(8): 1926–1933.

Van Den Bree MBM, Shelton K, Bonner A, Moss S, Thomas H, Taylor PJ. (2009) A longitudinal population-based study of factors in adolescence predicting homelessness in young adulthood. *J Adolesc Health* **45**(6): 571–578.

Chapter 19

The Dying Adolescent

Michael Stevens, Julie Dunsmore and John Collins

'Please see me, hear me, talk, laugh and cry with me... and maybe remember me.' (16 year old speaking on what she wanted from her doctors in the weeks before her death).

1. Introduction

This chapter seeks to provide guidance, support, and encouragement to physicians and other health carers who find themselves in the challenging situation of caring for a dying adolescent.

There are many successful styles of working with such patients and there are challenges involved in caring for young people who are dying or who have a serious medical condition for which the long term outlook is poor. However, opportunities to be involved in such care should be welcomed rather than avoided.

2. Definition of Palliative Care

Palliative care has been defined by the WHO as 'the active total care of patients whose disease is not responsive to curative treatment'. Control of pain, of other symptoms and addressing psychological, social and spiritual problems, are paramount. Palliative care is the achievement of the best quality of life for patients and their families. Palliative Care Australia expands the WHO definition, adding that palliative care:

- Provides relief from pain and other distressing symptoms.
- Affirms life and regards dying as a normal process.
- Intends neither to hasten nor postpone death.
- Integrates the psychological and spiritual aspects of patient care.
- Offers a support system to help patients live as actively as possible until death.
- Offers a support system to help the family cope during the patient's illness and in their own bereavement.
- Uses a team approach to address the needs of patients and their families, including bereavement counselling, if indicated.
- Will enhance quality of life, and may also positively influence the course of illness.
- Is applicable early in the course of illness, occurs in conjunction with other therapies that are intended to prolong life, such as chemotherapy or radiation therapy, and includes those investigations needed to better understand and manage distressing clinical complications.

2.1. *The Nature of Palliative Care in Young People*

A position paper from the United Kingdom first published in 1997 by the Royal College of Paediatrics and Child Health and the Association for Children's Palliative Care, defines palliative care as: 'an active and total approach to the care of children, embracing physical, emotional, social, and spiritual elements'. Four groups of life-limiting conditions in which young people might need palliative care were defined.

Group 1: life-threatening conditions for which curative treatment may be feasible but may fail. Palliative care may be necessary during periods of prognostic uncertainty and when treatment fails, for example cancer and cardiac anomalies.

Group 2: conditions in which there may be long periods of intensive treatment aimed at prolonging life and still allowing participation in many normal childhood activities, but premature death is still possible, for example cystic fibrosis and muscular dystrophy.

Group 3: progressive conditions without curative treatment options, in which treatment is exclusively palliative and may commonly extend over many years, for example the mucopolysaccharidoses.

Group 4: conditions with severe neurological disability which may cause weakness and susceptibility to health complications, and may deteriorate unpredictably, but which are not considered progressive, for example severe cerebral palsy.

3. Towards Effective Communication with Adolescents

Effective communication underpins successful intervention in seriously ill or dying adolescents.

3.1. *How Adolescents Think*

At times of increased arousal, including anxiety, fear, and pain, a young person may regress to earlier patterns of behaviour, and temporarily disconnect from being able to see the long-term implications of decisions or actions. Anger or silence may be ways of masking fear, and however unsatisfactory, as ways of regaining power in a situation where power and control may be rapidly evaporating.

Adolescents tend to think in absolutes, and may not initially understand that treatment in some cases may be a trial and error process with a need for constant review. One should be careful when declaring how long a planned treatment will last. Promises of outcomes that may not be deliverable should be avoided. Providing opportunities on a regular basis to talk through treatment plans and the likely effects of treatment is important to the establishment of trust, and can reduce anxiety about the 'what ifs'.

3.2. *What Helps*

Effective communication is interactive, with provision of ample opportunities for questions and feedback. Always continue to ascertain the adolescent's understanding of information provided. Adolescents may not ask questions or go back over information that has been given because the content is unavoidably confronting, or for fear of being seen as stupid. Information should be conveyed in plain language, and honestly.

3.3. *What May Not Help*

An impersonal or detached manner, avoidance of eye contact, excessive use of medical jargon, not providing time for one-to-one discussions, or appearing uncomfortable about spending time with the patient all work against the development of establishing a sound professional relationship with the patient.

4. Control of Symptoms as the First Step to Effective Palliative Care

4.1. *Managing Pain*

Pain may be caused by progression of the underlying disease, by unwanted and cumulative side-effects of toxic therapies, by some medical procedures, or by combinations of all of these. Pain is always influenced by cognitive and emotional factors, and these factors must be included when assessing pain. Important principles of pain control include use of the appropriate analgesic, regular reassessment of pain, management of opioid side-effects, non-pharmacological methods as deemed helpful, and psychosocial and spiritual support to ameliorate the patient's emotional and existential distress.

Pain management should follow guidelines produced by the WHO, in combination with individual knowledge of the patient and his or her family. Use of non-opioid analgesics, opioid analgesics, and adjuvant analgesics should be based on the WHO analgesic ladder which emphasises pain intensity rather than aetiologic factors as the guide to choice of analgesic. It is important that the young person be an active partner in plans for pain management. For example, if the pain medication causes unwanted sedation, the young person may elect to defer the next dose until after visiting hours. Concerns that pain management may shorten life or cause addiction should be listened for, and addressed.

4.2. *Managing Other Distressing Symptoms*

The most commonly reported symptoms are lack of energy, pain, drowsiness, nausea, cough, lack of appetite, and psychological symptoms such as feeling sad, nervous, or irritable, or worrying about what will it be like to die. Such symptoms cause high distress in more than one-third of patients. Effective symptom management in young people under palliative care will be assisted by the ongoing development and validation of instruments to measure and assess the intensity of symptoms and the effects of interventions aimed at controlling these.

5. Implications of Life Threatening Illnesses for Early, Middle and Late Adolescence

These developmental stages are described fully in Chapter 3. Age-related differences between these stages may be evident in the effects of a life-threatening illness.

5.1. *Early Adolescence*

Younger adolescents often have concerns about how their physical appearance is affected and about the effects of their illness on their mobility. Privacy can be all-important. Protection rackets (the parent protecting the young person, and the young person protecting the parent) are common in this age group; hence the need is to find out how they would like issues and treatment plans discussed, and whom to involve.

5.2. *Middle Adolescence*

At this stage adolescents may have significant concerns about being attractive to peers. Illness can adversely affect social standing within peer groups. The middle adolescent's sense of invincibility is high, and the threat of death is often denied — 'It won't happen to me' — which may lead to significant non-compliance with treatment. Issues related to control may be more prevalent.

5.3. *Late Adolescence*

Older adolescents and young adults most often focus on how their illness is a threat to their social, emotional, and economic future. It can interfere with the formation of intimate relationships, and older adolescents and young adults frequently raise concerns about future dependency on parents or spouses. Reproductive and sexual intimacy issues frequently need to be addressed. Older adolescents will often identify goals that they wish to achieve, so that flexibility with treatment and care choices becomes an important consideration in end of life care planning.

6. Losses Mourned by Adolescents with Terminal Conditions

Not all of the losses mourned are directly related to the process of having a chronic or debilitating illness.

6.1. *Health*

Young people describe losing a perception by others that they are healthy, independent, in control, and not unreasonably vulnerable to physical harm or emotional upset, and instead, being perceived as precious, or even more difficult, as someone to be avoided.

6.2. *Pre-Diagnosis Person*

Adolescents grieve for their former healthy selves, because they can no longer live in the style they had previously. The emotional and social changes challenge their view of who they are.

6.3. *Pre-Diagnosis Family*

Life in the family is no longer the way it used to be. There is often a plea for life to return to the way it was. Roles within the family may change, and expectations of how different family members respond to a crisis may be challenged.

6.4. *Body Image*

Both the illness and the side-effects of treatment cruelly alter the young person's body image, especially through changes in appearance and prowess.

6.5. *Independence and Relationships with Parents*

All the implications of being seriously ill compel the young person to become dependent again on parents and other authority figures. Young people may describe a sense of abandonment when parents leave them in hospital. Many young people confide how important their relationship with their parents is in reducing their anxiety about 'what next'? They feel that their parents will advocate for them and help keep them safe.

6.6. *Relationships with Siblings*

Siblings may express a wish to take the place of their brother or sister who is dying, wanting to stop their ill sibling's pain, and sometimes feeling that their death would be easier for the family to deal with. Siblings of ill adolescents may also experience feelings of hostility and guilt. They may be resentful or even angry because of all the attention given to their brother or sister. There may be guilt because of an irrational conviction that they have caused the illness, helplessness because of not being able to make things right, and possibly an obligation to make up to the parents later for the loss of the deceased sibling. Siblings are often overlooked or not included in family discussions about treatment and palliative care. Such exclusion may have significant effects on their future emotional and social health.

6.7. *Relationships with Girlfriends/Boyfriends*

Ill adolescents frequently prefer to break off friendships rather than risk causing their friends embarrassment or pain, or risk being abandoned.

The terminally ill young person may choose to break off a relationship to try to protect the partner from the pain of separation occasioned by death. They may fear that someone may stay with them only because of pity. Sometimes special friendships are not valued or even acknowledged by their own family. A hierarchy of grief may exist where one person, or the family, is considered to have the most rights to contact with the young person who is dying. Discussion with the young person who is facing death, about their wish to have visits, or under what circumstances, is an important part of care planning.

6.8. *School Life*

Young people report feeling upset by missing out on day-to-day life at school. Concern about dropping behind in schoolwork and missing out on rites of passage such as the school play, school formal, and graduation may cause distress. The care plan can provide an opportunity to do some innovative problem solving with a young person around some of these anxieties, and improve his or her sense of mastery.

6.9. *Uncertainty About the Future*

Terminally ill adolescents mourn the loss of the future as well as of the past. They may fear becoming a burden to their parents, and worry about their parents' well-being after they have died. Seriously ill young people describe being left in a limbo of uncertainty about long-term survival, often for many years after diagnosis and commencement of therapy. Acknowledgement of this reality by family, friends, or partner may help lessen anxiety in the young person, and help prevent feelings of having no capacity to reach or even recognise potential in his/her life.

6.10. *Hope*

Young people who have been told that they soon may die frequently report that others start to treat them as if they were already dead. Hope is an essential ingredient for living successfully. Their hopes may not necessarily be for a cure or magical recovery, but more often for joy and success with the challenges of living, and being remembered after their death. It is important to focus not on what one can no longer do, but rather, on what one can do.

7. Provision of Bad News

Most adolescents living with a life-threatening illness describe their willingness to confront the illness directly. An overwhelming majority categorically state that they would want to be informed of adverse events in their management, and most importantly, if they were dying. When asked whom they would prefer to provide them with bad news, about half say that it should be the doctor, about a third say their parents and their doctor together, and a minority their parents alone. Adolescents often comment on whether they think the news meant anything to the caregiver who provided it.

8. Avoiding Collusion

As the young person's condition deteriorates, it becomes more challenging for the physician to maintain good and frank communication with the patient because of the concern that sharing bad news with their patient will erode already depleted stores of hope. It becomes easier to report to the parents or the patient's partner, and leave the responsibility with them for passing the information on to the patient. A process may develop in which mutual agreement is reached to edit or even withhold significant information from the patient. Such collusion is inappropriate and ultimately damaging to all involved. Strive to keep channels of communication with the patient open, and preserve the young person's trust.

9. End-of-Life Care Planning — Finding the Right Words: from DNR to AND

As the death of the young person draws closer, health carers will be required to assist the family in making important decisions about end-of-life care. One of the authors (JC) has been instrumental in a collaborative project with local services to improve communication about end-of-life choices by changing the language used, the process for documentation, options for support at home and the role of paramedics in end-of-life care. The term 'Do Not Resuscitate' (DNR) has been changed to 'Allow a Natural Death' (AND), in end-of-life decision-making discussions. Supportive phrases such as 'continuing care' have been included. These changes permit a positive rather than negative approach when determining the level of support sought by the patient and family for the natural dying process. *The form to document discussions held with families about end-of-life care and allowing AND is available on application to the authors.*

10. Caring for the Young Person's Family, Friends, Partner, and Oneself

The death of a teenager or young adult is perceived as highly unnatural, and also highly threatening. Bereavement following the young person's death may be prolonged. Unfortunately there is a perception in our society that such a death is best quickly forgotten, and that there must be something wrong with a person who fails to achieve this. These attitudes will only cause added difficulty for those mourning the deceased young person. Criticism by family members about the way a person grieves or deals with his or her loss adversely affects recovery, and may lead to the development of complex mental health disorders.

The health professional needs to remember that caring for oneself is also important. Feelings of helplessness and frustration when faced with the tragedy of a young person's imminent death are not uncommon. Certain patients may trigger memories of losses and times of helplessness in the professional's own life. Strong bonds may be formed with patients and their loved ones. Dealing with life and death on a daily basis may take its toll if strategies are not actively put into place. Acknowledgement of the challenges that health professionals face in their work with a dying adolescent is the first step towards dealing with the effects of work. Techniques to assist with winding down psychologically at a working day's end and leaving work at work, support from significant individuals and regular opportunities for rest and recreation, will all assist. Sometimes acknowledgement of the effects of a particular young person on the professional becomes very important. What we do with the deceased young person's legacy has important ramifications for how we deal with the realities of working in this field. This may mean taking time to honour the deceased young person by attending the funeral or by taking some quiet time to acknowledge the death and the human connection that had been made.

It is also important to acknowledge times when antagonism towards the patient may be experienced, when the young person's frustration spills over into what may be seen as demanding behaviour, rage about what is happening, and issuing of blame because he or she cannot be cured. Difficulties may have arisen during the final phase of the young person's illness because of differing views about treatment strategies and management within the team. Such reactions are not uncommon. Ideally such disagreements should be discussed and resolved if possible earlier in the patient's management. Concerns about issues such as these should be addressed by discussing them with a trusted colleague, or by seeking out a mentor.

11. Caring for the Dying Adolescent — 10 Key Points

1. Remember the four Cs: *connect, communicate, care, consent.* Strive to maintain effective communication with the young person throughout his or her illness. Humour and honesty both allow for more trusting and open communication.
2. You cannot do it all. *Embrace a team approach* to management.
3. Recognise that the *young person has a right to participate* in decisions about his or her treatment and care.
4. Consider the young person's symptoms in both the physical domain and the *broader psychosocial and existential/spiritual* domains.
5. Young people *have many and varied aspects of their lives* and personalities that give them their identity. For example some still see themselves as school or college students, even if they have had to discontinue study. Acknowledge this.
6. *Promote resilience.* Three factors known to promote resilience in adolescents can be incorporated into care. First, connection to family: makes it easier for family and friends to visit and support them.

Secondly, connection to peers and community: advocate for flexible visiting opportunities with peers and support the young person's access to social media, the internet and mobile phones. Thirdly, a sense of contributing and being valued: what are they good at and what gives them joy?

7. *Is the setting of care appropriate?* There may not be an age-appropriate shared hospital room available, but a photo board and other belongings around the young person may be helpful. Be open to the option of the young person dying somewhere other than in hospital.
8. *Protect the young person's dignity and privacy.*
9. *Reaching agreement about being permitted to die a natural death* is preferable to reaching agreement about not being resuscitated.
10. Be *willing to advocate* on behalf of the dying young person: he or she may be counting on you to do this for them.

References

Baum D, Curtis H, Elson S *et al.* (1997) *A guide to the development of children's palliative care services.* 1st ed. ACT/RCPCH, Bristol.

Bisset M, Hutton S, Kelly D. (2008) Palliation and end of life care issues. In: Kelly D, Gibson F (eds.), *Cancer care for adolescents and young adults*, pp. 192–213. Blackwell Publishing Ltd, Carlton.

Collins JJ. (2010) Paediatric palliative medicine: Symptom control in life-threatening illness in children. In: Hanks G, Cherny NI, Christakis NA, Fallon M, Kaasa S, Portenoy RK (eds.), *Oxford textbook of palliative medicine 4th ed*, pp. 1337–1350. Oxford University Press, Oxford.

Collins JJ, Stevens MM, Berde CB. (2008) Pediatric cancer pain. In: Sykes N, Bennett MI, Yuan CS (eds.), *Clinical pain management 2nd ed*, pp. 345–358. Hodder Arnold, London.

Dunsmore J, Quine S. (1996) Information, support, and decision-making needs and preferences of adolescents with cancer. *J Psychosoc Oncol* **13**(4): 39–56.

Hain R. (2005) Whose dying is it anyway? Palliative care in adolescence. In: Eden TOB, Barr RD, Bleyer A, Whiteson M (eds.), *Cancer and the adolescent 2nd ed*, p. 204. Blackwell Publishing Ltd, Carlton.

Jones BL, Parker-Raley J, Higgerson R, Christie LM, Legett S, Greathouse J. (2008) Finding the right words: Using the terms allow natural death (AND) and do not resuscitate (DNR) in pediatric palliative care. *J Healthcare Qual* **30**(5): 55–63.

Palliative and end of life care glossary of terms (2008). Palliative Care Australia. Available online at: http://www.palliativecare.org.au/Portals/46/PCA%20-glossary.pdf (accessed November 27, 2011).

Stevens MM, Dunsmore JC. (1996.) Helping adolescents who are coping with a life-threatening illness, along with their siblings, peers and parents. In: Corr CA, Balk DE (eds.), *Handbook of adolescent death and bereavement*, pp. 329–353. Springer, New York.

Stevens MM, Dunsmore JC, Bennett DL, Young AJ. (2009) Adolescents living with life-threatening illnesses. In: Balk DE, Corr CA (eds.), *Adolescent encounters with death, bereavement, and coping*, pp. 115–140. Springer, New York.

Chapter 20

Disorders of Puberty

Ann Maguire and Kate Steinbeck

1. Introduction

Puberty is the time between the first rise in gonadal hormones in the blood (testosterone and oestradiol) and the achievement of full reproductive capacity. Disorders of puberty are primarily when puberty occurs too early, too late or not at all. There should be clinical suspicion if the sequence of pubertal events fails to progress or if the sequence is out of the expected order (Chapter 1). Investigation and management is the realm of the paediatric or adolescent endocrinologist but all clinicians need to understand when they should refer and when regular observation without intervention is indicated.

2. Delayed and Absent Puberty

Delayed puberty is defined as no pubertal changes by 13 years in girls and 14 years in boys.

2.1. *Intact Hypothalamic–Pituitary–Gonadal Axis (Functional Abnormality) (see Table 1)*

The most common cause is constitutional delay of growth and puberty, which is also known as maturational delay. Pubertal delay can also occur

Table 1:   Hypogonadotropic disorders of puberty.

Functional:
  Constitutional (sporadic or familial); more common in males
  Chronic illness
  Malnutrition
  Excessive exercise

Hypothalamic disorders: Usually associated with other hormone defects
  Congenital hypothalamic syndromes: Kallmann, Bardet-Biedl, Prader Willi, CHARGE
  Hamartomas and other vascular lesions
  Iron excess; thalassaemia
  Trauma
  Tumour: craniopharyngioma, meningioma
  Irradiation

Pituitary disorders: Usually associated with other hormone defects
  Congenital
  Tumours: non functioning
  Tumours: functioning — prolactinoma, Cushing's disease

in malnutrition, which may be intentional as in eating disorders and non-intentional as in elite level exercise, or if a chronic illness is severe or inadequately managed. In this setting the inhibition of gonadotropin releasing hormone release can be seen as an evolutionary protective effect to ensure that calories are not wasted on physical growth or development, which are non-essential for survival.

2.1.1. *Constitutional Delay of Growth and Puberty diagnosis*

This is a diagnosis of exclusion. It is more common in boys than girls and there is often a family history of pubertal delay. Bone age X-ray of the hand and wrist to assess skeletal maturation must be performed and will lag behind chronological age by 2–4 years. Diagnostic work up should exclude hormonal deficiencies, occult systemic illness and chromosomal disorders associated with delayed puberty. CDGP and other functional abnormalities of the HPG axis are difficult to differentiate from permanent hypogonadotropic hypogonadism. Dynamic testing using GnRH/GnRH agonist stimulation is often not helpful and no single test can distinguish between the two conditions with a high level of sensitivity and specificity. The longer the delay the more likely an abnormality exists. Only the demonstration of a complete recovery can truly distinguish CDGP from HH.

2.1.2. *Treatment*

Treatment is often not required for CDGP and expectant observation is used in most mild cases. In extreme cases or if the adolescent is experiencing psychosocial distress due to delayed puberty, low dose, short courses of testosterone or an oestrogen may be used, but only after full endocrine assessment. The rationale is that the artificial gonadal steroid rise, known as priming, triggers GnRH activity and increased growth hormone secretion. More prolonged therapy, as described in Section 2.6 is used if pubertal progression does not occur or if there is osteoporosis present.

2.2. *Abnormalities of the Hypothalamus* (see Table 1)

Secondary sexual characteristics will be absent. Cryptorchidism (failure of testicular descent) is common in HH and intra-abdominal placement further compromises testicular function. There may be evidence of other pituitary hormone deficits as a result of thyrotropin releasing hormone, corticotropin releasing hormone, GHRH and antidiuretic hormone deficiency, and hyperprolactinaemia due to pituitary stalk damage. If there is extensive hypothalamic damage as may occur with tumours, then sleep disturbances, hyperphagia, and rage attacks may be present. Kallmann syndrome is associated with anosmia. Coloboma, **h**eart defects, choanal **a**tresia, **r**etardation (growth and intellectual) and **g**enital and **e**ar defects may be seen in the CHARGE syndrome. The hypothalamus is damaged by irradiation and survivors of childhood cancer who have received cranial irradiation may fail to enter puberty.

2.2.1. *Diagnosis*

Gonadotropins (luteinising hormone and follicle stimulating hormone) and gonadal hormone levels are low, because of absent GnRH stimulation. Imaging studies are mandatory, with MRI preferred.

2.2.2. *Treatment*

If the condition has been diagnosed in childhood, hormone developmental therapy should be commenced at the time of normal puberty, no later than 12 years and the doses of other pituitary hormone therapy adjusted for the pubertal growth spurt.

2.3. *Abnormalities of the Pituitary* (see Table 1)

It may be difficult to distinguish between hypothalamic and pituitary damage, particularly with tumours. LH, FSH, and gonadal hormones will be low, there may be other associated pituitary hormone defects and brain imaging is essential. HDT is the same as for hypothalamic or gonadal abnormalities.

2.4. *Abnormalities of the Gonads* (see Table 2)

2.4.1. *Diagnosis*

Elevated gonadotropins (FSH and LH) and low oestradiol or testosterone indicate primary gonadal deficiency. Clinically there will be absence of secondary sexual characteristics, except for pubic and axillary hair which may develop under the influence of adrenal androgens if the hypothalamic–pituitary–adrenal axis is intact. Testicles will be small (<3 ml if the

Table 2:   Hypergonadotropic disorders of puberty.

Congenital
    Klinefelter syndrome (XXY)
    Turner syndrome (XO, XX/XO mosaic & isochrome X)
Acquired
    Bilateral torsion
    Infection; mumps orchitis
    Testicular trauma
    Chemotherapy
    Surgical removal
    Radiation
    Autoimmune

condition presents before the time of normal puberty) and soft. Primary amenorrhoea may be the presenting symptom in females. Hot flushes are uncommon in females who have primary gonadal failure in adolescence. A pelvic ultrasound will show pre-pubertal uterine dimensions (uterus smaller than the cervix) and ovaries may be difficult to visualise. Uterine growth will occur with HDT. As with secondary and tertiary hypogonadism partial states of deficiency may exist.

2.4.2. *Klinefelter syndrome*

This occurs in 1 in 500–1000 births. Nowadays many of these boys are diagnosed with prenatal karyotyping for the detection of Down syndrome and other aneuploidies. If the diagnosis is not made antenatally then clinical presentations in childhood and adolescence may include learning difficulties, tall stature with disproportionately long limbs, failure to progress through puberty, gynaecomastia and small (<3 ml) testicles. The most common presenting feature of KS in adulthood is infertility. The adult KS patient is at greater risk of autoimmune disease, chronic lung disease, breast cancer and germ cell tumours, depression, osteoporosis (if androgen therapy is not instituted or maintained), and varicose veins. Thus endocrine follow up is lifelong.

2.4.3. *Turner syndrome*

This occurs in 1 in 3000–5000 births, with a much higher prevalence at conception, and it is the commonest sex chromosome disorder in females. Signs and symptoms vary with presentation age. Short stature, failure to enter puberty or primary amenorrhoea are presenting features in adolescence. Neck webbing, low set ears, low hairline, short fourth metacarpal, co-arctation of the aorta, bicuspid aortic valve, and renal tract anomalies (including duplex collecting system, single kidney, horseshoe kidney) may be present. Additional morbidities include conductive and neurosensory deafness, autoimmune hypothyroidism, coeliac disease, inflammatory bowel disease, elevated liver transaminases and cirrhosis of the liver, kyphoscoliosis, learning and social difficulties, early appearance of cardiovascular risk factors (dyslipidaemia and hypertension) and osteoporosis (especially if hormone replacement is inadequate or not maintained). Aortic dilatation can occur, even in the absence of aortic valve disease and regular monitoring using cardiac echo or MRI is required throughout adult life. Given the potential for spontaneous fertility in mosaic Turner syndrome and the success of assisted reproduction with egg donation it is vital to be aware of the risk of aortic dissection with dilatation in pregnancy, and the need for rigorous blood pressure control at all times. The life expectancy in TS remains significantly lower than the general female population.

2.5. *Other Causes of Primary Amenorrhoea*

Absence of menarche will accompany the absence of puberty of any aetiology. If there is normal female secondary sexual development, confirmed by normal gonadotropins and oestradiol, consider Mullerian agenesis or imperforate hymen. Both are ultrasound diagnoses. In Mullerian agenesis the fallopian tubes, uterus, and upper third of vagina are absent. A functional vagina may be achieved by graduated dilator therapy so that vaginoplasty may not always be required. Androgen insensitivity syndrome in its complete form may present as primary amenorrhoea. Gonads are usually in the inguinal canal and only the lower third of the vagina is present, with absent Mullerian structures on pelvic ultrasound. Gonadotropins and testosterone are elevated and the karyotype is 46XY. The treatment is gonadectomy, oestrogen only HDT, and vaginal dilation therapy. The gender identity is female.

2.6. *Hormone Developmental Therapy*

HDT is used to initiate and maintain maturation. Therapeutic preparations of GnRH, LH, and FSH have short half-lives and are degraded by gut peptidases, so must be given parenterally. Hence, testosterone or oestrogen compounds are used for pubertal induction regardless of whether the aetiology is primary or secondary or tertiary hypogonadism. Pubertal change should be monitored clinically using Tanner or similar staging, as well as by plasma testosterone and oestradiol (if the oestrogen chosen is detectable on plasma assay). Additionally, in primary gonadal failure, suppression of elevated FSH (female) and LH (male) can be used to determine adequacy of replacement. Aim for high normal range levels as suppression into the low normal range may not be possible without over-replacement.

2.6.1. *The principles of Hormone Developmental Therapy*

- Take no less than two years to complete pubertal induction.
- Start at one quarter or less of the full adult replacement dose.
- Do not increase the dose under six months.
- Emphasise that HDT is for life in males and until the age of natural menopause in females.
- There are minimal published data on HDT in adolescents and adults in their reproductive years. Adverse findings for hormone replacement therapy in post-menopausal females *cannot* be extrapolated to adolescents and young adults.

2.6.2. *Females*

Oral oestradiol valerate or oestradiol gel or patches may be used. Using these preparations plasma oestradiol can be measured to monitor dosage regimens, unlike the oestrogen compounds in the oral contraceptive pill. Unopposed oestrogen therapy will cause endometrial hyperplasia and the risk of endometrial cancer. Thus a progestogen (progesterone like compound) must be added to the regimen by the last quarter of the puberty induction or earlier if menstrual bleeding occurs. If menses are desired then cyclical progestogen (7–10 cycle days) and continuous oestrogen are used. If menses are not desired, use continuous oral progestogen combined with continuous oestrogen in one of the formulations above. The continuous dosing regimen maintains an atrophic, thin endometrium for as long as it is used and if adherence is satisfactory, most users will not have breakthrough bleeding.

2.6.3. *Males*

Commence induction of puberty with oral testosterone undecanoate or testosterone patch or gel at a reduced dose. Oral TU is absorbed through the intestinal lymphatics and thus avoids first pass through the liver. Oral TU at maximum dose is unlikely to achieve normal young adult testosterone levels and in the last third or half of pubertal induction a switch should be made to parenteral therapy. Injectable TU lasts approximately 12 weeks, but testosterone levels should be checked immediately prior to the next injection so that time between injections can be reduced if the testosterone nadir is too low. Testosterone pellets last 5–6 months but require sterile insertion by trochar. Availability is a limitation for use. Older preparations of testosterone should be avoided as stable testosterone levels are unlikely to be achieved with depot esters, and oral compounds are more likely to be hepatotoxic.

3. Early Puberty

Signs of puberty that occur before the age of eight in females or nine in males are abnormal, and require specialist investigation and treatment.

3.1. *True Central (Gonadotropin Dependent) Precocious Puberty*

This condition is when the normal events of puberty commence early, with gonadotropins and gonadal hormones rising in a normal pubertal manner (Chapter 1). In males there will be testicular enlargement due to FSH stimulation, unlike in other forms of precocious puberty when the testes remain small. In 80% of females, but in only 20% of males, CPP occurs in the absence of a central lesion or abnormality. Central abnormalities include hydrocephalus, irradiation, surgery, infection, hamartomas, gliomas, and pinealomas, some of which have significant additional morbidity and mortality.

3.1.1. *Diagnosis*

The diagnosis of CPP may be clear from baseline measurement of LH, FSH, and oestradiol or testosterone if all the hormones are in the pubertal range. If baseline bloods are not diagnostic then GnRH stimulation testing should be performed. Elevated peak levels of LH and FSH (with LH being more prominent than FSH) supports the diagnosis of CPP. *Cranial imaging is mandatory in confirmed CPP.*

3.1.2. *Treatment*

The treatment aim is to avoid psychosocial disturbance as a result of rising hormones, a physical body asynchronous with peers and short adult height as a result of premature fusion of the epiphyses under the influence of oestradiol or testosterone (aromatised to oestradiol). The therapy is with GnRH agonists, using long lasting depot preparations. GnRH agonists down regulate GnRH receptors after a brief period of stimulation. GnRH antagonists which are free of significant adverse side effects are not yet widely available. GnRH agonists are continued until an age where puberty is acceptable and the adolescent is agreeable to stop treatment.

The increased prevalence of overweight and obesity in females is thought to contribute to an increased incidence of borderline cases of CPP in 7–8 year olds, which often do not require therapy but always require investigation. CPP is seen more frequently than expected in female international adoptees and adopting parents should be counselled about the possibility. True CPP can also be seen in long standing severe primary hypothyroidism when excess TRH stimulates GnRH receptors. The treatment is to ensure adequate thyroxine replacement $\pm$ GnRH agonist therapy if puberty is well established.

3.2. *Gonadotropin Independent Precocious Puberty (also known as Pseudo or Non-Central Precocious Puberty)*

3.2.1. *Isosexual*

The physical changes of puberty are consistent with gender. However, LH and FSH levels are suppressed and testosterone or oestradiol are above pre-pubertal levels. Causes include testotoxicosis, McCune Albright Syndrome, congenital adrenal hyperplasia, and androgen or oestrogen of non-gonadal origin (tumour or exogenous).

Testotoxicosis (also known as familial male precocious puberty) is an autosomal dominant abnormality of the LH receptor, with pubertal changes occurring as early as the first year of life. Inhibitors of steroidogenesis and anti-androgens are the mainstays of treatment.

MAS in its full form includes polyostotic fibrous dysplasia, *café au lait* skin lesions, and autonomous endocrine gland function as a result of a G protein receptor defect. The FSH receptor is commonly affected, resulting in elevated oestradiol levels. Treatment includes inhibitors of steroidogenesis and anti-oestrogens.

3.2.2. *Contrasexual*

The physical changes of puberty are of the opposite gender. In this situation LH and FSH are again suppressed and testosterone or oestradiol are above the pre-pubertal range in females and males respectively. This rare condition is generally the result of a gonadal or adrenal tumour.

3.2.3. *Endocrine disruptors*

These are synthetic chemicals which when absorbed block or mimic endogenous hormone function. Xeno-oestrogens have been implicated in both early puberty and later reproductive abnormalities. Diethylstilbestrol, once given to treat threatened miscarriage and which induces vaginal cancers in offspring, is the best described example of an endocrine disruptor.

4. Other Abnormal Pubertal Events

4.1. *Gynaecomastia*

Breast enlargement occurs in up to 80% of males in Tanner Stages 3 and 4. It may be tender, unilateral or bilateral, and is often asymmetric. Adolescents may be concerned that it is cancer or be socially embarrassed, making them reluctant to take part in sports. Gynaecomastia needs to be distinguished from adipose tissue. The presence of a mass of firmer tissue centred beneath the areolae suggests true glandular breast tissue rather than adipose tissue. Ultrasound may assist in making this differentiation in obese males. Male hypogonadism, particularly Klinefelter syndrome should be considered. Thyrotoxicosis, oestrogen secreting tumours, anabolic steroid abuse, and chronic marijuana use should be excluded.

Gynaecomastia typically resolves spontaneously within six months to two years. In severe cases surgery may be indicated. Although aromatase inhibitors have been used in clinical trials, gynaecomastia is not an approved indication for their use and these would not be considered standard therapy for what is usually a benign condition.

4.2. *Female Hirsutism*

This is the appearance of terminal hair on the face or trunk and is different to secondary sexual hair and the thickening of limb and eyebrow hair seen in normal female puberty. If associated with oligomenorrhea and *without* virilisation, hirsutism may indicate polycystic ovaries or late onset congenital adrenal hyperplasia and requires further endocrine assessment. Hirsutism *with* virilisation, which includes loss of female characteristics (breasts and body fat), clitoromegaly, balding and deepening of the voice usually indicates an adrenal or ovarian tumour, and requires *urgent* endocrine investigation.

4.3. *Premature Pubarche*

This is the early appearance of pubic and axillary hair in either sex, often accompanied by increased body odour and seborrhoea due to adrenarche. Endocrine investigation is required to exclude CAH or other abnormal androgen production. The usual findings are slightly advanced bone age and sometimes mildly elevated DHEA and DHEAS. No treatment is generally required. Polycystic ovarian syndrome is a potential sequelae. Premature pubarche is more common in low birth weight infants and metformin has been used to treat female patients in a research setting. This is not currently considered to be standard therapy.

4.4. *Premature Thelarche*

This is isolated breast development occurring before the age of normal puberty. It is diagnosed in the presence of pre-pubertal FSH, LH, and oestradiol, and with no evidence of maturation of the uterus or ovaries on pelvic ultrasound. Growth velocity and bone age should not be significantly increased. Premature thelarche may represent hypersensitivity to endogenous oestradiol, temporarily increased ovarian steroid secretion due to an ovarian cyst or a mild, fluctuating variant of CPP. Endocrine disruptors and ingested oestrogen also need to be considered in the diagnostic work up.

It is essential that if a diagnosis of premature thelarche or adrenarche is made that there is follow up through puberty, and beyond in females, to ensure that there are no reproductive sequelae.

5. Transition to Adult Care

5.1. *Ongoing Medical Management*

Adolescents who require induction of puberty will need ongoing HDT. For females this will be until the age of normal menopause and for males lifelong. The goal is to maintain oestradiol and testosterone levels in the normal adult range. The risks of not taking therapy for ovarian insufficiency far outweigh the risks of exogenous hormone replacement in females. Expert opinion is that the adverse effects of prolonged use of HRT in the post-menopausal female do not apply to hypogonadal females in their reproductive years. This should be clearly discussed with the young woman. Advice should include the need to take both oestrogen and progestogen compounds to avoid the risk of endometrial hyperplasia and advice given regarding usual surveillance for breast cancer. Oral HDT should be ceased before anything but minor surgery to reduce the risks of deep venous thrombosis and pulmonary emboli.

5.2. *Potential Long Term Health Implications*

Early puberty is associated with higher risks of breast cancer, eating disorders, and depression. Later puberty is associated with higher risk of osteopaenia and anxiety disorders.

References

Ambler GR. (2009) Androgen therapy for delayed male puberty. *Curr Opin Endocrinol Diabetes Obes* **16**(3): 232–239.

Bojesen A, Gravholt C.H. (2007) Klinefelter syndrome in clinical practice. *Nat Clin Pract Urol* **4**(4): 192–204.

Carel J-C, Leger J. (2008) Clinical practice. Precocious puberty. *N Engl J Med* **358**(22): 2366–2377.

Davenport ML. (2010) Approach to the patient with turner syndrome. *J Clin Endocrinol Metab* **95**(4): 1487–1495.

Divasta AD, Gordon CM. (2010) Hormone replacement therapy and the adolescent. *Curr Opin Obstet Gynecol* **22**(5): 363–368.

Gordon CM. (2010) Clinical practice. Functional hypothalamic amenorrhea. *N Engl J Med* **363**(4): 365–371.

Ibanez L, Diaz R, Lopez-Bermejo A, Marcos MV. (2009) Clinical spectrum of premature pubarche: Links to metabolic syndrome and ovarian hyperandrogenism. *Rev Endocr Metab Disord* **10**(1): 63–76.

Isidori AM, Giannetta E, Lenzi A. (2008) Male hypogonadism. *Pituitary* **11**(2): 171–180.

Nordt CA, Divasta AD. Gynecomastia in adolescents. *Curr Opin Pediatr* **20**(4): 375–382.

Practice Committee of American Society for Reproductive Medicine. (2008) Current evaluation of amenorrhea. *Fertil Steril* **90**(5): S219–225.

Ranke MB. (2003) In: Karger, AG (ed.), 3rd revised and extended edition, Switzerland. *Diagnostics of Endocrine Function in Children and Adolescents.*

Chapter 21

The Deaf Adolescent

Eric Weiselberg

1. Introduction

Worldwide, there are approximately 278 million people with a moderate to profound hearing loss. In the United States, the incidence of congenital deafness and hearing loss is 2–3 out of 1000 births. Of the 28 million people in the United States with hearing loss, 15%–17% manifest before 19 years of age. Deaf adolescents have the same developmental tasks as normal adolescents. Protective factors to enter adulthood successfully include positive self-esteem and attitude, communication skills, education, a supportive family and community, and access to age-appropriate health care. Without these in place, the adolescent is at risk for life-long high-risk behaviours. While these goals are the same for all adolescents, this chapter will highlight some of the barriers that the deaf adolescent may face in order to achieve his or her optimal potential.

2. Definitions

Deaf, with an uppercase D, signifies a cultural identity of someone who identifies with other members of the Deaf community and who may use sign language for communication. The term deaf, with lowercase d, indicates the audiologic situation of severe to profound hearing loss. Such persons may not identify as members of the Deaf community, may use spoken language, and may prefer the terms hearing-loss, hard-of-hearing, or hearing impaired. For the purpose of this chapter, the term d/Deaf will be used to signify both meanings.

3. Aetiology

Over 100 genes have been identified that cause hearing loss (for an up-to-date listing, see the Hereditary Hearing Loss Homepage at http://hereditaryhearingloss.org/). At least 50% of deafness is genetic, with 77%–88% autosomal recessive, 10%–20% autosomal dominant, 1%–2% X-linked, and mitochondrial deafness 1%–20% depending on the population. Seventy percent to 80% of genetic causes are non-syndromic. There are about 400 syndromes that include hearing loss, including Down, Treacher Collins, Stickler, Noonan, BOR, CHARGE, Goldenhar, and Mitochondrial (ototoxicity) syndromes which are typically represented among deaf individuals. While detailed discussion can be found elsewhere, some common genetic causes, such as Connexin 26 and Waardenburg syndrome, and others that have a medical impact on adolescence and adulthood are discussed in this chapter.

3.1. *Connexin 26*

The most common form of non-syndromic deafness is caused by mutations in the Connexin 26 (GJB2) gene located on chromosome 13q11. Connexin 26 is part of a gap junction responsible for ion transport and potassium homeostasis within the cochlea. Many mutations have been identified, with 35delG the most common, having a carrier rate of 1:51 in Europe. Diagnostic mutation analysis is available, and identification avoids costly investigations and concerns for syndromic causes of deafness.

3.2. *Waardenburg Syndrome*

Waardenburg syndrome is one of the more common syndromic causes of congenital deafness. It is autosomal dominant, although there can be great heterogeneity in presentation within families. Classic features include heterochromic irides or brilliant pale blue irides, and white forelock or premature greying. There are two main types and two rarer forms. WS type I, in addition to the classic features, has dystopia canthorum (wide inner canthal distance). WS type II does not have the displaced inner canthi. More rare is WS type III (Klein–Waardenburg) which is associated with limb anomalies, and WS type IV (Shah–Waardenburg) with Hirschsprung disease.

3.3. *Usher Syndrome*

Usher syndrome is perhaps the one genetic cause of deafness that impacts most on adolescent development. US consists of deafness and retinitis pigmentosa making it the leading cause of deaf–blindness. There are three types: US Type I (40%) has congenital deafness, early onset RP and vestibular dysfunction; US Type II (57%) consists of less severe hearing loss with later onset RP; US Type III (3%) has variable hearing loss. Only US Type I will be discussed here. The RP begins early with destruction of the retinal rod cells and loss of night vision in early childhood. By late childhood/early adolescence the cone cells deteriorate, and blind spots (scotoma) begin to develop in the peripheral vision and by adolescence the visual fields can be significantly limited. US Type I can impact on every part of adolescent development, including body image acceptance, independence, and peer relationships. With worsening visual fields, individuals may be considered clumsy, bad at sports, or snobby for 'ignoring' friends. Keeping up with classroom or social discussions can be difficult because of the difficulty in tracking signed conversations. Socialising and mobility can be affected by the limited visual fields and night blindness. The adolescent may be ostracised for being 'different' or may self-isolate. Diagnosis is made by establishing a negative response on an electroretinogram. Personnel skilled in US issues should convey the diagnosis, for terms such as 'you will go blind' should not be used as individuals may have many years of useful vision ahead. The diagnosis is certainly devastating for the family and the adolescent, with literature reports of significant risk for depression and suicidal ideation. Orientation and mobility services should be offered to help with classroom functioning and daily living skills. Opportunities to meet other youth with US should be encouraged, through agencies such as the Helen Keller National Center in the United States.

3.4. *Jervell and Lange-Nielsen Syndrome*

Jervell and Lange-Nielsen syndrome, an infrequent but important aetiology, has congenital deafness and prolonged QT, which can lead to sudden death. Individuals are prone to *torsades de pointes* (a distinctive type of ventricular tachycardia), which may spontaneously revert to normal sinus rhythm. During short attacks, the individual may have palpitations and sweating, and during longer attacks, seizure-like episodes or syncope may occur. If the *torsades de pointes* continue, it may lead to ventricular fibrillation and sudden death. Precipitating events include physical or stressful stimuli, supposedly due to the release of catecholamines, and events can also occur during menses or sleep. Other precipitating factors include severe hypokalaemia, hypocalcaemia, or hypomagnesaemia. Treatment with beta-blockers is used to protect against the surges of catecholamine that can occur during stress. Automated internal cardiac defibrillators have become the mainstay of treatment. The KVLQT1 gene, which involves potassium ion transport, will be a focus for future therapy.

3.5. *Alport Syndrome*

Alport syndrome involves mutations in genes that code for collagen (COL4A3, COL4A4, COL4A5) and results in hearing loss and progressive nephritis. The renal disease begins with haematuria and can lead to end-stage renal disease before 30 years of age in the juvenile form, or after 30 in the adult form. AS is genetically heterogeneous, with 80% X-linked (although females can have a mild presentation), 15% autosomal recessive and the remainder autosomal dominant. The hearing loss is not congenital, but variably progressive starting in childhood or adolescence. The concern for the practitioner is the invariable progressive renal disease, leading to the need for dialysis or renal transplantation.

3.6. *Congenital Rubella Syndrome*

First described by Sir Norman Gregg of Australia in 1941, congenital rubella syndrome has been a leading cause of deafness worldwide, especially during times of epidemics. When exposed during the first trimester, there is a 90% risk of foetal teratogenicity, which chiefly includes deafness, congenital cataracts, and heart disease (often a patent ductus arteriosus) depending on when during the pregnancy the foetus was exposed. Of importance, however, is that there are late manifestations, including Type I diabetes (20%), type II diabetes (22%), thyroid disease (19%), glaucoma (making CRS the second most common cause of deaf-blindness after Usher syndrome), heart disease (pulmonic stenosis), early menopause, short stature, and subacute panencephalopathy. With the introduction of the rubella vaccine in 1969, the Centers for Disease Control announced in 2004 that rubella was no longer endemic in the United States. Worldwide, as of 2009, 130 countries (67%) offer the rubella vaccine. However in many countries the vaccine is given only to females, allowing the rubella virus to stay endemic within males, and capable of producing CRS in susceptible females. Therefore, CRS remains a significant cause of deafness and developmental disabilities, especially in developing countries. The practitioner needs to be vigilant for signs of CRS among deaf children and adults from these areas of the world, and monitor for the late manifestations.

4. Deaf Identity Development

The d/Deaf adolescent faces the same developmental tasks as does the hearing (Chapter 3). However, the d/Deaf teen also faces the challenges of discovering him/herself as a deaf person. Glickman and Carey have proposed four Deaf Identity Development identities, based on cultural and racial development theory.

4.1. *Hearing*

Hearing refers to the view of one's deafness as a medical disability and thereby comparing oneself to the hearing majority for one's sense of normalcy. Individuals who maintain a hearing identity often do not use the term "Deaf" but rather 'hearing-impaired' or 'hearing-loss' implying a negative or less-than comparison to the hearing.

4.2. *Immersion*

Immersion identity signifies individuals who are immersed into the Deaf world, view other members of the Deaf community for their sense of identity, use sign language for communication, and reject notions of hearing as being superior.

4.3. *Bicultural*

Bicultural identity indicates those that are at ease in either the Deaf or hearing world.

4.4. *Marginal*

Marginal indicates those that do not identify with either Deaf or hearing, and lack a focus of normalcy. As over 90% of deaf children are born into hearing families, the overwhelming majority of whom do not sign regularly in the home, many children and adolescents are at risk of feeling marginalised, with development of poor self-esteem, isolation, peer rejection, and maladaptive behaviours.

The trend in the US and other developed countries is for mainstreaming students away from specialised schools for the deaf with presently about 75% of American students attending mainstreamed schools. Although the goal of this approach is to assimilate the deaf with the majority hearing community, schools for the deaf were historically the places for people to develop a Deaf identity. Acceptance in a mainstreamed classroom may be difficult for the deaf adolescent, with feelings of isolation and rejection by not having a cohort of similar individuals. Feeling different, or being perceived as different, is a breeding ground for marginalisation.

Cochlear implants do not automatically make the transition to mainstreamed class easier. There has been much discussion, especially within the Deaf community, that having a cochlear implant may further marginalise an individual and interfere with the development of a positive Deaf identity. Although there are many success stories, it is important to note that the benefits from having a cochlear implant vary greatly, from understanding speech, to being an adjunct to speech reading or to help recognise environmental sounds, but not making an individual hearing. Those adolescents with cochlear implants who maintain a bicultural identity, who have exposure to Deaf individuals as role models, and maintain the use of sign language when with other Deaf individuals, have the most positive attitudes and success. Identity development can be further compounded, such as being oral deaf (use voice and speech–read), latent (adult-onset) deaf, Deaf of Deaf (parents), hearing children of Deaf adults (Coda), Black Deaf, Gay Lesbian Bisexual Transgendered Deaf, Asian Deaf, and so on.

5. Psychosocial risks

There is a paucity of research on the risk behaviours of the d/Deaf, partly due to the difficulty in formulating standardised methodologies. However, not only does the d/Deaf adolescent have the same issues of risk-taking behaviours and emotional concerns as the hearing, but they are faced with issues of family and peer acceptance, isolation, communication barriers, and the identity developmental tasks described above that can affect one's psychological well-being. One study found that Dutch deaf children had a 2.6 times higher rate of emotional and behavioural problems compared to hearing peers, which was felt to be associated with poor parent–child communication. Those with positive mother-infant attachment, which can be influenced by ease of communication such that can occur with deaf children of deaf parents, showed fewer psychosocial risks, and were offered emotional support and coping skills, reinforcing the idea that d/Deaf adolescents should be connected with other d/Deaf individuals. Furthermore, the development of a positive cultural identity, with ease of communication and self-expression, may protect against negative behaviours.

In regard to typical adolescent risk behaviours, the d/Deaf adolescent may be faced with misinformation secondary to communication barriers and difficulty accessing confidential health care. About 50% of d/Deaf adolescent high school students have a lifetime prevalence of risky alcohol use and about 20% report illicit substance use, as well as significant multiple substance use. However, the deaf may be less likely to be asked about alcohol and cigarette use during physician visits than hearing peers.

A study of Deaf college students revealed that the most common source of sexual information was friends. Furthermore, the majority of individuals experienced coitarche between 15–18 years of age, used withdrawal as the most common method of birth control, did not use a condom in almost 70% of the most recent sexual encounters and 31% of the female responders reported being a victim of forced sex. Compared to hearing adolescents, the deaf show significant lack of HIV/AIDS knowledge and have difficulty receiving appropriate HIV/AIDS medical information.

6. Transitioning to Adulthood

Transitioning to adulthood entails moving from the school environment to the workplace, from home to community living, and achieving economic and social responsibilities of adulthood. For the d/Deaf adolescent this also involves access to health care and independence, which, because of societal situations, may involve additional barriers. One developmental hallmark of adolescent independence is obtaining a driver's license. In the United States, the deaf are able to obtain a driver's license, though individual states may differ in restrictions. In New York, for example, deaf drivers are restricted to the use of hearing aids or the use of full-view rear mirrors. Although there are reports of the deaf being able to obtain a commercial driver's license, US Federal regulations prohibit the issuance of a commercial license if hearing is worse than 40 dB or the individual is unable to hear whispered speech at five feet (150 cm). Similarly, the deaf can obtain a driver's license in many developed countries, however, there are at least 26 countries that prohibit the deaf from driving. For complete information, local motor vehicle regulations should be reviewed.

6.1. *Health Access*

Adolescents receive health information at school, from family, health professionals, friends, the media, and through 'incidental exposure' to the world around them. The deaf individual may not have the advantage of such incidental learning due to limited access to television, radio, family conversations, out-of-classroom discussions, public service announcements, and general 'background noise'. This leaves the d/Deaf adolescent at a severe disadvantage and at risk for misinformation and confusion.

For Deaf individuals who use sign language, access to physicians requires qualified sign language interpreters. Similarly, those with cochlear implants or who sometimes use voice for communication, may also require interpreters as they may depend on their native sign language for medical discussions. Written information is often inappropriate as the average reading level of the deaf high school student is at a 4.5 grade level. The Americans with Disabilities Act of 1990 requires the provision of qualified sign language interpreters for health care visits. Other countries have adopted similar laws such as the Australian Disability Discrimination Act of 1992 and the UK's Equality Act of 2010. However according to the World Federation of the Deaf, 29 of their 68 member states do not have any laws governing the use of sign language inter- preters. Health access also involves telecommunications. Advances in technology, including text-messaging and web-based video, have allowed for the ease of telecommunication among deaf people and between the deaf and hearing. Telecommunication access is mandated under the ADA, which has established relay operator centres to facilitate calls between deaf who use teletypewriter devices and the hearing. As the deaf now have access to videophones for ease of sign language telecommunication, Video Relay Service has also been established in the US and other coun- tries, including Australia.

6.2. *Higher Education and Employment*

The first public school for the deaf was established in France in 1755 by the Abbé de l'Épée. The first American school for the deaf was established in 1817 and the first college, now known as Gallaudet University, was established in Washington DC in 1864. During the 19th century, schools for the deaf were established throughout the US. These schools were much more than centres for learning, as these were the heart of Deaf cul- ture, allowing sign language to flourish, and for Deaf people to meet, socialise, marry, have children, and form a community. Towards the later part of the 20th century, there has been a shift for deaf students to be mainstreamed. The impact of mainstreaming on the deaf adolescent's

Deaf identity development has been a concern, especially within the Deaf community, for fear that these adolescents would become marginalised. Positive exposure to Deaf culture appears to be protective in establishing positive self-esteem and endorses a more bicultural identity.

Post-secondary education options include college/university education, vocational training, or joining the workforce. Anti-discrimination laws, such as the ADA, allow for educational opportunities within mainstreamed higher education. However, in spite of these opportunities, the deaf remain at a disadvantage. In the UK, the deaf are three times more likely to be unemployed than the hearing. Among deaf graduates, about 15% are under-employed and 5% unemployed. Feelings of marginalisation can persist in the workplace, with d/Deaf individuals not being included in the social aspects of office life, including work break discussions, work-related social gatherings, and even staff meetings. For quality of life, the d/Deaf adult should also be afforded access to Deaf cultural opportunities, gatherings, clubs and events.

Deaf adolescents face the same developmental goals as do their hearing peers, and providers need to address the psychosocial behaviours and risks that define this life stage. In addition, emphasis needs to be placed on the unique challenges that d/Deaf adolescents face on their journey to becoming healthy productive adults.

References

Banatvala JE. (2004) Rubella. *The Lancet (British edition)* **363**(9415): 1127.

Berman BA, Streja L, Guthmann DS. (2010) Alcohol and other substance use among deaf and hard of hearing youth. *J D Educ* **40**(2): 99–124.

Bisol CA, Sperb TM, Brewer TH, Kato SK, Shor-Posner G. (2008) HIV/AIDS knowledge and health-related attitudes and behaviors among deaf and hearing adolescents in southern Brazil. *Am Ann Deaf* **153**(4): 349–356.

Coll KM, Cutler MM, Thobro P, Haas R, Powell S. (2009) An exploratory study of psychosocial risk behaviors of adolescents who are deaf or hard of hearing: Comparisons and recommendations. *Am Ann Deaf* **154**(1): 30–35.

Dourmishev AL, Dourmishev LA, Schwartz RA, Janniger CK. (1999) Waardenburg syndrome. *Int J Dermatol* **38**(9): 656–663.

Glickman NS, Carey JC. (1993) Measuring deaf cultural identities: A preliminary investigation. *Rehabil Psychol* **38**(4): 275–283.

Joseph JM, Sawyer R, Desmond S. (1995) Sexual knowledge, behavior and sources of information among deaf and hard of hearing college students. *Am Ann Deaf,* **140**(4): 338–345.

Kemperman MH, Hoefsloot LH, Cremers CWRJ. (2002) Hearing loss and connexin 26. *J R Soc Med* **95**(4): 171–177.

Mason A, Mason M. (2007) Psychologic impact of deafness on the child and adolescent. *Prim Care* **34**(2): 407–426.

Nance WE (2003) The genetics of deafness. *Ment Retard Dev Disabil Res Rev* **9**(2): 109–119.

Olusanya BO, Ruben RJ, Parving A. (2006) Reducing the burden of communication disorders in the developing world: An opportunity for the Millennium Development Project. *JAMA* **296**(4): 441–444.

Punch R, Hyde M, Power D. (2007) Career and workplace experiences of Australian University graduates who are deaf or hard of hearing. *J Deaf Stud Deaf Educ* **12**(4): 504–517.

Schroedel JG, Geyer PD. (2000) Long-term career attainments of deaf and hard of hearing college graduates: Results from a 15-year follow-up survey. *Am Ann Deaf* **145**(4): 303–314.

Tamaskar P, Malia T, Stern C, Gorenflo D, Meador H, Zazove P. (2000) Preventive attitudes and beliefs of deaf and hard-of-hearing individuals. *Arch Fam Med* **9**(6): 518–925.

Van Eldik T, Treffers PD, Veerman JW, Verhulst FC. (2004) Mental health problems of deaf Dutch children as indicated by parents' responses to the child behavior checklist. *Am Ann Deaf* **148**(5): 390–395.

Weiselberg EC, Leigh IW. (2011) Medical and psychosocial considerations for the deaf adolescent. In: Fisher MM, Alderman EM, Kreipe RE, Rosenfeld WD (eds.), *Textbook of Adolescent Health Care* 1st ed, pp. 1581–1588. American Academy of Pediatrics, Illinois, USA.

World Health Organization *Deafness* and hearing impairment fact sheet. Available online at: www.who.int/mediacentre/factsheets/fs300/en/index. html (accessed February 19, 2011).

Chapter 22

The Adolescent and Young Adult with Intellectual Disability and Complex Health Needs

Helen Somerville and Cameron Ly

1. Introduction

Many adolescents and young adults with developmental disabilities have a complex set of medical problems, as well as significant psychosocial and daily care needs. Young people with a lifelong disability need significant support as they transition from paediatric (child and family centred services) to adult centred health services. In the past three decades, there has been a social revolution leading to a major demographic shift, with the deinstitutionalisation of people with disabilities.

1.1. *Demedicalisation*

In the same period, a hiatus for training of health care providers for this population has been created. Conversely, advances in medical diagnosis and treatments have led to a markedly reduced neonatal and infant mortality, and survival well beyond childhood. Major improvements in the management of complex health problems have resulted in a significant increase in longevity in this population.

Clinical changes to the health care team are compounded by associated needs in the provision of home-based health care and personal services. Suitable equipment, home modifications, and provisions of appropriate activity and social programs are all mandatory to address quality of life issues. Meeting the support and respite/accommodation needs of the person with intellectual disability and family/care givers is challenging.

1.2. *Legal Rights and Advocacy*

Individual and systemic change has resulted in an ongoing debate about models of care and service delivery. Comprehensive, specialised health care particularly for adolescents and young adults at both primary and tertiary levels is still evolving. Transition from the paediatric setting with clear case coordination by paediatrician and family doctor to the adult system with its silos of individual specialities and sub-specialisation within many specialties is challenging for the young person with complex health needs. Guardianship status may require review when a young person reaches the legal age of adulthood. Clinicians need to be aware of the relevant legislation before situations related to decision making and consent arise. Clinicians may also find and themselves needing to take over the role of patient advocate from ageing or exhausted parents, and of an educator for new carers.

1.3. *A Change in Attitudes to Disability*

Disability as a social issue and the notion of normalisation whilst well intended, has led to less than expected improvements in health and quality of life. However, multidisciplinary specialised health care is now evolving for this population. Community participation and services with an individual focus are developing apace. Up to 10% of children under the age of 14 years live with a disability and now most reach adulthood. In developing countries, there are also improvements in survival. This cohort of new adults with complex conditions has not previously been seen in adult health settings. Many will experience earlier onset of the diseases of ageing in their third and fourth decades.

Three common conditions, spina bifida, cerebral palsy, and Down syndrome are discussed in this chapter to highlight some of the specific adolescent and transition needs of developmental disability.

2. Spina Bifida

SB is a congenital neural tube defect caused by failure of the embryonic neural tube to close, resulting in potential damage to the exposed part of the spinal cord and nerves. There are four main types: Spina bifida *occulta,* myelomeningocele, meningocele, and lipomeningocele. A meningocele is a posterior meningeal cyst and as no nerve tissue is involved neurological sequelae are unlikely. Tethered cord (Section 2.4) may occur.

The SB defect usually involves three cell layers — the neural tissue, the vertebrae, and the skin. The most common and most severe type of open SB is myelomeningocele. There is usually an Arnold–Chiari malformation and hydrocephalus present in this most common form of spina bifida. The most common site of the defect is the lumbosacral region. Despite surgical intervention, associated syringomyelia can result in slow neurological decline over years, presumably due to atrophy of the spinal cord.

2.1. *Infancy and Childhood*

Neural tube defects are the most common and complex congenital defects affecting the central nervous system, and occur in 1 in 1000 pregnancies. NTD are associated with lower socio-ecomonic groups, poverty, famine, poor diet, and refugee status. Diabetes, chronic alcoholism, anticonvulsant medications (especially sodium valproate) and anorexia nervosa are risk factors, and SB is more common in teenage pregnancy. The availability of folate for the rapidly dividing cells of the embryo in the first few weeks of pregnancy is important in the aetiology of this condition. The metabolism of folate is genetically determined and hence the genetic nature of this condition. Fresh fruit and green leafy vegetables are the main dietary source of folate, with countries varying in the fortification of foods. It is recommended when planning a pregnancy that an additional daily 0.5 mg of folate is taken orally, and for those at higher risk of NTD 5 mg folate daily is recommended. The risk for future pregnancies, when a previous child has SB, is of the order of 1 in 20.

2.2. *Growth and Development*

Height growth can be compromised by the neurological deficit. Early onset of puberty can occur with hydrocephalus even when a shunt is inserted in the neonatal period. Girls are more commonly affected than boys.

2.3. *Spina Bifida Occulta*

This is the most common asymptomatic type, although presentation of low back pain and potential tethering of the spinal cord can occur during young adulthood. However, observational radiographic studies do not demonstrate a correlation between spina bifida occulta and non-specific low back pain.

2.4. *Tethered Cord*

In SB the spinal cord usually finishes at the site of the lesion and may be further fixed by fatty tissue or scar tissue. The spinal cord may be put on the stretch with growth, including during adolescence. Common symptoms include persistent lower back pain, that may worsen during sitting and which is relieved by changing position, deterioration of motor or sensory function in lower limbs, or unexplained change in continence or sexual functioning. Treatment is surgical release of the tethered cord.

2.5. *Myelomeningocele*

This is the most common type associated with physical disabilities and cognitive impairments, and which persists throughout life despite efforts to surgically close the defect after birth.

2.5.1. *Neurological impairments*

- Neurogenic bladder which results in incontinence and pelvi–ureteric reflux. Urinary tract infections are common. Renal failure, secondary to pelvi–ureteric reflux and renal calculi, can occur.
- Neurogenic bowel resulting in constipation and sometimes incontinence.
- Sexual dysfunction.
- Paralysis or motor weakness from the level of the lesion distally.

- Loss of sensation from the level of the lesion distally (touch, pain, and proprioception). Pressure ulcers are common, particularly the skin over the sacrum, upper thigh, heel and malleoli.
- Epilepsy which may be generalised, absence seizures or tonic–clonic seizures (10% affected). Shunt function should be checked if a patient presents with a first seizure.
- Visual disturbances include optic atrophy, strabismus, amblyopia and lateral nystagmus (cerebellar involvement) and sixth nerve palsy (blocked shunt or brain stem dysfunction). Optimising vision is important for the improvement of overall disability.

2.5.2. *Hydrocephalus*

Hydrocephalus, the excessive accumulation of cerebrospinal fluid in the ventricular system, occurs in 90% of SB patients. The treatment is usually a ventriculo–peritoneal shunt with a small pressure relief valve to drain the excessive cerebrospinal fluid into the abdominal cavity. Shunt obstruction is not uncommon. Headache, nausea, vomiting, blurred vision and neck pain are all common symptoms of a blocked shunt. The symptoms of shunt dysfunction can also be non-specific and mimic viral illnesses or even a hangover.

2.5.3. *Latex allergy*

This occurs in up to 85% of SB patients and varies from a mild local reaction to anaphylaxis. Early exposure and disease propensity are aetiological factors.

2.5.4. *Other management issues in myelomeningocele*

Cognition: patients with myelomeningocele can initially appear quite sociable and appear to have reasonable intellect, but cognitive impairments related to hydrocephalus are characteristic and must be accommodated in the treatment of all patients with this condition. The cognitive impairments include poor short term memory, reduced initiation skills which can lead to poor compliance, concentration and attention defects combined with easy distractibility, problems with task management so that many aspects of self management are compromised, and difficulties with executive function so that reasoning, problem solving and risk assessment difficulties are life-long. If there are difficulties with treatment compliance or integration into the workforce, then a neuro-psychological assessment may be helpful.

Routine renal and bladder management: the upper urinary tracts should be monitored with annual renal tract ultrasounds to exclude renal calculi or hydronephrosis, as well as measuring serum creatinine to exclude renal impairment. Renal failure was previously a major cause of death in patients with SB. A baseline urodynamic study should be performed by an adult urologist to monitor the lower urinary tract in those patients who undergo transition from paediatric to adult services. If there are high intravesical pressures or the presence of detrusor-sphincter dyssynergia causing pelvi–ureteric reflux, then oxybutynin should be initiated and closely monitored thereafter. In such cases, intermittent catheterisation should be the aim, although a suprapubic catheter or ileal conduit may be required.

Routine bowel management: a regular bowel regimen should be established together with education about healthy eating and good nutrition, so that patients can avoid severe constipation and faecal impaction.

Skin: patients should be encouraged to check their skin in the mirror daily, so treatment can be initiated early. Strategies to relieve pressure are most important, for example a tilt-in-space wheelchair. Nails should be kept short and regular podiatry reviews are useful.

Mobility: the majority use a wheelchair, but those who can stand and walk should be encouraged to continue this practice for as long as possible, albeit for exercise. Stretching reduces contractures.

Home modifications and equipment: an occupational therapist can assess the needs of a patient with SB in order to maintain independence.

2.5.5. *Psychosocial and quality of life aspects*

It is important to understand the psychosocial issues associated with the treatment of patients with SB and ideally, an *interdisciplinary* model should be used and common goals of treatment set amongst all the clinicians and therapists for a particular patient. The psychosocial issues that must be discussed with the patient include smoking, alcohol and drug use, family support, and accommodation (including government housing). Strong clinician advocacy is often required in order to obtain appropriate housing. Behaviour and adherence with therapy (Chapter 11) should be discussed and regularly reviewed given the acknowledged cognitive deficiencies. Finding an identity in life and struggling with body image can often result in depression, anxiety and eating disorders. Screening for major depression and anxiety disorders should be done in routine consultation. Finding suitable employment is important, provided there is the cognitive capacity to cope with the demands and stress of work. Despite the disability, many patients can drive a car, which maintains their independence and improves QOL. Recreational activities provide stimulation and further enhance QOL. Many young people with SB are involved in wheelchair sports. Youth development including peer support programs, education, advocacy, and policy can promote the health of patients with SB. Education is important to discuss relationships and sexual dysfunction and to reduce the risk of sexually transmitted diseases.

Most patients with SB have severe physical disability and complex care needs in the context of mild to moderate cognitive impairment. This is a particular challenge during the years of transition from paediatrics to adult services, requiring an interdisciplinary model of care to resolve complicated bio–psychosocial issues. The case below illustrates what can happen if transition is not effective.

Case Study: Rob is a 23 year old male with SB. He has an incomplete paraplegia, a ventriculo–peritoneal shunt, and a below knee amputation (as a result of osteomyelitis). He is single, living at home with his parents and socially isolated. He is relatively independent, uses a wheelchair, and drives. He is currently unemployed on a disability pension. Rob has had 12 hospital admissions in the past 12 months with pressure ulcers, cellulitis, and osteomyelitis. He still has three sacral pressure ulcers. He is being showered three times per week at a local hospital by community nurses as his parents' bathroom and laundry need renovation. The first adult health care intervention, after having failed to make a previous transition to adult care, was to arrange specialist medical review and renal ultrasound, continence products and wheelchair repairs. A program to improve self-care and diet was instituted. He was referred to a community-based fitness program for spinal cord injured individuals in wheelchairs. A graded program to improve exercise and socialisation was commenced. He also needed assistance with his applications for emergency housing, home care and employment.

3. Cerebral Palsy

CP is a persistent but not unchanging disorder of movement and posture (Table 1). It is the most common physical disability of childhood with a worldwide incidence of 1 in 400 births. CP results from damage to the developing brain (before or after birth). The cause is often unknown but may be genetic, infective, or metabolic. Advances in imaging, genetics and other investigations necessitate periodic review of the diagnosis. Intellectual/learning disability of varying severity is present in a significant proportion. Survival into adulthood has increased in the past 2–3 decades and with survival age related problems which occur at an earlier age, such as degenerative arthritis.

3.1. *Associated Health Conditions*

- Epilepsy occurs in over 50% and is often refractory, with multiple anticonvulsants required.
- Gastro–oesophageal reflux disease and/or dysphagia which are often difficult to detect because of communication difficulties.
- Chronic lung disease often resulting from repeat episodes of aspiration.

Table 1: Classifications of cerebral palsy.

a) **Type** of motor disorder	Spasticity	70%–80%
	Dyskinetic (athetoid and/or dystonia)	10%–20%
	Ataxic	~10%
	Mixed	~10%
b) **Distribution** of motor disorder	Hemiplegia	
	Diplegia	
	Quadriplegia	
c) **Severity** of motor disorder	Gross motor function classification score	I–V

- Osteopenia/osteoporosis risk factors that include lack of weight bearing activity, vitamin D deficiency with limited sun exposure and anticonvulsant use.
- Disorders of hearing and vision which impact on communication and socialisation.

3.2. *Management Issues*

Difficulty in communication often complicates health care. Comprehensive portable health reports and assistance at consultations are mandatory for optimal care. Numerous assessment tools and interventions have been developed over the past two decades and are now readily available for the paediatric and younger adolescent age groups. Important management considerations for the adolescent and young adult with CP include:

- Access to medications which treat dystonia and spasticity such as botulinum toxin A, and oral and intrathecal baclofen which have maintained mobility and weight bearing for longer, and reduced the incidence of contractures.
- Expertise in, and access to, newer orthopaedic procedures in the adult system, as well as physiotherapy and occupational therapy interventions. These include muscle stretching and splints, single event multilevel surgery (SEMLS), hand surgery to maximise function and complex scoliosis surgery.
- Gastro–oesophageal reflux disease is common and treatable after appropriate investigations. Constipation is also common and treatable with diet, fluids, and physical activity.
- Optimal nutrition is essential and consideration of the introduction of enteral feeding should be part of regular review.
- Regular dental care and saliva management therapies can significantly improve QOL.
- Chest health assessment and management with the use of CT scanning to document chronic lung disease, video fluoroscopy to document aspiration, and advice regarding suitable dietary consistencies and use of nebulised hypertonic saline, regular antibiotics and physiotherapy all improve respiratory status.

- Bone health surveillance and treatment of osteopenia/osteoporosis.
- Menstrual management may be necessary with the achievement of healthy body weight and more regular cycling.
- A defined plan for the management of arthritis, contractures and pain, and the awareness of spinal cord compromise (especially in dystonic/athetoid CP) (Section 2.4).

3.3. *Psychosocial and Quality of Life Issues*

Alongside the health improvements are significant advances in mobility aids and equipment including electronic wheelchairs, car seating and modifications, and sophisticated communication and computer devices. Meaningful employment, suitable supported accommodation, and day and recreational and sporting programs are rapidly being developed. However, access to financial support for therapy, aids, accommodation, and specialised programs is often limited for the adult population with CP. This situation significantly impacts on independence and QOL for the adolescent or adult with CP, and may require strong advocacy from health professionals. Parents may have been their major advocates in the past, but many parents are ageing with degenerative conditions of their own and need to have the burden of care reduced or taken from them.

Psychological health supports are also fragmented and difficult to access and parental grief often resurfaces at the time of adolescence, further complicating the family relationships. Reduced independence and functional ability with age and restricted social and recreational access may result in significant depression in the young person. Comorbid mental health conditions are more common than in the general population and may require medication as well as counselling support. Drug side effects and interactions must be considered and may influence mood and cognition significantly.

3.4. *Ongoing Health Care Needs*

A number of authors have noted a significant decline in contact with health professionals once a person with CP approaches the end of schooling and mid- to late- adolescence. Funding for and access to experienced health professionals is limited. Multi and interdisciplinary clinics for young people transitioning from paediatric to adult services (with the general practitioner or primary care physician as case manager and assistance from transition coordinators, where available) is now accepted as the gold standard of care. Such clinics allow a clear pathway for access to specialist assessment and intervention. Development of adequate funding for equipment e.g. orthotics, employment or suitable accommodation settings, and psychosocial supports is now being recognised as a right for these young people. In many countries, access to these services is limited when a young person leaves paediatric care, and again requires advocacy from adult clinicians.

3.5. *Progressive Health Issues*

Progressive health issues include:

3.5.1. *Orthopaedic and musculoskeletal*

Progression through puberty and subsequent ageing is associated with residual (from childhood) and acquired musculoskeletal deformities. Spinal stenosis and spinal cord compression may appear. Signs and symptoms are often put down to ageing and neither adequately investigated nor managed. Loss of physical function and alterations in sphincter function deserve thorough evaluation as failure to diagnose and manage can significantly impact on health status and QOL. Mobility may decrease, chronic pain and contractures emerge, and osteoporosis and pathological fractures occur. Thorough and regular evaluation and management is vital to minimise loss of physical function and independence.

3.5.2. *Seizures*

Seizures may present at any age. Evaluation (or re-evaluation) and investigation of epilepsy management by an adult neurologist should be mandatory in late adolescence/early adulthood. The balance of seizure control, medication side effects, and QOL is a delicate one. The interactions of various medications and effects on other systems, for example anticonvulsants and bone health, need proactive management.

3.5.3. *Nutrition*

Under-nutrition, or over-nutrition with weight gain causing further deterioration in or impairment of physical health, may present in adolescence or adulthood. Tailored investigations and management often significantly improve QOL. Access to food via the parent/carer and use of food as a reward or comfort is an important factor in obesity in this population. Undernutrition may result if the young person does not receive the necessary assistance at mealtimes.

3.6. *Summary*

A smooth transition from multidisciplinary paediatric health, educational, and psychosocial services to hospital and/or community based adult services which provide medical, nursing, allied health, and vocational professionals will result in improved health and QOL outcomes for the adolescent and young adult with CP. The lack of skilled and knowledgeable staff about condition specific management may have to be faced. Decisions based on size or chronological age rather than developmental stage may result in young people being admitted to or placed in inappropriate environments. Medication errors can be common due to size discrepancy as adult doses may be applied according to age. The lack of suitably sized equipment is common in adult hospitals for young people who have disorders of growth associated with developmental disability. Based on chronological age, families may be excluded from communication with the health care teams, which can affect engagement and ongoing care within the adult service.

The pivotal role of the general practitioner or primary care physician as case manager, the evolving role of clinical nurse specialists, and the need for development of adult physician training programs with a developmental disability focus have been recognised in a number of countries. Faculties of health and social science also have an increasing focus on physical and intellectual disability, thus producing a work force with knowledge and expertise. Practical clinical experience is vital. Disability Medicine fits well into the curriculum for adult rehabilitation specialist training. Those who have trained in Rehabilitation Medicine have a clear understanding of consequences of loss of function, therapy options and equipment needs.

4. Down Syndrome

DS is the commonest identifiable cause of intellectual disability. Overall, DS occurs in 1 in 800 live births, but this reduces to 1 in 400 at a maternal age of 35 years onwards. Over 90% have Trisomy 21 with the remainder having mosaicism or translocation. The level of ID follows a bell shaped curve as for the normal population, with a shift to left.

4.1. *Puberty and Adolescence*

Puberty tends to occur at the same age as for the general population. Females often have regular menstrual cycles, but may have difficulty coping with menstruation (Chapter 50). While females have been considered to have sub-fertility, there are documented cases of pregnancy. Low birth weight, stillbirth, and a higher rate of congenital anomalies (particularly cardiac) are seen in DS pregnancies. Males may have cryptorchidism, small testicles, azospermia or oligospermia and reduced testosterone levels. There are however a few cases of confirmed fertility in DS males. Both males and females need contraceptive advice appropriate to their cognitive level and to their lifestyle, as well as how to reduce the risks of sexually transmitted infections with regular condom use. Counsellors expert in ID and sexuality are particularly needed, as young people with DS are usually highly sociable and engage in many activities which may place them at risk.

4.2. *Specific Health Issues and Associations*

These include:

- Thyroid dysfunction (hypo- or hyperthyroidism) in 30%.
- Congenital heart defects in 30% — most commonly septal defects.
- Epilepsy in 30% (may present at any age).
- Visual and auditory impairments.

- Gastrointestinal anomalies include duodenal atresia, Hirschprung's disease, coeliac disease, and gastro–oesophageal reflux disease.
- Obesity in DS increases with age. Diet and exercise programs and participation in organised sport is encouraged. Surveillance for Type 2 diabetes mellitus should be part of routine assessment.
- Obstructive sleep apnoea is common as a result of muscle hypotonia and facial dysmorphism, and this may be the reason for sleep disturbance.
- Immunodeficiency and skin disorders.
- Increased risk of leukaemia, acute myeloid and lymphoblastic, compared to age matched population.
- Depression and other mental health disorders.
- Atlanto-axial instability and ligamentous laxity have an increased incidence in Down syndrome with ageing. Any spinal cord symptom, such as loss of mobility, hand dysfunction, or sphincter problems necessitates immediate investigation.
- Early onset of cognitive decline, most often Alzheimer's type dementia.
- Premature menopause.

A planned annual screening is necessary to manage these associations adequately.

4.3. *Mental Health and Emotional Well-being*

The prevalence of a psychiatric disorder in people with DS is around 40%, twice that of the general population. The physical and emotional changes in adolescence are coupled with major lifestyle changes together with social and environmental changes. These include a move from school to vocational training and/or meaningful employment, changes in recreation and sporting options, and changes in family dynamics. Transition from the paediatric health service to the adult health system will require clear coordination but there is no empirical evidence for what works best. All these conspire to predispose the young person with DS to mental health issues, as they are likely to miss the support and social aspects of paediatric care.

Self-talk, imaginary friends, and fantasy are all common in young people with DS. However an increase or change in frequency, and a change in context or tone may indicate a developing problem. Often these symptoms are dismissed in the adult system.

Depression (with or without psychotic features) is often present in adolescence at a similar rate to that of the general population but often with quite different symptomatology in DS. *Bipolar disorder* may also be present in DS, possibly more often in those with *less* intellectual impairment. Treatment usually requires an anti-depressant and anti-psychotic medication as well as significant psychosocial support. *Anxiety disorders and obsessive compulsive disorder* both appear to be more common in DS, approximately 2–3 times that of the general population. These conditions require both long term support and counselling, and often long term medications.

5. Conclusion

The young person with a disability faces not only the usual challenges of adolescence but significant psychosocial and health issues for which appropriate services are still evolving. Many health issues of middle and old age present much earlier in this population. Multidisciplinary health clinics, appropriate psychosocial and community services, funding and targeted professional training programs need expansion and funding to ensure optimal health and QOL outcomes for this population.

References

American Academy for Cerebral Palsy and Developmental Medicine. (2007) Session E: Developmental pediatrics. *Dev Med Child Neurol* **49**(111): 21–24.

Australian Academy of Cerebral Palsy and Developmental Medicine. (2010) Abstracts of the 5th Biennial Conference of the Australasian Academy of Cerebral Palsy & Developmental Medicine. *Dev Med Child Neurol* **52**(2): 1–66.

Dicianno BE, Kurowski BG, Yang JMJ, Chancellor MB, Bejjani GK, Fairman AD, Lewis N, Sotirake J. (2008) Rehabilitation and medical management of the adult with spina bifida. *Am J Phys Med Rehabil* **87**(12): 1027–1050.

Friedman D, Holmbeck GN, Delucia C, Jandasek B, Zebracki K. (2009) Trajectories of autonomy development across the adolescent transition in children with spina bifida. *Rehabil Psychol* **54**(1): 16–27.

Goldstein M, Bax M *et al.* (2007) The definition and classification of cerebral palsy. *Dev Med Child Neurol* **49**(109): 1–44.

Mitchell LE, Adzick NS, Melchionne J, Pasquariello PS, Sutton LN, Whitehead AS. (2004) Spina bifida. *Lancet* **364**(9448): 1885–1895.

O'loughlin EV, Somerville HM, Somerville ER. (2009) Dealing with multisystem disease in people with a developmental disability. *Med J Aust* **190**(11): 616–617.

Prasher VP. (1999) Down syndrome and thyroid disorders: A review. *Downs Syndr Res Pract* **6**(1): 25–42.

Rosenbaum PL, Livingston MH, Palisano RJ, Galuppi BE, Russell DJ. (2007) Quality of life and health-related quality of life of adolescents with cerebral palsy. *Dev Med Child Neurol* **49**(7): 516–521.

Rowe DE, Jadhav AL. (2008) Care of the adolescent with spina bifida. *Pediatr Clin North Am* **55**(6): 1359–1374.

Chapter 23

Key Issues in Adolescent Obesity

Shirley Alexander, Alison G Hoppin and Louise A Baur

1. Introduction

Obesity is a major global public health concern, affecting all ages and increasing the risk of developing chronic illnesses such as Type 2 diabetes, cardiovascular disease, and certain cancers. Adolescence, a time of significant physiological and psychological change, is a vulnerable period for the development of obesity. Adolescent weight tracks strongly into adulthood; thus, it is not only vital that adolescents affected by obesity are appropriately treated, but also that preventive measures are promoted during this susceptible phase of growth.

2. Definitions

2.1. *Body Mass Index*

Obesity is defined as excessive body fat in relation to height to the degree that it may have an adverse effect on health. As it is not feasible to use direct measures of total body fat in clinical practice, BMI (weight/height^2; kg/m^2) is the widely accepted indirect measure. BMI varies dramatically during childhood and adolescence. Unlike in adults, there is insufficient evidence in children and adolescents to provide an absolute definition of BMI cutpoints that denote health-related overweight. A range of different definitions for overweight and obesity have arisen, creating some confusion in the literature. These include:

The BMI-for-age and sex percentile charts developed by the US Centers for Disease Control are recommended for clinical use in several countries to define degree of adiposity in children and adolescents (2–20 years). Overweight is defined as a BMI between the 85th and 95th percentile for age and sex, and obesity defined as a BMI ≥95th percentile for age and sex.

In 2000, the International Obesity Taskforce published a table of age- and sex specific cut-points based upon a compilation of nationally representative cross-sectional growth studies from a number of countries. The cut-points for overweight and obesity at 18 years accord with those used by the WHO to denote adult obesity. This definition is only for epidemiological use.

Several countries have developed their own BMI-for-age growth charts and these can be used clinically in order to chart and monitor an individual's BMI. In 2007, the WHO published the Growth Reference for 5–19 year olds.

2.2. *Waist Circumference and Waist-to-Height Ratio*

Waist circumference measured at the midpoint between the lower costal margin and the iliac crest, may be used as a proxy for abdominal obesity. In adolescents, waist circumference is strongly correlated with markers for comorbidities such as adverse lipid and glucose profiles, and hypertension. There are no internationally accepted criteria for high- or low-risk waist circumference in the adolescent age group; however, an adolescent whose waist circumference is within the adult at-risk range (men >94 cm, women >80 cm) would be considered at substantial risk of complications of obesity. Waist-to-height ratio can also be calculated: a ratio >0.5 is a strong predictor of metabolic complications of obesity for those aged six years or over. This measure is easy to calculate, does not require plotting, and is not sex specific.

3. Prevalence

Adolescent obesity prevalence trends have increased markedly since the 1970s. Rates vary depending on region, ethnicity and socioeconomic status. In Australia, one in four adolescents is overweight or obese, with higher rates in Indigenous young people and in those from more socially deprived areas. In Europe, prevalence ranges from 5% (Netherlands) to 25% (Malta), and in the US rates are as high as 35%. The prevalence is much lower in the Asia-Pacific and sub-Saharan Africa regions. Prevalence of abdominal obesity in adolescents is also high, with rates ranging from 41%–52% (depending on cut-points used) and no clear sex differentiation. Recent data from Europe, Asia, and North America suggest a levelling of prevalence rates over the past 10 years.

4. Aetiology and Risk Factors

Obesity ultimately results from a chronic energy imbalance, with energy intake exceeding energy expenditure. However, the aetiology of obesity is complex with interactions between genetic, metabolic, environmental, and behavioural factors, all of which contribute to varying degrees.

4.1. *Genetic Factors*

Single-gene mutations, such as congenital leptin deficiency, pro-opiomelanocortin deficiency and melanocortin 4 receptor mutations are very rare causes of obesity. Genetic syndromes with obesity as a manifestation are also extremely rare. The commonest is Prader-Willi syndrome which is generally diagnosed in early childhood. The most likely genetic cause of common obesity is polygenic, requiring favourable environmental conditions for full expression. Heritable factors are responsible for 45%–75% of the inter-individual variations in adiposity. The precise mechanisms and contributions to the development of obesity are yet to be ascertained.

Epigenetics and metabolic programming: there is increasing evidence that nutritional and environmental influences or exposure at critical periods in the development of a child can predispose to obesity and metabolic disease in later life. Gestational diabetes, maternal obesity, intrauterine growth retardation, and high birth weight are all associated with an increased risk of later obesity.

4.2. Risk Factors

4.2.1. Ethnicity

Hispanics, African Americans, South Asians, Indigenous and First Nation groups, Maoris and Pacific Islanders, and those of Mediterranean and Middle-Eastern descent appear to have greater susceptibility to developing obesity.

4.2.2. Screen time

Time spent watching television is directly related to the prevalence of obesity, is associated with an increased incidence of new cases of obesity as well as a decrease in remission rates of established obesity, and is a significant predictor of overweight and obesity in children and adolescents. Having a TV in the bedroom is an even greater obesity risk. Potential mechanisms for the association include increased exposure to food marketing, increased snacking on energy-dense food and drink whilst watching TV, displacement of physical activity, and/or reduction in basal metabolic rate. Evidence for associations between other small screen recreation activities and obesity is less well-established.

4.2.3. Sweetened beverages, nutritional intake, and eating patterns

Adolescent eating habits such as an increased frequency of eating away from home, an increased consumption of nutrient-poor, energy-dense foods, increased snacking behaviours, and inadequate fruit and vegetable consumption may all contribute to excessive weight gain. Irregular eating patterns, particularly skipping breakfast, are strongly associated with overweight and obesity. There is also an association between increased consumption of sugar-sweetened drinks and obesity.

4.2.4. Sleep duration

Shortened sleep duration is associated with obesity and insulin resistance. Potential underlying mechanisms include neuro-endocrine imbalance in leptin and ghrelin leading to alterations in appetite control, or an increased opportunity to eat while staying up late engaged in sedentary activities.

4.2.5. *Viral factors*

Recent evidence linking the presence of human adenovirus 36-specific antibodies to the prevalence and severity of obesity in children and adolescents raises the possibility of triggering or exacerbation by exposure to a virus.

4.2.6. *Environmental pollutants*

Endocrine disruptor chemicals (environmental pollutants with hormone-like activity that can disrupt endocrine signalling pathways such as phytoestrogens, bisphenol A and diethylstilbestrol) are postulated to contribute to the development of chronic diseases including obesity and T2DM.

4.2.7. *Endocrine disorders*

Endocrine disorders such as hypothyroidism, growth hormone deficiency, hypercortisolism and hypothalamic lesions may lead to obesity, but represent less than 1% of cases of adolescent obesity.

4.2.8. *Medications*

Glucocorticoids, anti-psychotics (particularly risperidone and olanzapine), anti-epileptics (sodium valproate), and insulin may contribute to weight gain. Short courses of glucocorticoids are less likely to have an effect on weight gain, and alternate day steroids for long-term use may reduce weight gain.

5. Obesity Complications

The health implications of obesity result from its medical and psychological comorbidities. Clinically important comorbidities of obesity seen during adolescence include the following:

5.1. *Obstructive Sleep Apnoea*

This occurs in about 5%–10% of children with obesity, and in up to 90% of obese adolescents with habitual snoring. When severe, obstructive sleep apnoea can cause right heart strain (cor pulmonale) and neuro–behavioural problems, including attention deficit disorder and poor school performance.

5.2. *Insulin Resistance*

Adolescents with obesity tend to be insulin resistant, particularly if there is a family history of T2DM, and the situation is further exacerbated by the normal insulin resistance of puberty. Impaired glucose tolerance or raised fasting glucose levels are seen in 10%–20% of adolescents with obesity. The overall prevalence of T2DM during adolescence is 1%–4% in most populations, with rates being much higher in certain racial and ethnic groups, including Native American, African American, and Hispanic populations. Fasting insulin levels are often elevated in children with obesity. However, measurements of fasting insulin are not sufficiently correlated with more precise measures of insulin resistance to be a good predictor of T2DM risk. Measurements of HbA1c, fasting plasma glucose, or an oral glucose tolerance test can be used as measures of diabetes risk (pre-diabetes) or diabetes mellitus, as shown in Table 1.

Table 1: Laboratory assessment for pre-diabetes and diabetes mellitus (American Diabetes Association 2011).

	Pre-diabetes	**Diabetes mellitus**
Fasting plasma glucose.	5.6–6.9 mmol/L (100–125 mg/dL).	≥7.0 mmol/L (126 mg/dL).
Hemoglobin A1c.	5.7%–6.4%.	≥6.5%.
Oral glucose tolerance test, plasma glucose level 2 hours after 75 gm glucose load.	7.8–11 mmol/L (140–199 mg/dL).	≥11.1 mmol/L (200 mg/dL).

5.3. *Hypertension*

Left ventricular hypertrophy and hypertension are significantly more common in obese adolescents, with the prevalence of hypertension increasing progressively with BMI. Adolescents with obesity are three times more likely to be hypertensive than those in lower weight ranges.

5.4. *Dyslipidaemia*

Up to 50% of obese adolescents may have some degree of dyslipidaemia. The most common lipid abnormality in overweight and obese adolescents is low high-density lipoprotein, but elevations of low-density lipoprotein and triglycerides are also associated with obesity, as these are in adults.

5.5. *Cardiovascular Disease*

The insulin resistance, dyslipidaemia, and hypertension that are associated with obesity during adolescence are all predictors of cardiovascular disease in adulthood. Higher BMI during adolescence is associated with coronary heart disease during adulthood, even within the range of BMIs that is considered normal during adolescence. Adolescents with obesity are more likely to develop early atherosclerotic changes in the aorta and cardiac vasculature and decreased arterial distensibility.

5.6. *Fatty Liver Disease*

Non-alcoholic fatty liver disease comprises infiltration of fats into the liver (hepatic steatosis), to fatty liver with inflammation (steatohepatitis), to steatohepatitis with significant fibrosis. The prevalence and severity of NAFLD varies by race, and is present in 10%–75% of obese adolescents. NAFLD is typically asymptomatic and often discovered because of a mild elevation of alanine aminotransferase. The natural history of paediatric NAFLD is not yet established, but current evidence suggests that a minority of adolescents with NAFLD develop progressive liver disease, leading to liver failure or transplantation, and this is most likely in patients with advanced fibrosis at diagnosis. Weight loss is the only established treatment for NAFLD and is generally effective.

5.7. *Polycystic Ovary Syndrome*

PCOS is associated with obesity, insulin resistance, and other elements of the metabolic syndrome and should be excluded in overweight female adolescents (Chapter 50).

5.8. *Other Physical Comorbidities*

These include tibia vara (Blount disease), slipped capital femoral epiphyses, gastro–oesophageal reflux disease, asthma, and idiopathic intracranial hypertension (pseudotumour cerebri).

5.9. *Depression and Social Exclusion*

The most common comorbidity in adolescent obesity is psychosocial. In most modern cultures, adolescents who are overweight or obese are confronted by overt or covert bias and social exclusion, even within the medical community. In part as a result of these social challenges, depression and poor self-esteem are common among overweight and obese adolescents, affecting up to 20%–30% of those with obesity. Conversely, there is some evidence that depression leads to obesity.

6. Clinical Assessment

The main purpose of the clinical assessment is to identify treatable causes of and complications of obesity and to identify underlying lifestyle and psychosocial factors that led to, maintain and/or act as barriers to the treatment of obesity.

6.1. *History*

When assessing an adolescent, interview the young person both with and without the parent/main carer present. This gives the young person the opportunity to be open, have a sense of recognition as an individual and highlight his/her concerns or priorities which may be very different from those of their parents. Be alert for symptoms of obesity complications.

6.2. *Physical Examination*

Serial measurements of BMI and waist circumference are the most useful anthropometric measures and can be used to monitor change over time. Adolescents with simple obesity may have generalised or abdominal obesity. Warning signs of secondary causes of obesity such as hypothyroidism, hypercortisolism and Prader-Willi syndrome include short stature, dysmorphic features and developmental delay. A graded assessment schedule is shown below in Table 2.

Table 2:   Evaluation for comorbidities of obesity in adolescents.

Test	Indications
Lipid profile.* Fasting glucose and insulin. +/− Haemoglobin A1c Alanine aminotransferase (ALT). Aspartate aminotransferase (AST).	All adolescents with obesity (>10 years, repeat every two years). (*also for overweight).
Blood pressure.	All adolescents with overweight or obesity.
Sleep study (polysomnogram).	Moderate to severe obesity and any symptoms suggestive of sleep apnoea (habitual snoring, mouth breathing, nocturnal enuresis).
Testosterone and sex hormone binding globulin (SHBG) or free testosterone.	Girls with abnormal menses or hirsutism.
Glucose tolerance test.	If fasting glucose >5.6 mmol/L, or Haemoglobin A1c >5.7%, or symptoms of diabetes.
Depression screen.	All adolescents with obesity.

7. Management

If left untreated, an obese adolescent is likely to become an obese adult with the increased risks of obesity-related comorbidities. Combined behavioural lifestyle intervention programs produce significant short and long term clinically meaningful weight reductions in adolescents.

General principles of management include:

- Accurate assessment of obesity and its complications.
- Defining treatment goals according to what is important to the young person and supported by parent/carer.
- Age appropriate intervention: consider consultation with the young person separately as well as with the parent/carer.
- Family involvement: encouraging behaviour change for all the family.
- Long term changes in diet, physical activity, and sedentary behaviour: reducing energy intake, encouraging healthier nutrition choices including drinking water instead of sweetened beverages, increasing activity levels by incorporating activity into daily living as well as increasing sporting activities and reducing screen time.

Although parental involvement is important, and parents are still the gatekeepers to the home food environment and enforcers of rules around screen time and activity, treatment success depends on engaging the adolescent with the process including motivation to change. This may be achieved using skills and strategies such as motivational interviewing, behaviour modification (via stimulus control) and goal setting. For some, weight-loss may not be the main goal but rather an improvement in self-esteem, and through this a sense of belonging in relation to their peers, as their ultimate desired outcome.

Desirable outcomes include an improvement in adiposity demonstrated by a slowing of weight gain, weight maintenance, or weight loss, and a reduction in waist circumference or waist-to-height ratio and reduction in medical and psychosocial comorbidities of obesity including reduced requirement for pharmacological treatment of complications, better peer relationships and improved family functioning.

7.1. *Conventional Approach*: *Lifestyle Interventions*

7.1.1. *Dietary management*

Eating habits become established early in childhood. Unhealthy dietary habits may become more prominent in the adolescent who is developing greater autonomy in food choices, along with increases in personal income. Thus the emphasis should be on developing the skills and knowledge to enable healthier dietary choices. Given a choice of prescriptive or non-prescriptive meal plans, adolescents appear to prefer the former. There is no evidence linking healthy eating plans aimed at weight loss with the development of an eating disorder. *Key dietary interventions* include eating breakfast, regular meals (not grazing) and eating meals at a table rather than in front of the television, reducing sugar-sweetened beverages, reducing portion size, and increasing vegetable and fruit intake.

7.1.2. *Physical activity and sedentary behaviour management*

Targeting sedentary behaviour may be as beneficial as aiming to increase physical activity. Furthermore, increasing incidental activity may be easier, and cheaper to implement than increasing organised activities. Choosing alternative active transport to and from school, taking the stairs instead of the lift, helping with household chores, and spending time outdoors with peers, can all contribute to healthier lifestyle habits. Encourage family activities, with parents acting as role models. Set rules/regulations around screen time. If contemplating an organised sport, find an activity that the young person enjoys and that fits with the family budget. Self-consciousness (wearing sports gear or having attained less physical prowess) and joint pain may limit physical activity.

7.2. *Non-Conventional Approaches*

For the majority of overweight or obese adolescents, conventional lifestyle interventions will form the foundation for treatment. However, in adolescents who are more severely affected, including those with obesity-related complications, adjuncts to lifestyle-modification programs may be considered to enhance weight loss attempts.

7.2.1. *Very low energy diets*

VLEDs provide as little as 800 kcal/day. Such diets may be used as partial supplementation, with the inclusion of normal food items. If VLEDs are used alone, they must be formulated to be nutritionally complete and provide a low carbohydrate (50 g/day of glucose) intake to induce ketosis. Evidence for use of VLEDs in adolescents is limited. Concerns as to whether such energy restriction may affect linear growth seem unfounded; however, the age of the young person and length of time of intervention should be taken into account when considering VLEDs. Problems with VLEDs include difficulties adhering to such a restricted eating pattern and palatability of the meal supplements.

7.2.2. *Pharmacotherapy*

Anti-obesity medications may have a role in the treatment of adolescent obesity, as an adjunct to a comprehensive lifestyle intervention program. Pharmacotherapy should be trialled prior to bariatric surgery, if such an option is being considered. Currently, there are few recommended medications for use in adolescents, and in many countries the use will be 'off label'.

Orlistat, a gastric and pancreatic lipase inhibitor, may be prescribed (120 mg three times a day with meals) under medical supervision. It is often not tolerated because of flatulence, steatorrhoea, faecal urgency, and faecal incontinence. Absorption of fat soluble vitamins A, D, E and K is reduced, and supplementation with a multivitamin is recommended.

Metformin may be prescribed in obese adolescents with clinical insulin resistance, including PCOS. When prescribing metformin, dosage is gradually increased, commencing with 500 mg daily, to a maximum of 2 g, and is taken with meals. Slow or extended release preparations are available that may assist with compliance and reduce the potential side effects (abdominal pain and diarrhoea). Patients should be monitored for potential Vitamin B12 malabsorption.

7.2.3. *Bariatric surgery*

Bariatric surgical procedures are either restrictive (gastric banding, sleeve gastrectomy) or malabsorptive (gastric bypass, biliopancreatic diversion), although that latter group also includes a degree of restriction. In adults, bariatric surgery can be highly effective, with significant and sustained reductions in BMI, and either resolution or significant improvement in obesity-related complications. Neuro-endocrine mechanisms play a role, as patients report a subjective decrease in appetite as well as an increase in postprandial satiety. The first randomised controlled trial in adolescents of laparoscopic adjustable gastric banding versus lifestyle intervention was published in 2010 and demonstrated a mean weight loss in the banding group of 34.6 kg compared with 3.6 kg in the lifestyle intervention group. The metabolic profile and quality of life were also improved, and thus bariatric surgery may be a considered option when non-surgical interventions have been unsuccessful. Seven of the 25 patients randomised in the surgical arm required revision procedures. Baur and Fitzgerald provide a summary of inclusion and exclusion criteria for surgery. Importantly, it is advisable that surgery should only be carried out by units with suitable expertise and facilities, after appropriate assessment and counselling of the young person and family, and in conjunction with attendance at a comprehensive weight management service to assist in implementation of lifestyle interventions pre- and post-operatively. Bariatric surgery is limited by cost and availability in the public health sector.

7.3. *Specific Treatment of Comorbidities*

The treatment of OSA consists of lifestyle intervention for weight loss, with the addition of tonsillectomy if tonsils are large, and continuous positive airways pressure ventilation during sleep. Compliance with CPAP is often low in adolescents but if used consistently has been shown to improve school performance.

The first line of treatment for insulin resistance is weight loss and increased physical activity. Metformin is second line and discussed in Section 7.2.2. The first-line treatment for PCOS is lifestyle modification. A 5%–7% weight loss may improve oligomenorrhoea. Other treatments for PCOS are discussed in Chapter 50. Orthopaedic intervention for slipped capital femoral epiphyses or Blount disease will be required. Treatment for gastro–oesophageal reflux, asthma, and severe depression are similar to that in adolescents of healthy body weight, but may be more refractory to treatment until weight loss is achieved.

8. Transition Planning

As obesity is a chronic disorder, it is important to consider, in a timely, coordinated fashion, transitioning strategies to adult services for the young person who is developing independence and managing their own care. This is particularly pertinent when the young person has not yet attained a healthy weight or has obesity-related complications requiring involvement of multiple services. The transition to young adulthood is a risk time for further weight gain due to:

- Reduction in physical activity and organised sports after leaving school.
- Share house or college campus living, and more meals in general eaten away from the family home.
- Increased alcohol intake.
- Less discretionary time for exercise if in full employment.
- Marriage and childbirth.

Clinical services for the management of obesity in adults generally focus on older age groups with established comorbidity. In addition, little research has been done on the optimal weight management approaches for young adults. Their lifestyle is much closer in type to that of adolescents, and concern about future ill health often remains low or non-existent.

9. Prevention Strategies

Public health prevention measures are essential to curb the obesity epidemic. Prevention strategies will be required at many levels to address the numerous elements contributing to the development of obesity. Therefore, coordinated efforts at an individual, local, national, and international level will be required. Clinicians have a role to play at the family level, by encouraging healthy lifestyle practices in families where there is a history of obesity and/or the metabolic syndrome. They should be very clear that puberty and adolescence are a risk time for weight gain. Some obesity prevention strategies that clinicians may choose to advocate for in their communities are:

- Regulation of the amount and type of food marketing directed to children and adolescents.

- Regulation of the types of food and drinks provided at schools via canteens and vending machines.
- Regulations limiting the type and number of fast food outlets within the immediate school environment.
- Development of school curricula encouraging healthy eating and physical activity.
- Provision of easily accessible recreation facilities such as gyms, parks and swimming pools.
- Availability of low cost fruit and vegetables in lower income areas.
- Provision of safe and affordable public transport.
- Urban planning that provides safe and walkable neighbourhoods.

References

Barr-Anderson DJ, Van Den Berg P, Neumark-Sztainer D, Story M. (2008) Characteristics associated with older adolescents who have a television in their bedrooms. *Pediatrics* **121**(4): 718–724.

Barshop NJ, Sirlin CB, Schwimmer JB, Lavine, JE. (2008) Review article: Epidemiology, pathogenesis and potential treatments of paediatric non-alcoholic fatty liver disease. *Aliment Pharmacol Ther* **28**(1): 13–24.

Baur LA, Fitzgerald DA. (2010) Recommendations for bariatric surgery in adolescents in Australia and New Zealand. *J Paediatr Child Health* **46**(12): 704–707.

Beebe DW, Byars KC. (2011) Adolescents with obstructive sleep apnea adhere poorly to positive airway pressure (PAP), but PAP users show improved attention and school performance. *PLoS ONE [Electronic Resource]* **6**(3): e16924.

Garnett SP, Baur LA, Cowell CT. (2008) Waist-to-height ratio: A simple option for determining excess central adiposity in young people. *Int J Obes* **32**(6): 1028–1030.

Greydanus DE, Bricker LA, Feucht C. (2011) Pharmacotherapy for obese adolescents. *Pediatr Clin North Am* **58**(1): 139–153.

Lee JM. (2008) Why young adults hold the key to assessing the obesity epidemic in children. *Arch Pediatr Adolesc Med* **162**(7): 682–687.

Niemeier HM, Raynor HA, Lloyd-Richardson EE, Rogers ML, Wing RR. (2006) Fast food consumption and breakfast skipping: Predictors of weight gain from adolescence to adulthood in a nationally representative sample. *J Adolesc Health* **39**(6): 842–849.

O'Brien PE, Sawyer SM, Laurie C, Brown WA, Skinner S, Veit F, Paul E, Burton PR, Mcgrice M, Anderson M, Dixon JB. (2010) Laparoscopic adjustable gastric banding in severely obese adolescents: A randomized trial. *JAMA* **303**(6): 519–526.

Sjoberg RL, Nilsson KW, Leppert J. (2005) Obesity, shame, and depression in school-aged children: A population-based study. *Pediatrics* **116**(3): e389–392.

Truby H, Baxter K, Elliott S, Warren J, Davies P, Batch J. (2011) Adolescents seeking weight management: Who is putting their hand up and what are they looking for? *J Paediatr Child Health* **47**(1–2): 2–4.

Chapter 24

Adolescents with Eating Disorders

Jorge L Pinzon, Gail Anderson and Simon Clarke

The incidence of all eating disorders is increasing, due to both a true increase and increased ascertainment. This chapter addresses eating disorders in the second decade. Over the last 20 years, there has been an increased recognition of the problem in 8–13 year olds.

1. Epidemiology

The point prevalence of anorexia nervosa is approximately 0.5%. Lifetime prevalence rates of 1.9% for full AN and 2.4% for partial AN have been reported in an Australian female twin cohort. The community point prevalence of bulimia nervosa is higher in adult women (1%), not nearly as high in adolescents and rarely seen in childhood. More commonly, there is a progression along a continuum from AN to BN as the patient gains or loses weight. The lifetime prevalence of BN is 3% of women and 90% of people suffering from eating disorders are female. Eating disorder not otherwise specified point prevalence is up to 5% of women, of whom over half have binge eating disorder. The prevalence of body dissatisfaction (Chapter 4) and other disordered eating syndromes is much higher.

2. Classification of Adolescent Eating Disorders and Disturbances

The two main classification schemes which have been used to diagnose eating disorders in children and young adolescents are the International Classification of Diseases and the Diagnostic and Statistical Manual for Mental Disorders which are shown in Tables 1 and 2. A potentially more suitable set of diagnostic criteria for eating disturbances in younger adolescents is the Great Ormond Street Children's Hospital classification shown in Table 3.

Table 1:   International Classification of Diseases — 10th edition (2004).

- Anorexia nervosa (F50.0).
- Atypical anorexia nervosa (F50.1).
- Bulimia nervosa (F50.2).
- Atypical bulimia nervosa (F50.3).
- Overeating associated with other psychological disturbances (F50.4).
- Vomiting associated with other psychological disturbances (F50.5).
- Other eating disorders (F50.8).
- Eating disorder, unspecified (F50.9).
- Feeding disorders of infancy and childhood.

Table 2:   Diagnostic and Statistical Manual for mental disorders — IV revised edition (2000).

- Anorexia nervosa (307.1):
    - Restrictive type.
    - Binge eating/purging type.
- Bulimia nervosa (307.51):
    - Purging type.
    - Non-purging type.
- Eating disorder not otherwise specified (307.50).
- Feeding disorders of infancy and early childhood (307.59):
    - Pica (307.52).
    - Rumination disorder (307.53).

Table 3:   Great Ormond Street classification.

- Anorexia nervosa (and atypical or subclinical forms).
- Bulimia nervosa (and atypical or subclinical forms).
- Food avoidance emotional disorder (FAED).
- Selective eating.
- Restrictive eating.
- Food refusal.
- Specific fear or phobia leading to avoidance of eating.
- Pervasive refusal syndrome.
- Appetite loss secondary to depression.

3. Developmental Perspectives

Prior to the onset of puberty, 20% of those diagnosed with an eating disorder are male, as opposed to 8% post puberty. Females are more vulnerable as they enter puberty with the corresponding pressures on body image, combined with dietary restraint and disordered eating behaviour. Younger adolescents tend to decompensate more rapidly, possibly due to physiological factors related to their linear growth and pubertal development. Sometimes younger adolescents are classified as partial AN by accepting at least one missing criteria from the DSM-IV, but they still have similar medical compromise to those with full AN. Their weight loss may be actually faster than those with full AN.

Malnutrition, a common hallmark of eating disorders, is harmful during the vulnerable period of adolescent brain development (Chapter 2). Cognitive changes occur with acute malnutrition of any aetiology, including reduced ability to complete tasks and obsessions around food. Significant brain change has been well documented during active AN, with reduced grey matter on MRI, particularly in temporo–parietal areas, when compared to age matched controls. These changes may not completely reverse with recovery. It has been suggested that these differences may play a role in causality since these brain areas are also involved with image of self.

4. Spectrum of Eating Disorders in Adolescents

4.1. *Anorexia Nervosa*

Young people with AN are characterised by a relentless pursuit of thinness, resulting in significant (25%) weight loss or a failure to gain weight during growth, a refusal to maintain a normal body weight and an extreme fear of gaining weight or becoming fat. There may be primary or secondary amenorrhoea present. AN is further divided into the binge eating/purging type or the restrictive type.

4.2. *Bulimia Nervosa*

BN occurs more frequently in the older adolescent and young adults. The features of BN are regular binge eating, occurring on average twice weekly for three months, together with regular use of extreme weight control measures including purging, fasting or excessive exercise to counteract the perceived and feared effects of overeating. Body weight in BN is usually in the normal to overweight range. Both AN and BN have, as part of their diagnostic criteria, an intense preoccupation with weight or shape issues as an expression of self worth.

4.3. *Eating Disorder Not Otherwise Specified*

EDNOS is a heterogeneous group that includes binge eating and other syndromes where the criteria for either AN or BN fail to be totally met. The greater majority of eating disordered patients fall within the EDNOS category and this can be problematic when attempting to assess prognostic outcome. Consider the obese adolescent who starves in order to lose weight rapidly, whose weight is now in the normal weight range but who is physiologically and medically compromised due to the rapidity of weight loss. Whilst not meeting the criteria for AN, this patient must be identified as EDNOS which provides little prognostic information.

5. Aetiology

Eating disorders have a significant heritability. Twin studies estimate that 55%–83% of the variance in AN, BN and Binge Eating Disorder is accounted for by genetic factors. No single gene, or group of genes with large effect have yet been identified as responsible for eating disorders. Rather it appears that a number of genes of moderate effect interact with environmental factors. Genetic linkage suggests associations with genes involved in the production of serotonin. Brain derived neurotropic factor and opioid systems may also contribute. The underlying endophenotype in eating disorders is one of an anxiety disorder which when subjected to various stresses leads to increasing perfectionism and starvation. The secondary effects of starvation then induce or exacerbate depression, anxiety, and obsessional thinking.

6. Prevention of Eating Disorders

Prevention is important because of the physical and psychological consequences, and the fact that established eating disorders are complex and difficult to treat and can have poor remission rates. There is often difficulty in accessing treatment coupled with an increasing incidence in younger age groups. Prevention programs would also likely benefit those with lesser degrees of disordered eating.

6.1. *Targeted Prevention*

The current evidence favours programs aimed at high-risk female participants. However programs may be better directed at mixed sex younger adolescents. Body dissatisfaction is emerging at an increasingly younger age in both sexes. Girls may benefit from boys understanding the result of weight related bullying, and involving both sexes might overcome the difficulty of identifying those at high risk given the high prevalence of abnormal attitudes and behaviours.

6.2. *Programs*

The ideal prevention program is interactive in style and focussed on student centred learning where critical thinking and content acquisition is enhanced. Perfectionism is only starting to reach its peak in 15 year olds and prevention programs may be best directed before or around this age.

Programs that teach media literacy may enable young people to effectively cope with the media messages being delivered, including those related to adolescent sexuality. A further challenge is to incorporate similar messages in obesity prevention programs, as the link between disordered eating and obesity is well established.

7. Assessment and Treatment of Eating Disorders

The assessment and management of eating disorders is best done by an experienced multidisciplinary team who have access to specialist inpatient, ambulatory care or community resources for ongoing management.

7.1. *Comorbid Medical Problems*

Medical problems associated with starvation or purging include

- Osteoporosis and amenorrhoea.
- Renal scarring and dehydration.
- Hair loss and other signs of protein calorie malnutrition including muscle wasting (cardiac and skeletal).
- Gastrointestinal bleeding.
- Bradycardia and other cardiac rhythm disturbances.
- Electrolyte disturbances (hypokalaemia, hypophosphataemia, hypomagnesaemia, and hypocalcaemia) may be present at diagnosis or *may occur as a consequence of refeeding*.
- Bone marrow suppression (anaemia, leucopaenia and thrombocytopaenia).

All of these changes largely revert with careful nutritional refeeding.

7.2. *Other Potential Medical Comorbidity*

There is a higher prevalence than expected of eating disorders in Type 1 diabetes. Patients may manipulate their insulin to produce weight loss and ketosis. Serious bacterial infection may occur with normal body temperature in patients with AN because of an impaired immune response. The secondary fatty liver of AN often results in abnormal liver function tests, which will resolve with weight gain.

7.3. *Comorbid Psychiatric Problems*

7.3.1. *Changes secondary to starvation*

These include increased anxiety, depression, irritability, and sleep disturbance. There are also cognitive changes with poor verbal memory and reduced attention span, as well as reduced alertness, comprehension, and judgment. Socially there is withdrawal, reduced sense of humour, feelings of social inadequacy, isolation, strained relationships and reduced sexual interest. The patient is preoccupied with food and meal planning, and has a tendency to hoard.

7.3.2. *Other psychiatric disorders*

Other psychiatric disorders may precede the development of the eating disorder including depression, anxiety, obsessive compulsive disorders, Asperger syndrome, post traumatic stress disorders or attention deficit disorders. The effects of starvation greatly exacerbate the depression and anxiety and make the patient more obsessive until nutritionally rehabilitated. The use of anti-depressants in the initial phase of the illness does not appear to be effective, perhaps because of the lack of serotonin substrate.

7.4. *Baseline Medical Investigations*

A full blood count, reticulocyte count, electrolytes, urea, creatinine, and liver function tests (including albumen), calcium, magnesium, and phosphorus should be done to assess the degree of metabolic disturbance. Fat soluble and water soluble vitamin levels may be indicated. LH, FSH and oestradiol levels will indicate the degree of hypothalamic suppression (Chapter 20). Thyroid function tests to exclude hyperthyroidism, dual energy X-ray absorptiometry for assessment of bone density and an ECG to exclude conduction abnormalities are all indicated.

7.5. *General Therapeutic Approaches*

The majority of adolescent patients will not require hospital admission and will be managed appropriately utilising medical management and Maudsley family based therapy in the case of AN. Psychological treatment for both inpatient and ambulatory care management may consist of cognitive behavioural therapy, interpersonal therapy, dialectical behaviour therapy, or specialist supportive clinical management. Ambulatory assessment and treatment teams are generally composed of a physician, psychiatrist, psychologist, nurse, social worker, and dietitian.

7.6. *Criteria for Hospital Admission*

The main reason for admission is medical instability as defined by any of the following: bradycardia (heart rate less than 50 beats per minute); hypotension (<80/40); ECG abnormalities such as a prolonged QTc interval >440 m sec; dehydration; hypothermia <35.5°C; significant electrolyte abnormalities; other critically abnormal pathology results; weight less than 75% of expected body weight in the presence or absence of medical instability. Comorbid medical problems such as Type 1 diabetes may lower the threshold for admission. Other criteria for admission are comorbid psychiatric problems that complicate ambulatory treatment, or severe family dysfunction or abuse.

7.7. *Inpatient Management*

Adolescents are best treated in dedicated adolescent wards, rather than being exposed to more chronic adult eating disordered patients with entrenched illness who are resistant to treatment. Adolescent teams will also be more experienced in the *earlier and more aggressive refeeding* and management required in this situation. The initial and invariable resistance should be met and countered by experienced staff with a clear rationale and care plan, including the objectives of the admission and the minimum healthy weight to be achieved prior to discharge. Both the parents and young person need reassurance throughout this process. The aim of admission should be a consistent weight gain of 1–1.5 kgs per week until at least 90% of expected weight is achieved. The closer the final discharge weight is to a minimum healthy, age appropriate BMI, the less the chance of readmissions.

7.7.1. *Acute medical management of the medically compromised patient*

The medically compromised adolescent who is bradycardic requires cardiac monitoring until the heart rate remains above 50 beats per minute, including overnight. Other initial objectives include the correction of hypothermia with judicious reheating (space blankets or overhead heaters), bed rest while hypotensive and adequate refeeding to reverse medical compromise.

7.7.2. *Refeeding*

Various regimens have been suggested. For the past 10 years at the Westmead Hospital campus in Australia, continous nasogastric tube feeding with a balanced carbohydrate, fat and protein supplement has been advocated during the first 24–48 hours of admission of a medically compromised adolescent. Tube feeds are weaned from continuous to overnight feeds and patients are encouraged to eat a prescribed oral diet during the day as soon as the patient's heart rate remains over 50 beats per minute overnight as well as during the day. Weight gain and return to a healthy body mass index is then encouraged by eating an oral diet only, without the long term help of supplement feeds. Routinely the patients are commenced on phosphate and vitamin supplements prior to commencing the refeeding process in order to prevent the occurrence of the refeeding syndrome, indicated by hypoglycaemia, hypophosphataemia, and oedema.

7.7.3. *Ward management*

Once medically stable, the full ward behavioural program is instituted. Nurses play a pivotal and demanding role in the administration of the program and in the consistent setting of limits. Nursing observations provide valuable insights into the interactional behaviours of patients with peers, staff, and family that are important in planning ongoing care. Historically, the emphasis has moved from strict to more lenient behavioural programs with clear expectations for the adolescent and their parents, but which also allow time away from the ward to practise safe eating with family and friends prior to discharge.

Behavioural programs (both inpatient and ambulatory) work best in the context of a multidisciplinary treatment approach. This approach, while supportive, also contains adolescent distress and eating disordered behaviours, strengthens team alliances, and limits functional impairment. Regular communication between members of the treating team is paramount, and clinical meetings are generally held between one and three times a week. Regular updates and communication with the family are vital, and are best done on a weekly basis by one specified team member.

7.8. *Family Based Treatment*

Family treatment (modelled on the Maudsley family based therapy) relies on actively involving the parents at the outset of treatment. This model is typically described as having three phases. The first phase of this type of treatment establishes a 'parents in charge' philosophy. The second phase encourages the adolescent to resume responsibility for their eating and weight recovery. In the third phase when weight is restored, the therapy shifts towards addressing more adolescent developmental issues and how these may have played a role in the evolution of the eating disorder.

8. Day Care Programs

Day programs for the management of eating disorders are also available in many parts of the world. The use of more comprehensive family based programs has reduced the rate of readmissions to hospital. There are however a number of patients who would gain more independence and benefit from a day-patient setting. These programs are considerably cheaper and less restrictive than hospital based programs and are likely to be most effective when patients are medically stable enough to attend.

9. Transition

Eating disorders are chronic illnesses which may take years, often decades, to be satisfactorily managed. As the young person progresses through adolescence, the treating team must alter their strategies to accommodate normal developmental changes. In particular, the need for increasing autonomy and independence must be addressed. The involvement of the family however remains critical, but this must now be achieved by respecting the young person's privacy while not letting the family relinquish control over the illness at too early a stage. The balance remains a fine one. If the eating disorder has not resolved or relapses at an age when transition to adult care is necessary, there also needs to be a comprehensive transitional care plan involving multidisciplinary handover to an appropriate adult based service. Such services may have a different focus or approach and both the relinquishing and receiving team must try to ensure that this is not a time when the young person declines further therapy.

10. Morbidity and Mortality

Adolescents, particularly those diagnosed in early adolescence, have a better prognosis and outcome than adults. Good outcomes are also associated with a shorter duration of illness at diagnosis. Most young adolescents with AN recover after one to five years of specialist treatment. Psychiatric comorbidity and somatisation are associated with chronicity of the disorder. Other poor prognostic indicators are a longer illness prodrome, later age at presentation, and lower BMI at presentation. The health-related burden of eating disorders in older adolescents and adults is as high as that of other major psychiatric disorders such as schizophrenia, and medical disorders such as hypertension. Anorexia has a mortality rate higher than that of any other psychiatric illness, and a suicide rate 1.5 times higher than that of major depression. The limitations in interpersonal functioning and the loss of valuable time at study or work add to the cost. Physically many never or only partially recover, with premature death from inanition. Five percent to 12% of eating disorder patients will die per decade.

References

Ackard DM, Fulkerson JA, Neumark-Sztainer D. (2007) Prevalence and utility of DSM IV eating disorder diagnostic criteria among youth. *Int J Eat Disord* **40**(5): 409–417.

Bravender T, Bryant-Waugh R, Herzog D, Katzman D, Kriepe RD, Lask B, Le Grange D, Lock J, Loeb KL, Marcus MD, Madden S, Nicholls D, O'Toole J, Pinhas L, Rome E, Sokol-Burger M, Wallin U, Zucker N, Workgroup for Classification of Eating Disorders In, C. & Adolescents. (2010) Classification of eating disturbance in children and adolescents: Proposed changes for the DSM-V. *Eur Eat Disord Rev* **18**(2): 79–89.

Fairburn CG, Cooper Z, Shafran R. (2003) Cognitive behaviour therapy for eating disorders: A "transdiagnostic" theory and treatment. *Behav Res Ther* **41**(5): 509–528.

Javaras KN, Laird NM, Reichborn-Kjennerud T, Bulik CM, Pope HG Jr, Hudson JI. (2008) Familiality and heritability of binge eating disorder: Results of a case-control family study and a twin study. *Int J Eat Disord* **41**(2): 174–179.

Kaye W. (2008) Neurobiology of anorexia and bulimia nervosa. *Physiol Behav* **94**(1): 121–135.

Kohn M, Madden S, Clarke S. (2011) Refeeding in anorexia nervosa: Increased safety and efficiency through understanding the pathophysology of protein calorie malnutrition. *Curr Opin Pediatrics* **23**(4): 390–394.

Lock J, Le Grange D, Agras WS, Moye A, Bryson SW, Jo B. (2010) Randomized clinical trial comparing family-based treatment with adolescent-focused individual therapy for adolescents with anorexia nervosa. *Arch Gen Psychiatry* **67**(10): 1025–1032.

Miller CA, Golden NH. (2010) An introduction to eating disorders: Clinical presentation, epidemiology, and prognosis. *Nutr Clin Pract* **25**(2): 110–115.

Nicholls D, Hudson L, Mahomed F. (2011) Managing anorexia nervosa. *Archives of Disease in Childhood,* **96**(10): 977–982.

Peebles R, Hardy KK, Wilson JL, Lock JD. (2010) Are diagnostic criteria for eating disorders markers of medical severity? *Pediatrics* **125**(5): e1193–1201.

Strober M, Freeman R, Morrell W. (1997) The long-term course of severe anorexia nervosa in adolescents: Survival analysis of recovery, relapse, and outcome predictors over 10–15 years in a prospective study. *Int J Eat Disord* **22**(4): 339–360.

Chapter 25

Adolescent Sexuality, Sexual and Reproductive Health

Melissa Kang, Rachel Skinner and Deborah Bateson

1. Introduction

Sexuality is a crucial aspect of adolescent development. The events of puberty bring sexuality into sharp focus at this stage of life. Despite, or perhaps because of, its biological, emotional, social, and cultural dimensions, adolescent sexuality remains a difficult entity for many societies to deal with. Social and cultural taboos can impact on health care, from the point of broaching the subject (history taking) to investigating and treating the range of health issues that can result from adolescent sexual development and associated behaviours. Legal and ethical issues may play a part in determining the outcomes of health-seeking.

Health professionals tend to focus on identifying 'risk' and promoting 'safety' within the fairly narrow parameters of pregnancy and sexually transmitted infections. National sexual health indicators in most countries focus on statistics such as teenage childbirth or pregnancy rates and STI incidences. While important, this focus ignores profound underlying processes associated with new experiences of sexual arousal, sexual attraction, and sexual identity formation.

2. Adolescent Sexual Identity and Sexual Behaviour

Human sexuality encompasses body image and function, sexual drives, gender and gender identity, sexual identity, attraction and orientation, relationship dynamics, family and cultural expectations, and personal values and belief systems.

2.1. *Puberty*

Puberty triggers not only physical maturation of the reproductive system, but a range of emotional and cognitive changes. Early experiences of sexual arousal and attraction may lead to sexual fantasies and dreams and solitary sexual behaviours such as masturbation. Preoccupation with bodily changes of puberty can be inextricably linked with body image and notions of one's own sexual attractiveness. Romantic and sexual attraction may involve people of the same or opposite sex, or both. All these experiences occur within a cultural context that will shape the individual's responses to them. For some, these experiences may go almost unnoticed or be perceived as positive and exciting, while for others, they can lead to worry or anxiety or harmful health behaviours. One of the goals of adolescent development is adjustment to all these changes resulting in healthy body image and sexual identity.

2.2. *Diversity in Sexuality Experiences*

Over a third of young people who are *same-sex attracted* realised their sexual differences before puberty. SSA young people do not necessarily identify as gay, lesbian, or bisexual and do not necessarily have sex at all, or have sex with people of the same sex. Those who are sexually active have sex younger than their non-SSA peers, have more sexual partners, are less likely to use condoms, and have higher rates of pregnancy and STIs. The majority of SSA people report experiences of homophobic abuse (verbal and physical) or exclusion, much of this occurring at school. Young people who are SSA experience higher levels of mental health problems, such as depression and suicidal thinking, and substance use. Young people with *chronic illness, disability, or from culturally and linguistically diverse backgrounds* may also have more difficulty with healthy sexual development for physical, emotional, and socio–cultural reasons.

2.3. *Partnered Sexual Behaviour*

This often starts in adolescence. There appears to be a typical trajectory of sexual behaviour involving kissing, sexual touching, and intercourse. Oral sex increasingly precedes or coincides with intercourse, whereas one or two generations ago, it was relatively uncommon among young people.

The *age of first vaginal intercourse* is of interest in public health because it has implications for rates of pregnancy and STIs. In Western countries, the age of first vaginal intercourse has fallen over the last several decades, while the age of marriage has risen. In many developing countries, the age of first intercourse for females is much younger than in Western countries because of early marriage. In countries in Latin America, and some middle-Eastern and Southeast Asian countries, age of first intercourse is later for women and men, and coincides with age of marriage. The median age of first vaginal intercourse in Western countries ranges from about 16–18 years. Most surveys of adolescent sexual behaviour do not enquire specifically about homosexual sexual practices.

3. Sexual History Taking in Young People

3.1. *Introduction*

Talking to young people about sex can be difficult for health professionals. Yet discussing sexuality and sexual behaviour is an appropriate part of a medical and psychosocial history, and young people believe that it is appropriate for doctors to discuss these issues with them.

The main barriers to sexual history taking include embarrassment on the part of the health professional, concern about the appropriateness of taking a sexual history, and concern about the patient's embarrassment. Young people, particularly younger adolescents, may fear confidentiality breaches if they bring up sexual health concerns. They are also more likely to be concerned about being judged and may not have the confidence to raise sexuality or sexual health concerns with doctors.

The health consultation, regardless of presenting problem, provides an important opportunity to discuss sexuality and offer sexual and preventive health advice. The young person should be made to feel that they have the right to confidential sexual health advice, as well as access to safe and effective contraception and to testing for STIs. Health professionals can use the consultation to acknowledge that adolescence is a time for exploring sexuality and that sexual attraction and experimentation can be confusing for some.

3.2. *General Guidelines for Taking a Sexual History*

It is essential to ensure privacy, by taking a sexual history in a private area and not with other persons present, unless the specific permission of the young person has been given. Explain confidentiality and its limits (Chapter 6).

- Normalise sexual history taking:
  'I ask all young people questions about sexuality and sexual health as part of a general assessment.'

- Ask permission:
  'I'd like to ask you a few questions about sexuality and relationships. If you are not comfortable answering you don't have to. Would it be OK if I start?'

- Using a third-person approach is one option:
  'Around your age some young people are becoming interested in sex and sexual relationships. Are any of the kids in your year at school having sex? What about in your group of friends? What about you — have you had any romantic or sexual relationships?'

- Do not assume heterosexual attraction, even if young person mentions an opposite sex partner:
  'Have your relationships/sexual partners been with/been male/s, female/s or both?'
  'Are you attracted mainly to males, females, both, unsure?'

Avoid questions such as 'Do you have a boyfriend/girlfriend?'

- Ask specifically about sexual practices and condom use but frame the
  questions first:
  *'I'm going to ask some very specific questions about sexual practices
  and condom use, this will help me assess your risk of STIs.'*
  *'In your current relationship/in the past 12 months when have you had
  sex has that involved [vaginal] intercourse/oral sex/anal sex?'*
  *'Do you and your partner use condoms when you have intercourse/
  oral sex/anal sex?'*

- Explore condom use:
  'Do you use condoms sometimes, mostly, always?'
  *'Do you or your partner have any difficulty talking about or using
  condoms? Is it easy for you or your partner to get hold of them? Are
  you and your partner comfortable with how to use them?*

- Explore contraception use further:
  *'Condoms can be an effective form of contraception, but I'd like to
  also ask whether you/your partner use any other form of contraception, if so what/how long have you used this form of contraception/do
  you find it easy to use?'*

- Ask about pregnancy:
  'Have you ever been pregnant? Have you ever made any one pregnant?'

- Explore the context of sex (this questioning will be guided to some
  extent by the responses above):
  *'Have any of your sexual encounters happened in situations where
  you've been drunk or under the influence of drugs or when you
  haven't felt in control of the situation for some other reason?'*

- Ask about unwanted sex:
  *'Have you ever been pressured or forced to have any type of sex that
  you didn't want? [Can you tell me a bit more about that?]'*

- Decide whether it might also be appropriate to enquire about
  exchanging sex for money or other commodities:
  *'Have you ever had sex in exchange for money or something else
  (such as food, shelter, drugs)? [Can you tell me a bit more about
  that?]'*

3.3. *Medico–Legal Obligations*

Medico–legal and ethical issues arise in adolescent health care generally, but can be particularly pertinent in consultations about sexual health. In Australia, legislation relevant to sexuality includes (but is not limited to) the age of consent to have intercourse, child protection legislation, and mandatory reporting, notification of communicable diseases including several STIs, confidentiality, consent to one's own medical treatment (including contraception and abortion), abortion laws, laws about sterilisation, and female genital mutilation.

In Australia, although the age of consent to have sex is 16 years in most jurisdictions, health professionals are able to treat sexually active young people under 16 confidentially. This includes prescribing contraception, or conducting STI screening if they believe the young person is competent to consent to their own treatment. There is only an obligation to report sexual abuse, not sexual activity itself.

4. Sexually Transmitted Infections

4.1. *Introduction*

Young people are more vulnerable to sexually transmitted infections for biological, behavioural, psychological, socio-cultural, and economic reasons. In adolescent women, exposed columnar epithelium on the cervix uteri increases the risk of infection with cervical pathogens, especially Chlamydia trachomatis. Cervical mucus in early adolescence is thinner than in older adolescents and adult women, which might allow pathogens to more readily penetrate mucosal sites or the upper genital tract.

Young people in Western countries are likely to have a greater number of sexual partners because of the increasing gap between sexual debut and marriage-equivalent relationships. Negotiating condom use is complicated by factors such as gendered power dynamics, perceptions of trust and 'cleanliness', as well as contextual factors such as alcohol and substance use. Access to condoms can be inhibited by cost and visibility (being seen obtaining or carrying them). Barriers to accessing STI testing and treatment which are more pertinent among young people include lack of knowledge, cost, and concerns about of confidentiality.

4.2. *Epidemiology and Clinical Presentation of STIs in Adolescence*

4.2.1. *Chlamydia*

In Western countries, chlamydia is the most common bacterial STI in young people. Chlamydia most typically causes cervicitis in women and urethritis in men, which can lead to vaginal or urethral discharge in women and men respectively, dysuria in both women and men, and lower abdominal pain or dyspareunia in women. However chlamydia is asymptomatic in up to 90% of women and 50% of men. Adolescent girls aged 15–19 have the highest incidence. It is estimated that 20% of untreated chlamydia in women leads to pelvic inflammatory disease, and that 20% of these women develop tubal infertility. Ectopic pregnancy is another complication of chlamydial PID. Complications in men are uncommon, but epididymitis in young sexually active men is largely attributable to chlamydial urethritis. Subgroups such as Indigenous Australian and African–American young people have much higher prevalence rates of chlamydia, as well as gonorrhoea, syphilis, and trichomoniasis.

4.2.2. *Genital herpes and human papillomavirus*

Genital herpes and human papillomavirus are the most prevalent of the viral STIs, although understanding epidemiologic patterns is hampered by the fact that these infections are not notifiable in many countries, including Australia, the US, and most European countries.

Genital HPV infections are the most prevalent STIs in the world. These are highest in young women and the association between some high risk subtypes of HPV infection and cancer of the cervix, vagina, vulva, penis, and anus are well documented. Other subtypes can cause benign condylomata acuminata (genital warts). Most HPV infection however is probably subclinical. The introduction of a quadrivalent vaccine against subtypes 6, 11, 16, and 18 has seen some decreases in the prevalence of external genital warts in young women and in heterosexual men.

HPV vaccination is most effective when the recipient is naïve to the HPV types covered by the vaccine. More than three quarters of new HPV infections occur during adolescence and young adulthood (15–24 year age group) hence vaccination is targeted to early adolescence prior to the onset of sexual activity. The recommended age for HPV vaccination, the funding arrangements, and delivery programs vary between countries and jurisdictions. Every effort should be made to identify adolescent and younger adult women who may not have been vaccinated against HPV and who may benefit from vaccination. It is important to keep in mind that vaccine effectiveness will reduce with increased exposure to HPV as occurs with increasing age.

The prevalence of genital herpes is difficult to gauge because of subclinical infection. It is however the dominant cause of genital ulcer disease in developed countries. The seroprevalence of HSV Type 2 increases with age. There has been an increase in genital herpes attributable to HSV Type 1 in young people in the past one to two decades. Reasons might include a decrease in childhood-acquired HSV 1 infection and an increase in oral–genital contact among young people. Prophylactic protein subunit vaccines have been under trial for the past several years.

4.2.3. *Hepatitis B Virus*

HBV is endemic in some parts of the world where infection is acquired in the perinatal period or early childhood. In Western countries, subgroups of young people from high prevalence countries may be at risk of sexually acquired HBV, as are indigenous young people and those who engage in high risk activities such as injecting drug use. Universal HBV vaccine is now given in most developed countries at birth or early childhood, however some young people may have missed this and should be offered the appropriate course (Chapter 33).

4.2.4. *Human Immunodeficiency Virus*

HIV prevalence among young people in developed countries remains low. However a significant proportion of those infected (predominantly men who have sex with men and, to a lesser extent, injecting drug users) acquire the infection before the age of 25. Indigenous people in countries such as Canada, the US, and Australia have higher rates of HIV that are acquired heterosexually or through sharing injecting equipment. Increases in heterosexually acquired HIV in some European countries are due to migration of people from high prevalence countries, particularly sub-Saharan Africa. HIV infection is associated with higher risk of acquisition of other STIs.

4.3. *Screening Asymptomatic Young People for STIs*

STI screening is guided by epidemiologic trends and specific risk behaviours. These will vary within and between countries and populations, including subpopulations of young people.

Many developed countries have implemented chlamydia screening programs or have national guidelines that recommend regular screening for chlamydia in sexually active young people. Asymptomatic chlamydia infection is a good candidate for screening as the prevalence is moderately high and the screening test is highly sensitive and specific, relatively cheap, and non-invasive. Nucleic acid amplification testing for chlamydia has replaced culture. NAAT can be performed on first void urine in men and women, self-collected vaginal or endocervical swabs in women, and urethral swabs in men. Nevertheless, achieving high uptake of regular screening in this population has proved difficult and innovative methods for promoting chlamydial screening are needed. Screening that occurs outside clinical settings (such as schools, universities, and sports clubs) has higher uptake. Gonorrhoea, syphilis, and HIV screening are useful in certain subpopulations, as is HBV screening. HPV and HSV are not amenable to screening. In the case of HPV, Pap tests are used to screen for cervical dysplasia due to HPV infection in women over 18 years. Screening for HPV DNA or HPV serology in asymptomatic individuals does not have clinical utility and is only used in research situations. HSV serology is of limited clinical utility and viral isolation is only feasible in active lesions.

4.4. *Management of STIs*

Antimicrobial therapy for some STIs will depend on local patterns of resistance, as well as the presence of symptoms and complications.

Table 1: Screening for STIs.

STI	Test type	Specimen	Comments
Chlamydia	NAAT	First void urine, self-collected vaginal swab, endocervical or urethral swab	
Gonorrhoea	NAAT	As above	
Syphilis	Serology (RPR or VDRL)	Blood	
Hepatitis B	Serology (HepBsAg) and HepBcAb	Blood	HepBsAb if need to check immunisation status.
HIV	Serology (HIV Ab)	Blood	

Uncomplicated or asymptomatic chlamydia infection is generally treated with an oral stat dose of 1g of azithromycin.

Contact tracing is an important aspect of STI control and management. How far back to trace contacts will depend on the infective agent and the young person's specific circumstances. Guidelines may vary between countries. In Australia, young people with a new diagnosis of chlamydia are asked to trace sexual contacts back six months, while for gonorrhoea it is about two months. Those with primary syphilis should trace contacts back for 3 months and secondary syphilis six months. Those newly diagnosed with HIV should trace contacts back to the last negative test or the onset of risk behaviours. Contact tracing for HSV and HPV is not routine.

5. Contraception in Adolescence

5.1. *Introduction*

While teenage girls may present requesting contraception, this usually occurs some months after they become sexually active, when they have established their first serious relationship. It is important to assess contraceptive needs in all teenagers, even those not yet sexually active. At first intercourse, most teenagers only use condoms, or a less effective form of contraception (like withdrawal). Risk of unintended pregnancy in adolescence is highest in the first six months of sexual activity. The National Surveys of Australian Secondary Students, HIV/AIDS and Sexual Health, have shown consistently that hormonal contraceptive use is more common in older teenagers than younger teenagers; similarly younger teenagers are more likely to use condoms than older teenagers. Younger teenagers tend to use condoms alone for pregnancy protection and then transition from condom use to hormonal contraception as they enter more established relationships. Among Australian school students, only 50% report use of hormonal contraceptives at their last sexual encounter, with about two thirds reporting condom use alone or in addition to hormonal contraception. This is despite a high level of knowledge about contraceptive options. While three quarters of teenage mothers did not intend pregnancy, about 50% were not using contraception when they conceived.

5.2. *Contraceptive Counselling*

Research has identified that attitudes and beliefs of sexually active teenage girls are important to pregnancy risk. For example, an adolescent's self-perception of their risk of pregnancy during unprotected sexual intercourse and of the potential impact of motherhood on their lives may influence their likelihood of an unplanned pregnancy. Those who perceive a low risk of pregnancy, or who consider that motherhood would have a positive impact on their lives may be more likely to become pregnant or a teenage parent. Some adolescent girls hold beliefs about infertility. These beliefs may be based on previous experiences of unprotected sexual encounters which did not result in pregnancy, experiences of irregular menses, use of drugs and alcohol, or a general sense of invulnerability. In addition, adolescents may also hold false beliefs about side effects of or limited efficacy of contraception.

Beliefs around pregnancy and motherhood should be explored and challenged in a constructive way. For example, guiding the adolescent to consider how they and their family would feel if they became pregnant, providing education about contraceptive efficacy and 'myth busting' about contraceptive misinformation may help.

Long acting reversible contraceptives, such as the contraceptive implant and injection, have been demonstrated to be more effective in the prevention of repeat teenage pregnancy, and are appropriate options for adolescents with low motivation to use contraception. Education about Emergency Contraception is also important as a 'back up plan' to regular contraception in these adolescents. EC can now be accessed through pharmacies in Australia, the UK, and the USA without a doctor's prescription, which provides for more rapid access and hence potentially greater efficacy. The International Consortium for Emergency Contraception database provides information about global access to EC.

Some adolescent girls may still consider teenage motherhood a logical and appropriate life choice, and it may not be possible or appropriate to change these beliefs. It may be more appropriate to ensure that they understand the importance of good prenatal and postnatal care.

In young heterosexual relationships, the responsibility for contraception is usually assumed to be that of the female partner, although not all couples actually discuss this role delineation. Many studies have found that pregnancy prevention is the main concern for both males and females who are sexually active, and STI prevention is of lesser concern. Ideally couples should be encouraged to attend a clinical assessment together, at least on one occasion, to encourage open discussion about roles and responsibilities. In addition, this consultation provides an opportunity for the male partner to access sexual health clinical services.

Cultural barriers may also prevent effective use of contraception. As an example, Indigenous Australian adolescent girls have greater challenges in negotiating condom use with partners, as condoms are often viewed as being associated with shame, a bad reputation, and coercion. Similar cultural barriers to condom and other contraceptive use are seen in many minority cultures within Western countries. These barriers often reflect the prevailing attitudes in the country of origin to sexual activity outside of marriage, and to the autonomy of women in sexual relationships. Cultural sensitivities must be explored in all young people who are at risk of unplanned pregnancy.

5.3. *Contraceptive Options*

The range of contraceptive options that are safe, effective, and appropriate for young women from the time of menarche is similar to that for older adults. However accessibility varies by method, youth awareness, knowledge, cost, availability, and convenience. Contraceptive choice may also be influenced by concerns about perceived risks such as cancer, or side-effects such as weight gain. *Young people under 20 years of age have a higher chance of contraceptive failure in the first year of use than do older women.* Continuation is likely to be increased when the young person's concerns are addressed. Some young people may choose a method based on its additional benefits, for example on acne, painful periods, or irregular periods.

As for women of all ages, a *medical history* should be taken to ensure that the young woman is medically eligible to use a particular method of contraception. The World Health Organization Medical Eligibility Criteria and UK Medical Eligibility Criteria for contraceptive use provide evidence-based guidance on method eligibility. Other countries including the US and Australia have developed their own guidelines for local use. A *follow-up consultation* approximately three months after a method is started is a useful way of consolidating information and ensuring that all concerns have been addressed.

A young person who is a *legal minor* may need to be deemed competent to consent to treatment in many legal jurisdictions before contraceptive treatment can be prescribed or administered without parental consent. A young person, especially one with an *intellectual disability*, may require additional counselling with appropriate resources, such as visual aids, to assist in the decision making process. For minors in many countries, consent for procedures which will result in sterilisation (tubal ligation or vasectomy or hysterectomy) is only available through a strict legal process whereby a court is required to give consent. With the increased availability of LARCs for the control of menstrual bleeding and highly effective non-user dependent contraception, this legal recourse is extremely unusual.

Contraceptive methods which require daily action such as the contraceptive pill and those which are coitally-dependent such as condoms have higher typical failure rates than methods which are administered less frequently. LARCs have the highest effectiveness, making them a suitable choice for young people wishing to avoid an unintended pregnancy. Adolescents who choose an effective form of contraception such as a contraceptive pill or implant should also be advised to combine these with a barrier such as a male or female condom, given the high risk of STI in this age group. If contraception is required *prior to menarche*, then non-hormonal methods are generally advised rather than the regular use of a hormonal method.

5.4. *Hormonal Contraceptives*

5.4.1. *Combined oral contraceptive pill*

The combined OCP is the preferred choice for many young women. It has a failure rate of approximately 0.3% when used perfectly, with less than one woman in a hundred falling pregnant in a year. In typical use the failure rate can be up to 9%. It is safe to initiate from the time of menarche and is sometimes used in young teenagers for its non-contraceptive benefits such as menstrual regulation or acne control. There are many different pill types available with various combinations of oestrogen and progestogen hormones. Some adolescents and young adults may have a contraindication to the use of an oestrogen-containing pill, including those with a history of venous thromboembolism or migraine with aura. Contraceptive pill choice will be determined by a combination of cost, side-effects, and possibly by added non-contraceptive benefits. The progestogen-only pill is usually not a preferred option for adolescents and young adults because it has to be taken within a three-hour timeframe each day. All young women using the pill as contraception need to know how to manage missed pills, what to do if they have acute gastroenteritis, how to access emergency contraception and that the pill does not protect against STIs.

Many young women find it useful to skip their withdrawal bleeds by skipping the placebo or sugar pills for three months or even longer in a so called 'extended regimen'. Reducing the hormone-free break from seven to four or even fewer days may reduce the risk of break-through ovulation and improve contraceptive effectiveness.

5.4.2. *Vaginal ring*

The vaginal ring is a flexible device which releases a combination of oestrogen and progestogen hormones for absorption through the vaginal mucosa into the systemic circulation. The ring is placed in the vagina, usually for a three week period, then removed for a week in order to induce a 'ring free' bleed. A new ring is used each month, although longer-acting rings have also been developed which may enhance continuation rates as well as improve affordability. The ring does not require any fitting and young women who feel comfortable with the idea of the ring may find this a convenient way to provide effective contraception. The failure rate for the vaginal ring is quoted at the same rate as the contraceptive pill. The ring does not provide protection against STIs but can be used concurrently with a condom.

5.4.3. *Transdermal combined contraceptive patch*

The combined contraceptive patch is available in several countries, although not currently in Australia, and provides an effective contraceptive option which is administered once weekly. The patch, like the combined pill and vaginal ring, contains oestrogen so general contraindications to oestrogen also apply. Young women may find this method convenient although some may have concerns about its visibility and may have problems with adhesiveness and skin irritation. Remembering to change at set times may also be challenging although SMS technology via a mobile phone may be helpful.

5.4.4. *Contraceptive implant*

There are several implants available worldwide comprising of one or more subdermal rods which release contraceptive hormones over a specified period of time. In Australia the only implant available is a single etonogestrel-releasing rod, which provides up to three years of highly effective contraception. Other implants include a two-rod levonorgestrel-releasing silicone device. The main mechanism of action is the inhibition of ovulation. The circulating levels of oestradiol remain at a sufficient level to cause no negative effect on bone density in adolescent women. The implant must be both inserted and removed by a trained health professional and should be easily palpable in the inner aspect of the non-dominant arm. Since the need for frequent action on the part of the user is removed, the implant offers highly effective contraception. The implant is also immediately reversible on removal so if a young person has unwanted side-effects she can be reassured that these will disappear on removal of the rod. Common side effects include unpredictable vaginal bleeding and this can lead to early discontinuation. It is important to exclude other causes of vaginal bleeding, particularly Chlamydial cervicitis in young women. Evidence for effective management of implant-related bleeding is scarce, but in practice the addition of an oestrogen-containing contraceptive pill can provide some immediate relief from troublesome bleeding.

5.4.5. *Contraceptive long acting injection*

The long-acting injection has been used for several decades and contains a variety of hormonal constituents. In Australia the depot-medroxyprogesterone acetate injection is administered on a three-monthly basis into the gluteal or deltoid muscle. The injection provides effective contraception although its efficacy will be reduced if the young women presents late for an injection. The injection mainly works by inhibiting ovulation by suppression of gonadotropins. The effect of progestogen-only contraceptive injections on the bone health of adolescents has been a subject of intense debate. Research studies suggest that there is a small loss of bone mineral density which is usually recovered after method discontinuation although the long-term sequelae are unknown. For this reason the injection is not advised as a first-line method for adolescents. Young women may experience side effects such as weight gain, acne, and unpredictable bleeding although the bleeding will tend to settle over time. Young people also need to be aware that the injection is not immediately reversible and it may take up to a year to return to the previous level of fertility.

5.4.6. *Levonorgestrel-releasing intrauterine system*

The LNG-IUS provides highly effective contraception for up to five years and whilst not historically a first-line option for adolescents, its use in this age group is increasing worldwide. The stem of the device releases a small amount of progestogen hormone which acts locally within the uterus to provide highly effective contraception. The added effect of reduction in menstrual blood loss can also be advantageous for young women with heavy menstrual bleeding. The LNG-IUS requires both insertion and removal by a trained health professional. While insertion may be more difficult and associated with increased pain in adolescents, insertion is generally feasible in the primary care setting. Young women may experience a higher explusion rate than older parous women.

Previous concerns in relation to infection risk have been dispelled in recent years. The main risk of infection for a woman with an IUS is related to the insertion itself, a risk which remains elevated for the first 20 days after the procedure. Thereafter a young woman's risk of infection is related to her own personal risk of an STI. It is increasingly understood that having an IUS *in situ* does not in itself increase the risk of developing PID and has no long term effect on fertility. However, an LNG-IUS is generally not advised as a first line choice for someone at high risk of STI acquisition although it can be combined with condoms for those in new relationships. A smaller size hormone releasing IUS is currently under trial in several countries and may have particular applicability for younger women.

5.4.7. *Copper Intrauterine Devices*

These have been used for several decades as an effective non-hormonal form of contraception. These are not generally a first line method of contraception for adolescents for similar reasons as the LNG-IUS, but may have a small role for those who choose not to use contraceptive hormones or in whom these hormones are contraindicated. The copper IUD provides highly effective reversible contraception for up to ten years. The device is associated with heavier and often more painful menses, but this side effect is offset by a lack of any hormonally related risks or side effects.

5.4.8. *Post coital emergency contraception*

Emergency contraception may be used up to five days after unprotected intercourse or contraceptive failure in order to reduce the chance of an unintended pregnancy. The commonest method comprises a single 1.5 mg dose of levonorgestrel taken as soon as possible after unprotected sex. A safety statement from the WHO states that the LNG-EC method primarily works by delaying or inhibiting ovulation and that it does not act to disrupt an established pregnancy. When taken within 24 to 48 hours of intercourse it can prevent up to 85% of expected pregnancies with efficacy declining over time. It may be used more than once in a cycle, and has no known teratogenic effects on an established pregnancy. Consideration of an advanced supply may be useful for some adolescents. This strategy has not been shown as yet to significantly reduce the rate of unintended pregnancies amongst teenagers, or to have an unintended negative effect on regular contraceptive use.

A newer oral form of emergency contraception, the selective progesterone receptor modulator, ulipristal acetate, is available in some countries. Ulipristal acetate has been shown to be at least as effective as the LNG-EC and has proven effectiveness up to 120 hours after unprotected intercourse.

A copper IUD inserted within five days of unprotected sex can also be used as an effective form of emergency contraception although access to this method within a short time frame may be limited.

5.5. *Barrier Methods*

Male and female condoms are less effective than most other methods of contraception for the prevention of pregnancy due to their coital dependence. Despite this, condoms are a popular choice since these can be easily purchased without the intervention of a health professional, have minimal if any risks or side effects, and are generally affordable. Male and female condoms are also the only form of contraception which provides effective protection against STIs and thus can also be doubled up with pills, rings, or LARCs for dual STI and pregnancy protection. Male condoms are commonly made of latex and young people need to know about correct use, to use them with water-based lubricant if needed and that they come in different sizes. Non-latex condoms are also available for those with latex allergy. Female condoms made of polyurethane are also available. Cost, limited availability as well as acceptability issues appear to limit their use although this may change with the development of newer prototypes.

6. Pregnancy in Adolescence

6.1. *Introduction*

Adolescent pregnancy is generally defined as pregnancy occurring under the age of 20 years. However, there are significant differences in the social, developmental, and health implications of young people who give birth across the teenage years. For example, a teenage mother of 18–19 years of age may be married, have planned her pregnancy, have a home life which is stable and well supported. In many cultures, this would be considered as a normal transition to adult life and responsibilities. In Australia, and other wealthy developed nations, this same teenager may not be married, however may still have completed high school education, have a stable partner and have decided to start a family. While she would be considered a young mother compared to the average age of parenting, with appropriate support of her partner and family, she is likely to have a healthy child and to be able to cope with the responsibilities of parenting. On the other hand, a younger teenager of 13–14 years of age who falls pregnant and decides to keep her baby, out of choice or circumstance, is much more likely to be exposed to a range of adverse experiences, for herself and for her child, than the older teenager.

In general, younger teenagers (under 16 years) and older teenagers with pre-existing vulnerabilities who give birth are of the greatest concern for health professionals and public health policy makers. It is these two categories of teenage parents and their children who are at higher risk of physical, psychosocial, and economic adversities.

6.2. *Epidemiology of Adolescent Pregnancy and Fertility*

6.2.1. *Incidence of teenage pregnancy and fertility*

The incidence of teenage pregnancy is defined as the number of pregnancies per 1,000 adolescent females per year. This includes miscarriages, abortions, live births, and still births. The teenage birth rate is termed the teenage fertility rate, and this does not include pregnancies ending in abortion or miscarriage.

Generally the rate of miscarriage is low in the teenage years, and induced abortion is high, particularly in wealthy developed nations. In Australia, the ratio of induced abortions to live births in the teenage years is over one, meaning that most pregnancies end in abortion. This ratio is generally higher in countries with lower teenage fertility rates. Teenage pregnancy rates (including abortions) are more difficult to measure as abortions are not always notified to data registers, unlike births, where most developed countries keep accurate data for all births. Although abortions are legal in many developed countries, there is still a stigma associated with the procedure; thus the reluctance to legislate for mandatory notification of abortions. In Australia, only a few states and territories require notification of abortions to a central register. In the rest, statistics on abortions are calculated indirectly using data where hospital discharges or medical procedures are recorded. These calculations are likely to be under-estimates.

In most wealthy developed nations, the TFR has dropped dramatically in the past 40 years. In Australia, the TFR (15–19 years) in the early 1970s was as high as 50 per 1,000 per year. The TFR dropped progressively until 10 years ago, and has remained stable at about 16–17 per 1,000 per year.

Australia's TFR is lower than in the US and the UK, but higher than in most other OECD nations. Lower TFR in wealthy nations is considered to be related to better universal access to education and economic security, as much as it is considered to be related to free and easy access to contraception, and abortion.

Within wealthy developed nations, there are geographical areas and ethnic and cultural groups who have higher rates of teenage births. In Australia, this is particularly the case for Indigenous teenagers for whom the TFR is four times that of non-Indigenous teenagers. Teenagers living in areas of social disadvantage and in rural areas also have higher fertility rates than better off, urban teenagers.

6.2.2. *Correlates of teenage pregnancy and fertility*

Teenagers who engage in risky sexual behaviour are more likely to have a teenage pregnancy. Risky sexual behaviour leading to pregnancy includes early age of sexual intercourse debut, high number of lifetime partners, and inconsistent use of contraceptives. In addition, over one half of teenage pregnancies occur within six months of first experience of vaginal intercourse, suggesting that hormonal contraceptives are not used or used inconsistently by these sexually active teenagers. Teenagers who have a pregnancy are also more likely to report having had an unwanted sexual experience in the past. Considering these risky sexual behaviours, it is not surprising that pregnant teens are at high risk of STI, such as chlamydia. The prevalence of chlamydia in teenagers attending an antenatal clinic is many fold higher than in a school population (>20% versus <5%).

Teenage mothers are also more likely to have engaged in other risky behaviour, such as substance use. They are also much more likely to smoke cigarettes than non-parenting teenagers.

Adolescent girls are more likely than adult women to report depressive symptoms before the birth and to experience postnatal depression after the birth. Behavioural problems in childhood and adolescence, such as oppositional and conduct disorders and aggressive and delinquent behaviour, are also more commonly a precursor to teenage pregnancy and birth. Teenage mothers have less stable romantic relationships, and are more likely to be single mothers than are adult mothers. Domestic violence is also much more common among parents who have had a child as a teenager. Similarly, children of teenage parents are more likely to experience abuse. Teenage mothers are more likely to have dropped out of school than their adult counterparts. They are also less likely to ever achieve the same level of education as their non-pregnant peers, and are more likely to be on lifelong welfare.

Many of these correlates of teenage parenthood also exist for teenage fathers, although the relationships are not as strong. This is likely to be because the father of a child born to a teenage mother is generally older and may not have dropped out of school or work. In addition, these relationships have a high risk of separation; and thus the care of the child falls largely on the teenage mother.

6.3. *Medico–Legal Implications of Pregnancy in Adolescence*

6.3.1. *Pregnancy in a minor*

Teenagers who fall pregnant may require consideration as to whether they have been the victim of an abusive sexual relationship. In many jurisdictions of Australia and elsewhere, sexual activity under the age of 16 is against the law; however if sexual activity is consensual and there is no risk of harm suspected, there is no need to report this to welfare authorities. If a teenager has had a sexual relationship with an older person, then concerns regarding the possibility of sexual abuse or assault must be considered. Coercive relationships in this setting can be difficult to determine as most adolescent mothers fall pregnant to an older partner, often a young adult, and describe a caring consensual relationship. Mature minor status of an adolescent mother under 16 years needs to be carefully considered in this setting, and these relationships often need to be monitored. A risk assessment based on the vulnerability of the young mother and the history of the partner should be made, hence the need for involvement of welfare services.

6.3.2. *Adolescent abortion*

Most jurisdictions have laws relating to abortion, and the circumstances in which a medical practitioner can provide a legal abortion. Abortion in Australia is widely available in most jurisdictions where it can be demonstrated that the pregnancy presents a psychological risk to the mother. In the case of an adolescent minor who wishes to access an abortion, this generally requires the consent of a parent or guardian. However, some jurisdictions provide for assessment of mature minor status when under the age of 16 years.

6.4. *Adolescent Parenting*

6.4.1. *Clinical care of the pregnant teenager and young mother*

Pregnant adolescents need specific clinical care which differs from that of pregnant adults. They have much lower antenatal clinic attendance, most likely due to the unplanned nature of their pregnancy (not being aware they are pregnant until later in pregnancy), lack of independent transport options, and poorer planning skills. They have higher rates of obstetric risk factors, such as anaemia, smoking, pre-eclampsia, urinary tract infection, and STIs. Antenatal services for adolescents must be pro-active, and include home visitation if necessary. Screening for STIs (in particular chlamydial infection) should be included in routine antenatal screening procedures. Antenatal iron and folate supplementation is essential, as are interventions to reduce smoking and substance use. Interventions to reduce smoking or substance use in pregnant teenagers should be oriented around psychosocial and counselling approaches rather than pharmacotherapies. Educational interventions around parenting, breastfeeding, and post-partum contraception should begin in the antenatal period.

In the immediate postnatal period, intensive support for breast feeding should commence, as the rate of breast-feeding drops dramatically within the first month or two post-partum. Ideally before discharge from the postnatal ward, a long-acting contraceptive should be considered, and pregnancy intentions explored. Return to sexual activity within the first six weeks is high (around 50% of teenage mothers) and few of these young mothers access contraception at the time of resumption of sexual activity. Rapid repeat teenage pregnancy (within two years of the first pregnancy), occurrs in at least one third of these adolescent mothers, and LARCs significantly delay the second pregnancy. Use of the OCP is generally no more effective than either condoms or no contraception in delaying the second pregnancy.

6.4.2. *Improving outcomes*

Adolescent parents and their children are susceptible to adverse outcomes. Appropriate prenatal education, supporting the early diagnosis of pregnancy and implementing antenatal care tailored to the needs of adolescents are helpful. Antenatal care of adolescents involves more intensive medical screening and psychosocial assessment and support. This may be facilitated through a dedicated adolescent antenatal clinic, which also provides support into the post natal period. Community based programs to promote effective parenting strategies, improve coping strategies, support vulnerable relationships, and identify situations of risk are essential. Regular home visitation programs using midwives in the antenatal and postnatal period have demonstrated improved outcomes for adolescent mothers and their offspring.

It is recommended that these nurses visit the home of the pregnant teenager and provide antenatal health education and support and then continue to maintain regular home visits in the post-partum period for at least two years. This longer term approach is likely to aid the reduction of adverse outcomes such as abuse, emergency department presentations, and under-diagnosis of other compromises to maternal and child well-being. It is important that the home visitation is undertaken by a trained nurse rather than a paraprofessional, as they are better able to evaluate situations of risk.

7. Summary

The approach to the sexual and reproductive clinical care of adolescents has similarities to that of adults, but there are important differences. The sexual and reproductive health care of young people requires an understanding of the broad range of factors influencing young people's sexual behaviour. It requires an understanding of adolescent sexual and psychosocial development within the context of an individual young person's social and cultural environment. Doctors who care for young people must have skills in sexual history taking, skills in the eliciting of beliefs which may influence sexual risk and prevention, and skills in assessment of competence. Doctors must be adept at engaging young people, ensuring confidentiality within limits and express a non-judgmental approach. They must also be able to communicate sexual health promotion messages and provide brief sexual health promotion interventions which engage young people. These skills are of equal importance as a thorough understanding of the epidemiology, pathophysiology and management of sexually transmissible diseases in young people. Expertise in the range of contraceptive options available for teenagers is essential.

References

Bearinger LH, Sieving RE, Ferguson J, Sharma V. (2007) Global perspectives on the sexual and reproductive health of adolescents: Patterns, prevention, and potential. *Lancet* **369**(9568): 1220–1231.

Contraceptive choices for young people. Faculty of Sexual and Reproductive Healthcare. Available online at: http://www.fsrh.org/pdfs/ceuGuidance YoungPeople2010.pdf.2011.

UK Medical Eligibility Criteria for contraceptive use (2009). Faculty of Sexual and Reproductive Healthcare. Available online at: http://www.fsrh.org/pdfs/ UKMEC2009.pdf. (accessed 25 July 2011).

Hillier L, Jones T, Monagle M, Overton N, Gahan L, Blackman J, Mitchell A. (2010) Writing themselves in 3 (WTI3). *The third national study on the sexual health and wellbeing of same sex attracted and gender questioning young people.* Monograph series no. 78 Available online at: www.latrobe. edu.au/ssay/atleast/downloads/wti3_web_sml.pdf.

Holmes K, Sparling F, Stamm W, Piot P, Wasserheit J, Corey L, Cohen M. (2008) *Sexually Transmitted Diseases*, 4th ed. McGraw, USA.

Kang M, Cannon B, Remond L, Quine S. (2009) 'Is it normal to feel these questions ...?': A content analysis of the health concerns of adolescent girls writing to a magazine. *Fam Pract* **26**(3): 196–203.

Marston C, King E. (2006) Factors that shape young people's sexual behaviour: A systematic review. *Lancet* **368**(9547): 1581–1586.

Moore S, Rosenthal D. (2006) *Sexuality in Adolescence: Current trends.* Routledge, East Sussex.

Sexual Health & Family Planning Australia (2012) *Contraception: An Australian Clinical Practice Handbook*, 3rd ed. Family Planning Association, New South Wales, Victoria and Queensland.

Skinner SR, Smith J, Fenwick J, Fyfe S, Hendriks J. (2008) Perceptions and experiences of first sexual intercourse in Australian adolescent females. *J Adolesc Health* **43**(6): 593–599.

Smith A, Agius P, Mitchell A, Barrett C, Pitts M. (2009) *Secondary students and sexual health 2008.* Results of the 4th National survey of Australian secondary students, HIV/AIDs and sexual health. Monograph series no. 70. Australian Research Centre in Sex Health and Society, Latrobe University.

Trussell J. (2011) Contraceptive failure in the United States. *Contraception* **83**(5): 397–404.

World Health Organization Medical eligibility criteria for contraceptive use 2009. 4th edition. [online] Available online at: http://www.who.int/reproductive-health/publications/family_planning/9789241563888/en/index.html (accessed 2011 25 July).

Chapter 26

Physical Activity and Sports Medicine

Carolyn Broderick and Damien McKay

1. Introduction

The physiological parameters associated with sports performance improve markedly during adolescence, but so too does the risk of musculoskeletal injury. Unique injury patterns are observed in adolescents that reflect the changes occurring in the growing skeleton. The benefits of physical activity during adolescence far outweigh the risks but it is important to be aware that this is a time of skeletal vulnerability and training regimens should reflect this.

2. Benefits of Sports Participation and Physical Activity in Adolescence

Sports participation and physical activity in adolescence is associated with physical and psychological benefits. It may also play a role in the prevention of a number of adult-onset diseases. Despite the increasing evidence to support this, a marked decline in physical activity occurs in the adolescent years and is more pronounced in girls than in boys. Boys are more active than girls in every age group.

2.1. *Improved Performance*

2.1.1. *Changes with maturation*

Many aspects of youth sports performance including strength, aerobic, and anaerobic fitness improve during adolescence. Changes in these physiological parameters more closely mirror biological age than chronological age with peak increases occurring at or around the time of the adolescent growth spurt. A pubertal spurt in aerobic power (VO_{2peak}) and strength occurs at the time of peak height velocity and peak weight velocity respectively.

2.1.2. *Relative age effect*

An interesting phenomenon in adolescent sport which has been observed worldwide is the impact of an adolescent's birth date on their subsequent sports performance — the so called 'relative age effect'. Those born closer to the cutoff dates for sport are over-represented in many elite sports. The advantage conferred by advanced maturity (and therefore improved strength and aerobic capacity) at a young age, is perpetuated by these adolescents being selected for representative and higher level teams where they have access to more resources and better coaching.

2.1.3. *Changes with training*

Improvements in cardio–respiratory fitness which result from physical activity have both short and long term benefits. Short term improvements in aerobic capacity and strength can be achieved in adolescents undertaking an appropriate training program. In the pre-pubertal years, strength training results in improvement in strength without any significant muscle hypertrophy and is thought to be the result of improved motor coordination and neural adaptations which increase motor unit activation and recruitment. In the later adolescent years improvements in muscle strength are associated with muscle hypertrophy (more marked in males than females). Similarly, while improvements in aerobic fitness occur with training in the pre-pubertal years, these are of a smaller magnitude than those observed in adolescents or young adults undertaking similar training regimens. There is a moderate correlation between sports participation in adolescence and physical activity in adult life; that is, active adolescents are more likely to become active adults.

2.2. *Bone Health*

Approximately one third to a quarter of bone mineral accrual occurs during the adolescent years and longitudinal studies have shown that bone mineral accrual during these years is greater in physically active adolescents than in the inactive. Inactivity during the adolescent years may result in failure to realise genetic potential for peak bone mass.

2.3. *Psychosocial Well-being*

Participation in organised sport can have psychological and social benefits with involvement in team sports being beneficial in promoting social competency and skills. Physical activity has also been shown to be effective in the prevention of depression in an adolescent population. There is also a positive relationship between physical activity and self-esteem.

2.4. *Disease Prevention and Treatment*

Physical inactivity has been identified as a primary risk factor for a number of diseases including Type 2 diabetes, cardiovascular disease and malignant disease, in particular breast and colorectal cancer.

There is also a growing body of evidence that exercise prescription should form part of the routine medical management of a number of chronic diseases which affect adolescents including cystic fibrosis, insulin resistance (pre-diabetes), Type 2 diabetes, juvenile idiopathic arthritis and malignant disease.

3. Musculoskeletal Injury

Adolescence is a time of skeletal vulnerability. The rate of injury from participation in sport and exercise increases with both chronological age and pubertal stage. This increase in injury risk is due to the unique properties of the growing musculoskeletal system and may also be influenced by increases in physical performance under the influence of puberty hormones, and increased risk taking behaviours.

3.1. *The Adolescent Musculoskeletal System*

During adolescence a number of unique anatomical, physiological, biomechanical, and psychological factors have the potential to influence injury risk (Table 1). In particular, numerous tissue property changes make the adolescent athlete more susceptible to injury. One of the most significant changes seen during skeletal maturation is the increased rate of production of growth cartilage at epiphyses (growth plates responsible for longitudinal growth) and apophyses (tendon-growth plate interfaces). Growth cartilage is thicker and more fragile during peak growth, thus increasing the risk of injury from sheer, tensile, or compressive forces. The relative vulnerability of these epiphyses and apophyses produce unique patterns of both acute and overuse injury.

Table 1: Unique characteristics of the adolescent athlete.

Anatomical

Articular cartilage weaker compared with adults.
Growth plate thicker and more fragile during adolescence.
Bone mineral density decreases during peak linear growth.
Increases in muscle mass precede increase in bone mass.
Possible reduction in flexibility during peak growth.

Physiological

Increase in strength with age.
Increase in anaerobic power with age.
Increase in aerobic capacity with age.

Biomechanical

Increased force required to move limbs with age.

Psychological

Increased risk taking behaviour.

3.2. *Effect of Maturation on Injury Risk*

Although injury incidence increases with chronological age and pubertal stage in many sports, the effect of maturational status (level of biological maturity compared to age matched peers) on injury rate remains unclear. Maturational status does however influence injury patterns. Biologically immature adolescents sustain higher rates of growth-related overuse injuries than acute injuries, and also appear to have a higher incidence of major injury causing significant loss of playing time.

3.3. *Issues Relating to Size and Pubertal Status Mismatch in Adolescent Sport*

An area of concern, particularly for parents of late maturing adolescents in contact or collision sports, is when adolescents of differing pubertal status compete against one another. One would expect that a smaller individual with lower aerobic fitness and strength is at greater risk of injury than their stronger, more mature opponent of the same chronological age, although there is currently no evidence to support this.

3.4. *Common Acute Injuries in Adolescents*

3.4.1. *Acute fractures, including avulsion fractures*

Adolescents display unique patterns of acute musculoskeletal injury. Rather than the acute muscle tears or ligamentous injuries commonly seen in the adult athlete, adolescent athletes more commonly sustain acute injuries to bone and in particular the growth plate as this is the weakest part of the bone–tendon–muscle unit during adolescence. The peak period of fracture risk in adolescents coincides with the adolescent growth spurt in both sexes, which may be due to a relative decrease in bone mineral content during peak growth and the relative fragility of the growth plate during peak growth. Together with the increased forces placed on growing bone as a result of increased speed and power seen at the time of the adolescent growth spurt, the adolescent athlete becomes vulnerable to two unique types of fracture: fractures through or involving the physeal plate, and avulsion fractures of the apophysis at the site of insertion of large powerful muscles. These avulsion fractures are particularly common in adolescence and occur most commonly at the hip and pelvis. Common examples include avulsion fractures of the anterior superior iliac spine (at the insertion of sartorius and tensor fasciae latae), the anterior inferior iliac spine (at the insertion of rectus femoris) and the ischial tuberosity (at the insertion of the hamstrings). Avulsion fractures also occur in the upper limbs of gymnasts and throwing athletes, particularly at the medial epicondylar apophysis, and the olecranon.

3.5. *Common Chronic and Overuse Injuries in Adolescents*

Whereas tendinopathy and peripheral stress fractures are common types of overuse injury seen in adult sporting populations, these patterns of injury are relatively uncommon in the adolescent population. The most common chronic musculoskeletal conditions seen in the adolescent are the osteochondroses.

3.5.1. *Osteochondroses*

The osteochondroses are a group of conditions that affect the maturing skeleton and articular cartilage. These are more common in boys than girls, and can be either intra-articular, physeal, or extra-articular. The more common osteochondroses are listed in Table 2.

The osteochondroses vary in their aetiology and frequency of occurrence. Although the causative factors are not fully understood, stress, ischaemia, and genetics may all be implicated. Traction apophysitis is the most common form seen in the adolescent population and also the most benign of the three types of osteochondroses, with infrequent associated complications. Management consists of relative rest, improving flexibility in the involved muscle-tendon unit and correction of biomechanical risk factors. Osteochondroses involving the

Table 2: Classification of osteochondroses.

Disorder	Site	Age (yrs)	Presentation
Physeal			
Scheuermann Disease.	Vertebral end plate.	13–17	Thoracic spine pain or kyphosis.
Distal Radial Physeal Injury.	Distal radial physis.	10–14	Dorsal wrist pain aggravated by excessive upper limb weight bearing.
Slipped Upper Capital Femoral Epiphysis.	Femoral epiphysis.	10–14	Acute or chronic hip, groin, medial thigh (or referred pain at the knee) in overweight, immature boys.
Intra-articular			
Osteochondritis Dissecans.	Knee.	10–14	Medial knee pain +/– locking and swelling in active adolescent.
Osteochondritis Dissecans.	Capitellum or radial head.	12–15	Lateral elbow pain +/– locking and swelling in the throwing athlete.
Freiberg's Infraction.	Metatarsal head.	13–18	Forefoot pain in active female athlete.
Extra-articular (Traction Apophysitis)			
Osgood–Schlatter Disease.	Tibial tuberosity.	10–14	Activity related knee pain most commonly in adolescent boys.
Sever Disease.	Calcaneus.	10–14	Activity related heel pain most commonly in adolescent boys.
Iselin Disease.	5th metatarsal.	10–14	Lateral foot pain in active adolescent boys.
	Navicular.	10–14	Medial foot pain in active adolescent boys.
Little Leaguer's Elbow.	Medial epicondyle.	11–14	Medial elbow pain in the throwing athlete.

physeal plate do have the potential for complication, mainly asymmetrical growth. As such it is important to identify these conditions early and manage appropriately.

3.5.2. *Spondylolysis*

Spondylolysis refers to a stress fracture or defect of the pars interarticularis of the lumbar vertebrae, which most commonly presents as low back pain aggravated by activity. It may also be the result of a congenital defect of the pars interarticularis. Spondylolysis is usually seen in adolescents who participate in sports involving lumbar spine extension, often in combination with rotation, such as ballet, gymnastics, bowling in cricket, and serving at tennis. Approximately 90% occur at L5 with the remainder usually occurring at L4. If there are bilateral defects of the pars interarticularis then slippage known as spondylolisthesis may occur. While there are no known predictors of slippage, the greatest risk for this appears to be at the time of the adolescent growth spurt.

Plain X-ray may be useful to confirm the diagnosis, with an oblique view most clearly demonstrating the presence of a spondylolysis. A lateral view is also beneficial as it will detect the presence and extent of a co-existent spondylolisthesis. MRI is used to help guide management, as it is useful in differentiating between a stress fracture, which has potential for bony healing as opposed to a congenital defect, which does not. MRI (due to its absence of ionising radiation) is now considered preferable to bone scan and reverse gantry CT, which were previously used to establish the age of the spondylolysis and the likelihood of bony union. Clinical outcomes are usually favourable even in the absence of bony union. MRI may also be useful in detecting an early stress reaction or fracture which may not be evident on plain X-ray.

Initial management requires rest from activities involving lumbar extension and physiotherapy to improve core strength to prevent recurrence by providing a dynamic brace for the spine. A brace to prevent hyperextension can be used in the adolescent who has pain with activities of daily living but there is no evidence that it reduces recovery time or improves the chance of bony union.

4. Joint Hyper-mobility Syndrome in Adolescents

4.1. *Clinical Presentation and Assessment*

Joint hyper-mobility is a common finding in adolescents, particularly females. It is more common in Asian populations and there is usually a family history of hyper-mobility. Joint hyper-mobility syndrome refers to a condition in which joint hyper-mobility is associated with joint pain involving more than four joints for more than three months. Other presentations of JHS include joint subluxations or dislocations and skin striae. Fatigue and poor exercise tolerance can be associated features. The most common joints involved are the knees, low back, and hands although other joints may be affected. If there is involvement of the hands and wrists, this commonly presents with handwriting fatigue, and poor handwriting. JHS has a number of overlapping traits with other heritable connective tissue diseases including Ehlers–Danlos syndrome. It is important to exclude other heritable connective tissue diseases before making the diagnosis. Adolescents presenting with clinical features of other heritable connective tissue diseases, such as recurrent fractures, heart murmurs, or chest wall deformities will require further investigations including echocardiography and DEXA scanning.

The Brighton score is the most widely used measure to report joint hyper-mobility although it is skewed towards the joints it includes, namely the hands, knees, elbows, and back. A Brighton score of $\geq 4/9$ is consistent with hyper-mobility. One point is scored for each side for apposition of thumbs to flexor aspect of forearm, extension of 5th finger $>90°$, and elbow and knee extension $>10°$ plus one point for palms flat to floor with forward flexion of trunk and knees extended. The diagnostic criteria for JHS, the Brighton criteria, are outlined in Table 3.

4.2. *Management Including Sport Recommendations*

The principles of management in JHS involve improving muscle strength including core strength and improving aerobic capacity with a regular aerobic exercise program. The use of orthotics in those with symptomatic pes planus is often necessary. Involvement of occupational therapists for handwriting assessment and support is also often required. Adolescents with JHS should be encouraged to take part in regular physical activity

Table 3: Brighton criteria (2000) for diagnosis of benign joint hyper-mobility syndrome. (*Diagnosis requires either both major criteria or 1 major and 2 minor or 4 minor criteria*).

Major criteria

Brighton score $\geq$4/9.
Arthralgia >3 months in >4 joints.

Minor criteria

Brighton score 1–3.
Arthralgia >3 months in 1–3 joints or back pain >3 months, spondylolysis/spondylolisthesis.
History of >1 joint dislocation/subluxation.
>3 soft tissue lesions (tendinosis, tenosynovitis, bursitis).
Marfanoid habitus.
Abnormal skin including striae.
Eye signs — lid laxity, myopia.
History of hernia, varicose veins, visceral prolapse.

and sports, excluding collision sports, where the risk of joint dislocation and subluxation is high.

5. Prevention of Injuries in Adolescents

5.1. *Prevention of Overtraining*

Unfortunately there is a lack of evidence-based guidelines to determine the threshold for overtraining in most adolescent sports. It is therefore necessary to rely on markers of overtraining to suggest that an adolescent's training load and volume are too high. These markers include excessive fatigue, amenorrhoea in females, recurrent musculoskeletal injuries, weight loss, and less obvious markers such as a lack of unstructured free time. Coaches involved in youth sport should be made aware of the potential hazards of overtraining during vulnerable periods of growth and should regulate training and competition loads during these periods.

5.2. *Protective Equipment*

The use of helmets in cycling, horse riding, and snow sports has been shown to reduce the incidence and severity of traumatic brain injury in children and adolescents. There is also good evidence for the use of ankle taping and bracing in reducing the incidence and severity of ankle injury in sport. The use of other items of protective equipment, while potentially effective, does not have the supportive body of evidence.

5.3. *Future Strategies*

Future strategies for injury prevention may include the introduction of weight for age categories in some youth sports including contact and collision sports such as the football codes. Matching players according to biological rather than chronological age has also been suggested although the logistics of classifying youth sport in this way is likely to be impracticable.

6. Potential Long Term Health Implications

The majority of musculoskeletal injuries presenting in adolescence do not cause long-term sequelae. Prolonged time out of sport and physical activity increases the risk of developing inactivity-related adult disease. Injuries have been cited as one of the major reasons for athletes to drop out of continued participation in sport and exercise and as such, appropriate identification and management of adolescent musculoskeletal injury is important.

References

Alexander CJ. (1976) Effect of growth rate on the strength of the growth plate-shaft junction. *Skeletal Radiol* **1**(2): 67–76.

Bailey DA, Mckay HA, Mirwald RL, Crocker PR, Faulkner RA. (1999) A six-year longitudinal study of the relationship of physical activity to bone mineral accrual in growing children: The university of saskatchewan bone mineral accrual study. *J Bone Miner Res* **14**(10): 1672–1679.

De Moor M, Beem A, Stubbe J, Boomsma D, De Geus E. (2006) Regular exercise, anxiety, depression and personality: A population-based study. *Prev Med* **42**(4): 273–279.

Grahame R, Bird HA, Child A. (2000) The revised (brighton 1998) criteria for the diagnosis of benign joint hypermobility syndrome (bjhs). *J Rheumatol* **27**(7): 1777–1779.

Kujala UM, Taimela S, Antti-Poika I, Orava S, Tuominen R, Myllynen P. (1995) Acute injuries in soccer, ice hockey, volleyball, basketball, judo, and karate: Analysis of national registry data. *Br Med J* **311**(7018): 1465–1468.

Le Gall F, Carling C, Reilly T. (2007) Biological maturity and injury in elite youth football. *Scand J Med Sci Sports* **17**(5): 564–572.

Le Gall F, Carling C, Reilly T, Vandewalle H, Church J, Rochcongar P. (2006) Incidence of injuries in elite french youth soccer players: A 10-season study. *Am J Sports Med* **34**(6): 928–938.

Michaud PA, Renaud A. & Narring F. (2001) Sports activities related to injuries? A survey among 9–19 year olds in switzerland. *Inj Prev* **7**(1): 41–45.

Morscher E. (1968) Growth cartilage and puberty. *Ann Radiol (Paris)* **11**(5): 351–356.

Musch J, Grondin S. (2001) Unequal competition as an impediment to personal development: A review of the relative age effect in sport. *Dev Rev* **21**(2): 147–167.

Tremblay MS, Inman JW, Willms JD. (2000) The relationship between physical activity, self-esteem, and academic achievement in 12-year-old children. *Pediatr Exerc Sci* **12**(3): 312–323.

Chapter 27

Depression and Anxiety

Sloane Madden

1. Introduction

Depression and anxiety disorders remain some of the most significant chronic illnesses affecting adolescents. Prevalence of anxiety disorders is between 5%–10% and of major depression around 4%–6%. Both major depression and anxiety disorders are twice as common in females. These disorders are highly treatable, with a growing evidence base supporting the safety and effectiveness of treatments including cognitive behavioural therapy and medication.

1.1. *Major Depressive Disorders*

Major depression is a serious neurobiological disorder with prominent mood, psychological, and physical symptoms. Major depression is characterised by disturbances in mood (sadness and irritability) with associated impairments in sleep, energy, concentration and appetite, decreased interest or pleasure, social withdrawal, feelings of guilt and worthlessness, psychomotor agitation or retardation, and suicidal ideation. It is distinguished from grief or sadness by its persistence, intensity, and functional impairment. Depression commonly co-occurs with other diagnoses including anxiety disorders, ADHD and substance abuse. Comorbid substance abuse is particularly common in depressed adolescents and young adults, with substance abuse leading to depressive symptoms or used as a form of self-medication.

1.2. *Anxiety and Anxiety Disorders*

Anxiety is a normal and useful emotion, important in maintaining safety and improving performance. Anxiety disorders are not simply too much anxiety, rather these are developmentally inappropriate concerns characterised by irrational fears and the avoidance of situations associated with these fears. Anxiety disorders lead to impairment of day-to-day functioning and are associated with prolonged and intense distress. In adolescents the most common presenting disorders are generalised anxiety disorder, social phobia, agoraphobia, and panic disorder.

When faced with feared situations adolescents may experience a variety of physical symptoms including a racing heart, difficulty in breathing, nausea, dizziness, sweating, and shaking. These symptoms resolve rapidly once the young person is away from the feared situation, which indirectly encourages avoidance. When seeing adolescents with anxiety disorders it is important to remember that one third of these young people will have two or more anxiety disorders, and that one third will also have a major depressive disorder.

1.2.1. *Generalised anxiety disorder*

Generalised anxiety disorder is the second most common anxiety disorder in adolescents with rates up to 5%. Generalised anxiety disorder is characterised by excessive worrying about future events, social acceptability, personal adequacy, and competency. Young people with generalised anxiety disorder often appear overly mature, attempting to carry out tasks and responsibilities perfectly. They regularly seek reassurance for their worries and doubts and are overly sensitive to criticism. They frequently present with a variety of physical symptoms.

1.2.2. *Social phobia*

Social phobia affects around 1% of adolescents. Social phobia is characterised by avoidance of social or performance situations for fear of being negatively judged or doing something embarrassing. While some adolescents may have very specific fears such as eating or writing in public, generally most will fear many different types of social situations. Commonly feared situations include public speaking or performing such as reading in class, social gatherings, and interactions with strangers. Untreated social phobia has a high association with substance abuse in late adolescence and adulthood.

1.2.3. *Post traumatic stress disorder*

PTSD involves the constant reliving of the traumatic event to which one has been exposed and avoidance of similar situations. Adolescents with PTSD experience nightmares, recurrent intrusive thoughts and flashbacks, which are the re-experience of the traumatic event as if actually there. They are chronically over aroused, reacting to situations of even minor threat with either explosive rage or complete shutdown. Events leading to PTSD in young people include physical and sexual abuse, witnessing of domestic violence, natural disasters such as fire, and transport accidents.

1.2.4. *Obsessive-compulsive disorder — a different type of anxiety*

While considered part of the anxiety disorder spectrum, OCD has a distinct pattern of aetiology, symptoms, treatment response, and longitudinal course that sets it aside from other anxiety disorders commonly seen in adolescents. OCD is now recognised as a common disorder, with prevalence ranging from 1–4%. OCD is characterised by the presence of persistent intrusive thoughts (obsessions) and repetitive behaviours, mental acts or rituals carried out to neutralise obsessional fears or reduce anxiety (compulsions). These thoughts and behaviours generate considerable distress, differentiating them from other repetitive or addictive behaviours such as gambling or substance abuse, which are experienced initially as pleasurable.

While the diagnosis of OCD in adults requires insight into the unrealistic and unhelpful nature of obsessions and compulsions, such insight is not required to make the diagnosis in adolescents. In more than 80% of cases OCD begins before adulthood, often with a chronic course. Commonly it starts around the time of puberty and is somewhat more likely to present in boys than in girls. When considering a diagnosis of OCD it is important to seek corroborative evidence, as many adolescents carry out their rituals in secret to avoid embarrassment.

Common obsessions include

- Contamination and germ fears.
- Fear of harming or harm befalling oneself or family.
- Sexual thoughts.
- Fear of having severe or lethal medical illnesses.
- Magical thinking regarding colours, lucky numbers, or other lucky objects.

Common compulsions include

- Hand washing or cleaning.
- Checking locks, windows, doors, and switches.
- Repetitive rituals, including tapping, counting, and reading.
- Symmetry or ordering rituals.
- Constant seeking of reassurance.

2. Aetiology

Genetics and environment both play a role. Studies of families have shown that young people with anxiety disorders or depression are much more likely to have parents or siblings with depressive or anxiety disorders. In adults, twin and adoption studies have confirmed a strong genetic contribution to both anxiety disorders and depression. What are inherited though are not specific disorders but rather the tendency towards anxiety and depression, which responds to and is shaped by life experiences.

3. Assessment

It is important to obtain information from a variety of sources including not only the adolescent but also their parents and school. Younger adolescents may lack both insight into the nature of their anxiety disorder as well as the capacity to describe their symptoms. Older adolescents may under report their symptoms as a result of embarrassment or in order to avoid treatment.

3.1. *Anxiety Disorders*

It is important to remember that many young people with anxiety focus on or complain of the physical symptoms of anxiety rather than the underlying worries leading to these feelings. Similarly some parents are reluctant to consider the possibility of a psychological disorder particularly when their adolescent is complaining of significant physical symptoms. Despite this it is important to rule out physical conditions including hyperthyroidism, asthma, epilepsy, hypoglycaemia, migraines and common causes of abdominal discomfort, nausea, and vomiting.

3.2. *Major Depression*

Many depressed adolescents present with irritability, anger, risk-taking, deteriorating school performance, and social withdrawal rather than sadness. Unlike adults who seem unable to enjoy any aspects of their life, adolescents will often appear to cheer up when spending time with their friends. This does not rule out a diagnosis of depression as the enjoyment young people experience in such instances is almost always less than when free of mood symptoms. As well as asking about physical and psychological symptoms of depression it is important to explore for the presence of elevated mood. Bipolar disorder often begins in adolescence and is characterised by the presence of depressive symptoms but also by periods of elevated mood including increased energy, decreased sleep, pressured loud speech, risk taking, and grandiosity. Depressed adolescents and young adults require an assessment for suicidal ideation and self-harm. This is addressed in Chapter 29.

4. Treatment

The treatment of adolescent anxiety disorders and depression falls into two broad categories, medication management and psychological therapies, of which cognitive behavioural therapy is the best supported by treatment studies. There is a growing body of evidence to support the use of interpersonal therapy in adolescent depression. In general psychological treatment would be seen as the treatment of first choice. Medication is reserved for young people who have failed to respond to or are unable to tolerate psychological treatment, or who are at significant risk due to thoughts of self-harm and suicide or who have comorbid psychiatric illnesses. Even when the decision to use medication is made, it is important that this is combined with psychological treatment to improve both acute outcomes and to reduce the risk of relapse particularly when medication is ceased.

4.1. *Cognitive Behavioural Therapy*

CBT is the first line treatment for adolescents with anxiety disorder, OCD, and mild to moderate depression. It is a talking based therapy arising from the link between thoughts, feelings, and behaviour. Central to CBT is the belief that thoughts influence behaviours and feelings, that unhelpful thoughts generating anxiety and depression can be identified and challenged, and that by replacing these thoughts with more realistic ones, behaviours and feelings can be changed. In practice CBT involves a clinician teaching adolescents coping skills to address anxiety symptoms as well as a chance to practise these skills to provide a sense of control over such symptoms. CBT generally involves five specific components:

- Psycho-education of the young person and their parents about the illness and its treatment.
- Somatic symptom management, including relaxation, controlled breathing, and monitoring of somatic symptoms.
- Cognitive restructuring which is about identifying and challenging negative thoughts.
- Exposure to an increasing hierarchy of feared situations.
- Relapse prevention plans.

Other elements that have been helpfully integrated with CBT include social skills training, problem solving, anger management, exercise, and pleasant events. CBT can be given on an individual or group basis and typically involves between 12 and 20 weekly sessions of between 30 and 60 minutes.

4.1.1. *CBT in anxiety*

CBT has been shown in a number of randomised controlled trials to be helpful in managing anxiety in adolescents and young adults when provided in either an individual or group format. With the exception of tailored programs for OCD, generic treatment programs which address all forms of anxiety have been shown to be most effective. The involvement of parents of younger adolescents in CBT treatment has been shown to improve outcomes, particularly when parents themselves are anxious. Efficacy has also been demonstrated for remote treatment delivery including self-help manuals and computer delivery.

4.1.2. *CBT in depression*

Trials in adolescent depression have shown CBT to be efficacious. Most evidence exists for CBT delivered in group settings, although evidence also supports individual CBT in adolescents with family involvement. CBT in addition to medication improves outcomes compared to medication alone.

4.2. *Interpersonal Therapy*

IPT focuses on addressing relationship issues between adolescents/young adults and significant others in their lives. While fewer studies of IPT than CBT have been carried out there is strong support for individual IPT with its efficacy shown to be equivalent to CBT.

4.3. *Selective Serotonin Reuptake Inhibitors*

In 2003 the UK Department of Health issued a warning to doctors against prescribing any SSRI except for fluoxetine in depressed adolescents under the age of 18 years. Following this in September 2004 the US Food and

Drug Administration mandated that a 'black box' warning be put on the label of all SSRIs indicating an increased risk of suicidal thoughts and behaviour in youth taking these medications. These warnings were based on a meta-analysis of 24 published and unpublished placebo controlled trials assessing the use of anti-depressants in the treatment of adolescents with depression. This analysis did not indicate an increased risk of suicidal thoughts in treatment trials of anxiety disorders or OCD. It is important to recognise that evidence for the efficacy of the SSRIs is greatest in the non-OCD anxiety disorders and OCD, and modest in adolescent depression.

Despite these concerns, SSRIs are the medications of choice in the treatment of both anxiety disorders and major depression in adolescents due to their overall demonstrated efficacy and safety.

4.3.1. *SSRIs in anxiety disorders*

Multiple randomised controlled trials in a variety of anxiety disorders including selective mutism, generalised anxiety disorder, social phobia, and separation anxiety disorder have shown the SSRIs (including paroxetine, fluoxetine, sertraline, fluvoxamine, and venlafaxine) to be significantly superior to placebo. All studies have demonstrated that SSRIs are well tolerated and safe. It is important to remember that effective SSRI doses in the treatment of anxiety disorders are higher than those recommended for depression. As in adults, SSRIs are not lethal in overdose. The evidence for the efficacy of SSRIs is similarly strong in the treatment of OCD. Interestingly the size of the treatment effect is modest and less than that seen for clomipramine, a serotonin specific tricyclic anti-depressant. Additionally there is evidence demonstrating increased efficacy of the combination of medication and CBT over either treatment alone.

4.3.2. *SSRIs in major depression*

The use of medication in depression has remained controversial since the link between suicidal thoughts and the SSRIs was first identified. Despite this there is increasing and strong evidence to support their use in adolescent depression particularly in moderate to severe depression. Strongest evidence exists for the efficacy of fluoxetine and escitalopram with some positive studies for sertraline and citalopram.

4.3.3. *Which SSRI?*

In major depression only fluoxetine and escitalopram have US FDA approval for their use in adolescents and it is advisable to start with one of these two anti-depressants. There is no empirical evidence that one SSRI is more effective than another. The main differences between medications revolve around their half-life. Fluoxetine has a half-life of up to two weeks, compared to one day or less for sertraline and fluvoxamine, which is particularly useful in adolescents where medication is often missed or forgotten. In young people care needs to be taken with agents with a short half-life, in particular paroxetine which has a half-life in adolescents of around 12 hours. Such agents have been associated with increased agitation, particularly in individuals with major depression or anxiety disorders with comorbid depression.

4.3.4. *SSRIs dosage and side effects*

Up to 80% of individuals will experience mild transient side effects, the most common of which are abdominal discomfort, headache, and sleep disturbance. While most side effects settle within three to four days, up to one in 12 adolescents will experience behavioural agitation or hypomania necessitating cessation of medication. This latter complication can be minimised by the use of low starting doses of medication with gradual increases in dosage as required. In general most adolescents would start on half the normal adult commencement dose. In most cases adolescents will need to be increased to a standard adult dose of medication. Two other important side effects in adolescents taking SSRIs are sexual dysfunction, and withdrawal symptoms with cessation of medication. While specific rates of sexual dysfunction in adolescents taking SSRIs are unclear, it is a clinically significant phenomenon, particularly in young males, who are unlikely to remain compliant with medication or discuss this problem should it occur. Withdrawal phenomena are experienced with rapid cessation of anti-depressant treatment and include agitation, restlessness, poor concentration, fatigue, and insomnia. Also of concern is the possible increased risk of relapse associated with the rapid cessation of medication. Ceasing medication over a period of around two weeks serves to reduce withdrawal symptoms.

Though SSRIs have been demonstrated to be efficacious in treating anxiety disorders and depression in the short-term, there is little evidence to guide clinicians with regard to their long-term efficacy. Based on the action of SSRIs in depression and anxiety disorders in adults, treatment for a minimum of 6–9 months is recommended.

4.3.5. *SSRIs and concurrent medical illness*

In general the SSRIs are safe in the chronically medically ill. The SSRIs are largely metabolised by the liver with their metabolites excreted by the kidneys. For this reason dosages should be reduced in individuals with renal and liver impairment. Theoretically SSRIs may decrease seizure threshold in epilepsy, although in practice this does not appear to be of significance. The SSRIs have no impact on cardiac conduction, heart rate, or blood pressure.

4.4. *Tricyclic Antidepressants*

TCAs were amongst the first medications successfully used in the treatment of major depression in adult patients and on the basis of this were prescribed to adolescents. Despite their efficacy in adults the most recent meta-analysis in the use of tricyclic anti-depressants showed that these were not efficacious in treating depression in adolescents. Hazell (1995) reviewed 12 double-blind randomised controlled trials of tricyclic anti-depressants in adolescents and found that these medications were no more effective than placebo. Trials of TCAs in adolescent anxiety disorders have mostly focused on school refusal. Evidence for the efficacy of TCAs remains equivocal, and at best these are a second line agent for the treatment of adolescent anxiety disorders, with use confined to specialist clinics. TCAs have been associated with unexplained sudden deaths in the US and are potentially lethal in overdose. The exception to this rule is the use of clomipramine in OCD (see 4.3.1).

4.5. *Benzodiazepines*

No controlled trials have demonstrated a significant difference between benzodiazepines and placebo in young people with anxiety disorders. Given problems of sedation, dependence, tolerance and withdrawal there is little role for benzodiazepines in the treatment of adolescent anxiety and no role in adolescent depression.

5. Conclusions

Major depression and anxiety disorders are common in adolescents and if left untreated cause significant impairment and distress and may persist into young adulthood. These respond well to treatment and the evidence is accumulating that CBT, medication, and other approaches can be helpful. There is a tendency for adolescents not to present with depressed mood or anxiety but with school refusal, physical symptoms, social withdrawal, and irritability.

References

Bridge JA, Iyengar S, Salary CB, Barbe RP, Birmaher B, Pincus HA, Ren L, Brent DA. (2007) Clinical response and risk for reported suicidal ideation and suicide attempts in pediatric antidepressant treatment. *JAMA* **297**(15): 1683–1696.

David-Ferdon C, Kaslow NJ. (2008) Evidence-based psychosocial treatments for child and adolescent depression. *J Clin Child Adolesc Psychol* **37**(1): 62–104.

Geller DA, Biederman J, Stewart SE, Mullin B, Martin A, Spencer T, Faraone SV. (2003) Which SSRI? A meta-analysis of pharmacotherapy trials in pediatric obsessive-compulsive disorder. *Am J Psychiatry* **160**(11): 1919–1928.

Hazell P, O'connell D, Heathcote D, Robertson J, Henry D. (1995) Efficacy of tricyclic drugs in treating child and adolescent depression: A meta-analysis. *BMJ* **310**(6984): 897–901.

Kodish I, Rockhill C, Ryan S, Varley C. (2011) Pharmacotherapy for anxiety disorders in children and adolescents. *Pediatr Clin North Am* **58**(1): 55–72.

Mann JJ, Emslie G, Baldessarini RJ, Beardslee W, Fawcett JA, Goodwin FK, Leon AC, Meltzer HY, Ryan ND, Shaffer D, Wagner KD. (2005) ACNP task force report on SSRIs and suicidal behavior in youth. *Neuropsychopharmacol* **31**(3): 473–492.

Rapee RM, Schniering CA, Hudson JL. (2009) Anxiety disorders during childhood and adolescence: Origins and treatment. *Ann Rev Clin Psychol* **5**: 311–341.

Smiga SM, Elliott GR. (2011) Psychopharmacology of depression in children and adolescents. *Pediatr Clin North Am* **58**(1): 155–171.

Turner CM. (2006) Cognitive-behavioural theory and therapy for obsessive-compulsive disorder in children and adolescents: Current status and future directions. *Clin Psychol Rev* **26**(7): 912–938.

Chapter 28

Assessment and Treatment of Psychotic Disorders in Adolescence

Jean Starling and Anthony Harris

1. Introduction

Psychotic disorders in adolescence are rare, with a prevalence of one in 500 18 year olds. About a third of adults with psychotic disorders report that their illness started before the age of 20 and the lifetime prevalence of all psychotic disorders in the adult population is 2%–3%. Schizophrenia has a lifetime morbid risk of 7.2 per 1000 and is a severe and chronic illness with a high burden of disease. However, all mental illnesses with psychotic symptoms impair emotional, cognitive, and social functioning. Furthermore, these disorders are highly stigmatised, making treatment and integration back into the community difficult.

Psychotic disorders, where a young person presents with thoughts or behaviour suggesting that they are out of touch with reality, are severe conditions associated with social and academic deterioration. These disorders may lead to long term handicap, particularly without early intervention. There is also an increased risk of suicide and harm to others, particularly when acutely unwell. Early and expert treatment is crucial, so prompt referral to psychiatric services is recommended, as is intensive treatment by a mental health team, including a psychiatrist, in the acute phase of the illness.

2. Assessment

2.1. *Symptoms*

- *Hallucinations*, or perceptions in the absence of a stimulus, most commonly auditory hallucinations, or hearing voices.
- *Delusions*, or fixed false beliefs, generally persecutory, where there is a belief of harm, or grandiose, with unrealistically elevated beliefs.
- Perceptual changes and odd or bizarre beliefs.
- Significant negative symptoms of reduced motivation, altered affect, altered sociability.
- Worsened cognitive performance in domains such as attention, concentration, memory, and planning.

These negative and cognitive symptoms best predict long term outcome and may precede the onset of hallucinations or delusions by many months. In addition changes in mood, anxiety, and levels of agitation are common and need to be enquired about.

2.2. *Obtaining a History*

Obtaining a history of psychotic symptoms can be difficult. Young people often avoid discussing such symptoms because they are *frightened of being seen as 'crazy'*. They need to be given a choice as to whether they would prefer to be seen alone or with the support of a trusted adult, often a parent. Starting the interview with a discussion of more neutral topics such as family, school, and friendships helps to build rapport and build up a picture of general functioning. The interviewer can then move on to ask about specific worries or concerns and explore those in more detail.

Asking about *symptoms of anxiety and depressed or elevated mood* is crucial, as is discussing thoughts of self-harm or suicide. Finally there needs to be *specific enquiries about psychotic symptoms*, where it is important to be neutral but direct, for example saying 'I am going to ask you some questions that seem really strange but are important to help me understand what is happening with your thoughts.' Examples of questions to use for a comprehensive assessment of psychotic symptoms are given in Table 1. A discussion of the rules of confidentiality is also important.

Table 1: A mental state assessment for psychotic symptoms.

	Interview questions	Rationale for questions
Appearance and behaviour	Observation at interview	Unusual behaviour or dress should be described and if possible understood during the interview
Insight	Could you tell me why you have come to see me? Do you think there is anything that you need help with?	If they understand that they are unwell and if they see the need for treatment co-operation is more likely
Mood-depression	Have you been feeling depressed or down recently? Have you lost interest in things you usually enjoy? Have you had problems sleeping? Have you had thoughts of hurting yourself? If yes to any of the above also ask about eating, agitation, concentration, guilty or hopeless thoughts and suicidal ideas or plans	Checking for a current and past history of depression and risk of self-harm or suicide
Mood-elevation	Have you ever had a period of time where you were feeling so good, excited or hyper that you felt out of control, or did worrying things? If yes ask for more details	A period of elevated mood may be part of bipolar disorder
Thought form	Observation of speech flow and association at interview	Thought disorder is often seen in psychosis and the type will help with diagnosis. Thought disorder is where thoughts are poorly connected. Speech can be also rushed in bipolar disorder or slowed in depression

(Continued)

Table 1: (*Continued*)

	Interview questions	Rationale for questions
Perceptual abnormalities — hallucinations	Did you ever hear things that other people couldn't such as noises or people's voices? If yes, what did you hear and how often? If voices, did they comment on what you were thinking or doing? How many voices did you hear? Were they talking to each other? Did you have visions or see things that other people couldn't? (ask for details) Also ask about tactile, olfactory and gustatory abnormalities	These questions ask about core psychotic symptoms. As hallucinations become more complicated (more often, say more things, more than one voice) a psychotic disorder is more likely.
Thought content — delusions	Start with "I would like to ask you about unusual experiences people sometimes have" Has it ever seemed that people were talking about you or taking special notice of you? Have you ever received special messages from the TV, radio, or other things around you? What about anyone trying to give you a hard time or hurt you? Have you ever felt that you were especially important or could do things that others could not? If yes to any get further details	As delusions become more complex (e.g. not just people looking at me but having an elaborate plan to hurt me) a psychotic disorder is more likely. Paranoid delusions are most likely in schizophrenia spectrum disorders, and grandiose delusions in bipolar disorder.
Cognitive functioning	Ask about current and past functioning at school including concentration, motivation, ability to learn and academic grades	Premorbid cognitive functioning affects prognosis, while deterioration is not only seen in psychotic disorders but also in depression.

2.3. *Other Assessments*

Understanding current academic and social functioning is crucial, in particular any deterioration. Past or family psychiatric history can be an important pointer for diagnosis. Parents can provide a developmental history including birth trauma or developmental abnormalities and can also describe symptoms that the young person is reluctant to talk about. Corroborative information from schools, health services, and other care agencies will be required. *It is rare for a psychotic disorder to exist in isolation in a young person.* Common comorbidities include substance misuse (ask about tobacco, cannabis, and stimulants), anxiety, depression, behavioural disorders, a history of trauma, or developmental disorders.

3. Making a Diagnosis

3.1. *Are Reported Symptoms Truly Psychotic?*

It is important to decide if the reported symptoms are truly psychotic or due to another disorder. For example a depressed teenager describing their own thoughts ruminating on what a failure they are, or an anxious adolescent seeing shadows by their bed and being convinced that burglars have broken into their house.

3.2. *Prodrome*

Symptoms may appear related to psychosis but do not meet full diagnostic criteria. Many psychotic disorders have a prodrome, with disturbances in mood, thoughts, and behaviour and some deterioration in functioning. However, some of these disturbances are non-specific. Early psychosis research has also identified 'psychotic-like experiences', which consist of bizarre experiences, persecutory ideas, and magical thinking. All but magical thinking increase the risk of later development of psychosis. Young adolescents with isolated symptoms at 11 years are 16 times more likely to have a diagnosis of schizophreniform disorder by the age of 26 years. Some trials show that early treatment can prevent transition to full blown illness.

3.3. *The Difficulties of Establishing a Diagnosis*

Even if it is clear that the young person meets criteria for a psychotic disorder, it can be difficult to make an accurate diagnosis early. The two most common psychotic disorders are schizophrenia and bipolar disorder.

In schizophrenia the prominent symptoms are hallucinations and/or delusions, with associated disturbed behaviour and deterioration in functioning. Schizophreniform disorder has the same symptoms but for a period of less than six months.

Bipolar disorder has mood symptoms as the predominant feature, with *mania* (at least one episode of severely elevated mood affecting all areas of functioning including sleep and cognition for a period of at least seven days) most prominent. Initial episodes of a bipolar disorder are *often depressive*, making it far more difficult to arrive at a diagnosis promptly. Initial diagnoses have poor reliability, with inaccuracy between observers and poor diagnostic stability over time.

Using the term 'early onset psychosis' initially is accurate and provides for more treatment flexibility. If there is a definite psychotic illness present, early treatment is crucial. The longer the duration of untreated psychosis the more difficult the symptoms are to treat and the greater the risk of long term disability.

4. Physical Investigations for Early Onset Psychosis

These are detailed in Table 2 and are performed to exclude treatable organic causes for psychosis, and as a baseline for preventing or managing side effects of treatment. A full physical examination is also essential, with particular emphasis on developmental or neurological abnormalities. Weight, height, blood pressure and pulse need to be recorded initially and monitored. There are also some acute autoimmune or inflammatory illnesses that mimic psychosis, especially when the onset is acute and could be a delirium. Appropriate general or subspecialty medical consultations are essential for these patients.

Table 2: The main investigations recommended at baseline assessment for early onset psychosis.

Investigation		Rationale
1. Blood tests	Full blood count	Detection of pre-existing haematological disorders such as anaemia, monitoring side effects of mood stabilisers
	Urea, electrolytes, liver function	Exclusion of pre-existing abnormalities (rare, but polydipsia can be seen in psychosis) Monitoring for side effects (some antipsychotics and antidepressants can cause hyponatraemia, mood stabilisers can impair liver function)
	Fasting glucose, cholesterol and triglycerides	Detection of insulin resistance or lipid abnormalities Initial and six monthly monitoring as most antipsychotics can cause weight gain and insulin resistance
	Thyroid function	Thyroid abnormalities can cause mood elevation or depression and are a side effect of lithium treatment
	Calcium levels	Abnormalities a rare cause of psychosis
	Prolactin	Exclusion of pre-treatment hyperprolactinaemia (e.g. due to pituitary tumour); to monitor possible antipsychotic induced hyperprolactinaemia
	Others including autoimmune and inflammatory screens	Used if illness very acute and autoimmune or inflammatory cause suspected
2. Brain imaging (Computerised Axial Tomography, Magnetic Resonance Imaging)		Exclusion of preexisting neuroanatomical lesions MRI preferable because of higher resolution image and less radiation exposure but noise and claustrophobia may not be tolerated, then CAT needed
3. Electroencephalogram		Exclusion of a seizure disorder
4. Urine drug screen		To rule out recent drug use, or identify illicit drugs taken recently

5. Management

5.1. *Risk Assessment*

It is crucial to assess for safety, both of the young person and the people they live with. Ideally assessment and treatment should occur while they remain at home with their family, but an *admission may be needed* if:

- There are concerns about risk of suicide.
- Aggression to others because of delusional beliefs.
- Exploitation by others while unwell.
- Homelessness.
- Exhaustion of carers, for example when a teenager has not slept for days and their family can no longer adequately supervise them.
- Physical symptoms such as fluctuating levels of consciousness that require urgent medical investigation.

Admission may need to be under a Mental Health Act if the consent of either the young person or their family cannot be obtained.

5.2. *Urgent Sedation*

Rapidly acting oral medication such as diazepam (5–10 mg), risperidone (0.5–1 mg) or olanzapine (2.5–5 mg) should be used. If orals are refused in a crisis, intramuscular or intravenous sedation using midazolam 5–10 mg or droperidol 5–10 mg is recommended. IV sedation should be avoided unless there are facilities to monitor oxygen saturation and provide airway maintenance and resuscitation if needed. IM or IV sedation usually requires physical restraint and is very distressing for the child and family. *The least coercive method of sedation is important because the first experience of mental health treatment can make the difference between ongoing compliance or avoidance of further treatment.*

5.3. *Next Step Medication*

If no emergency treatment is needed, medication decisions in early psychosis are based on controlling the psychosis and managing associated symptoms as shown in Fig. 1. If depression is the predominant

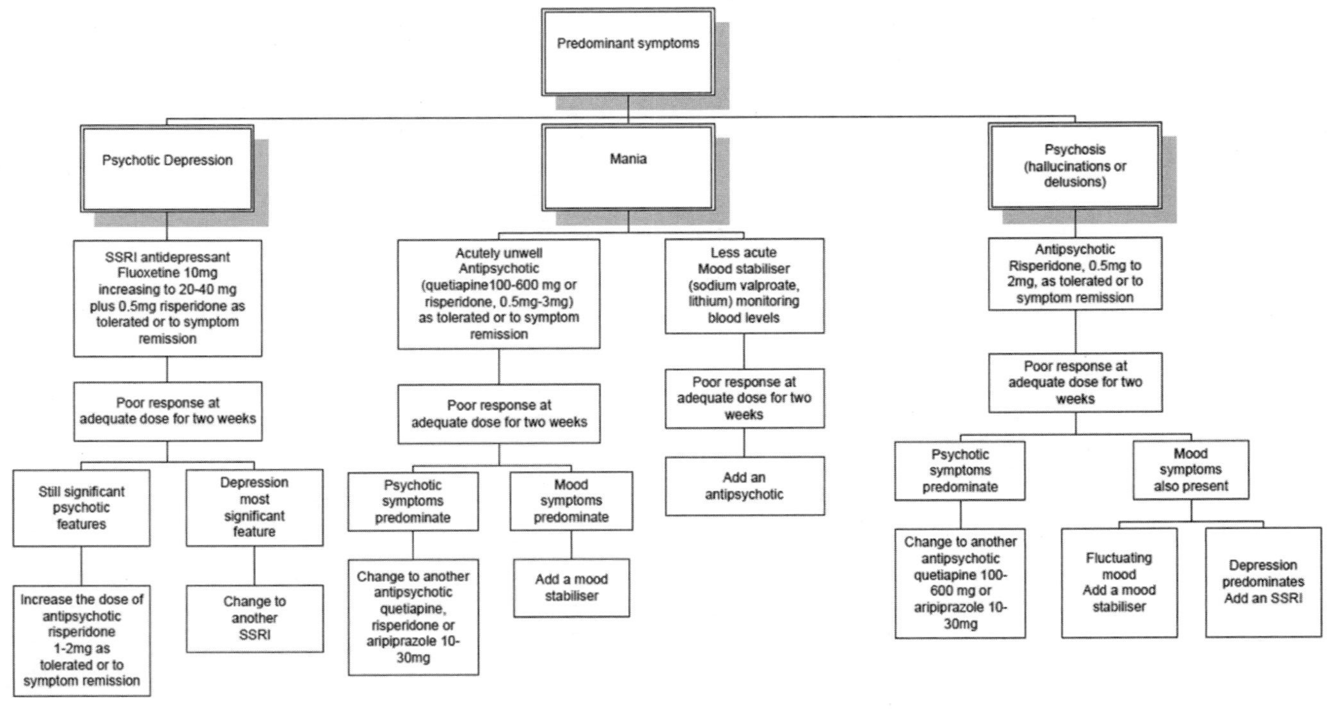

Fig. 1:   A treatment flow chart.

symptom and hallucinations or other psychotic symptoms are less prominent an anti-depressant should be trialled first, with a small dose of an anti-psychotic. When there is mania a mood stabiliser is more appropriate. If hallucinations or delusions are of most concern an anti-psychotic is used. Table 3 details side effects of the most commonly used anti-psychotic medications.

With any psychotropic medication it is important to 'Start Low and Go Slow' with dosage. This is to avoid side effects and maximise compliance with treatment. For more details about treatment with specific medications and their side effects see Tiffin's comprehensive review.

When there is no response to anti-psychotic medication after two weeks medication review is needed, as some response is usually seen in the positive psychotic symptoms by that time. If the maximum tolerable dose of a particular medication has been reached without effect a choice needs to be made about either changing medication or adding another medication class (Fig. 1). Failure to respond to two or more anti-psychotics trialled for an adequate time and at adequate doses should prompt referral to a specialist service for consideration of clozapine.

5.4. *Psychoeducation*

Psychoeducation is a structured way of providing information about psychotic disorders and their treatment for both young people and their families. There are manualised programs available, and evidence that psychoeducation reduces the rate of relapse in early psychosis. The ingredients of effective psychoeducation programs include:

- Providing information about the illness and treatment options.
- Offering a forum for the young person to discuss their illness and concerns, and
- Involving family members in the education process, whether with their children or in parent groups.

If successful, the rate of relapse is reduced by increased compliance with medication, reduction in maladaptive behaviours such as substance misuse, and early recognition of symptom return/deterioration. Coping skills and problem solving training can also be part of the education program.

Table 3: Common side effects of antipsychotic medications used in early onset psychosis.

Antipsychotic	Dose (mg)	Extra pyramidal side effects	Sedation	Weight	Prolactin	Postural hypotension	Potential disadvantages	Potential advantages
Risperidone	1–6 mg	++	++	++	+++	++	Galactorrhoea, sedation	Most data on use in adolescents (incl. in autism)
Quetiapine	200–800 mg	+	++	++	+	+	Initial sedation, often settles	Useful for psychosis with mood disorders or anxiety
Aripiprazole	10–30 mg	++	+	+	0	+	Initial agitation	Sedation, weight gain and elevated prolactin rare
Olanzapine	5–20 mg	+	+++	+++	+	+	Very significant weight gain, sedation. Not recommended long term	Sedating and calming when acutely unwell

5.5. *Cognitive Behavioural Therapy*

Some young people find CBT very helpful in understanding and managing their symptoms. The goals of CBT vary depending on the symptoms of concern, but can include coping strategies for psychotic experiences and managing low moods. Directly addressing the psychotic symptoms is best done in the recovery, rather than during the acute phase of treatment. Strategies include:

- Exploring and challenging delusional beliefs.
- Finding coping mechanisms to minimise the impact of hallucinations.
- Managing feelings of hopelessness and low mood using similar techniques to CBT for depression.

5.6. *Working with Families*

Initial work with families involves a psychoeducational approach, providing information about psychotic illnesses and how these affect thoughts and behaviours. Problem solving skills and communication strategies help families deal with difficult situations and reduce distress in the household. This reduces the risk of relapse, as well as preventing family estrangement.

6. Maintenance Medication and Side Effects

Long term use of anti-psychotic medication is recommended for at least 12 months after symptom remission to reduce relapse. Careful monitoring and management of side effects are essential. Weight gain and associated metabolic abnormalities are the most likely, but sedation and cognitive slowing can also cause distress.

Six monthly monitoring is required for:

- Involuntary movements.
- Weight, pulse rate and blood pressure.
- Fasting glucose and lipids.

Movement disorders including Parkinsonism and akathisia (restless legs) are less common with second generation anti-psychotic medications.

If these occur try small doses of an anti-cholinergic drug, for example benztropine 0.5 mg a day. Reducing the dose of the anti-psychotic is often more effective. Tardive dyskinesia, a rare chronic movement disorder, is often first seen as small movements in the face or fingers. Early identification is important as chronic TD may continue after medication is ceased. All mood stabilisers are teratogenic and this needs to be discussed with sexually active adolescents. The use of lithium requires clear instructions about the need to avoid dehydration, and to have regular lithium levels and thyroid function tests to monitor for possible toxicity.

7. Early Psychosis in Specific Populations

Young people with developmental disability, in particular pervasive developmental disorders, have an increased risk of psychosis but also are more likely to be wrongly diagnosed because of their eccentric behaviour and idiosyncratic interests. Those with a history of trauma may have intrusive memories or flashbacks that may seem psychotic but are part of the Post Traumatic Stress Disorder spectrum. Trauma itself is also a risk factor for the development of psychosis. Finally, drug use, in particular cannabis, psychostimulants and the hallucinogens, can precipitate a psychotic episode and increase the risk of relapse after recovery. Illicit drugs may also be used to self medicate distress in early onset psychosis, but ongoing use makes hallucinations and delusions less likely to respond to medication.

8. Services for Early Psychosis

While schools, general practitioners, paediatricians, and other health providers often identify young people at risk of psychosis, once early psychosis is identified it is essential that mental health services be involved. In Australia these services include Child and Adolescent Mental Health Services that are community based teams who see young people up to the age of 18, and Youth Mental Health Services, for ages 12–25 which include Headspace and Prevention and Early Intervention teams. All of these services use a case management model, with an allied health or nurse case manager and psychiatric consultation as needed. Some also provide assertive case management (a more intensive case management used for difficult to treat patients), drug and alcohol services, general health and sexual health services, or help with financial management, housing, and employment.

9. Recovery, Return to Education and Outcome

It is important to frame the interaction with the young person positively. Psychotic symptoms almost always remit within days to weeks, however negative symptoms (poor energy, motivation, and concentration) may continue for many months, particularly in the schizophrenia spectrum disorders. Returning to school may be difficult because of negative symptoms, cognitive difficulties, or the amount of time missed, including explaining any period of absence to others.

Options here include supported education programs, partial attendance for a period of time or special education placements. Some of these run jointly with mental health services while recovery continues. Liaison with an appropriate school counsellor is essential at this stage.

For those 15 years and older some of the Technical and Further Education providers such as TAFE (in NSW, Australia) provide support for students with disabilities. A day program or work preparation program may be needed for those whose recovery is slower. Additional evidence based interventions such as social skills training or cognitive remediation strategies may be very useful in the recovery process.

While the majority of symptoms improve in the first six months of treatment, improvement can continue for up to two years. The schizophrenia spectrum disorders tend to have the slowest response, the highest rate of residual deficits, and a lifelong risk of relapse is 80%–90%. A good prognosis is more likely with a rapid onset of psychotic symptoms, prominent mood symptoms, good social and educational functioning prior to the illness and a rapid response to initial treatment.

10. Transition to Adult Services

The youth specific mental health services are ideal for the adolescent population because they can continue with the same service into young adult life. After a psychotic episode some form of monitoring is essential for at least two years. When symptoms are stable, medication can be supervised by a general practitioner or family physician, sometimes with support from a psychologist or other mental health clinician. The identification of other stressful life transitions for example, tertiary education, moving out of home or new employment is important.

11. Case Study

Robbie was a 15 year old boy living with his parents and younger sister and in year 10 at high school. While never a keen student, he had lost interest over the last six months and his grades had fallen. He had also lost interest in sport (previously a favourite activity), and for the last two months had difficulty getting out of bed. The school counsellor had been concerned about depression and referred him to the local youth health service. When seen he was very distressed and described hearing two voices discussing his activities. He was also worried that the smoke detector in his bedroom was feeding information to a security agency. A provisional diagnosis of early onset psychosis was made after investigations ruled out organic disease. He was able to be treated at home with family support, and the symptoms responded to a small dose of risperidone. The community mental health team provided support and education to him and his family, and Robbie was able to gradually return to school as he recovered.

References

Addington J, Mccleery A, Collins A, Addington D. (2007) Family work in early psychosis. *J Fam Psychother* **17**(3–4): 137–153.

Barnes TRE, Leeson VC, Mutsatsa SH, Watt HC, Hutton SB, Joyce EM. (2008) Duration of untreated psychosis and social function: 1-year follow-up study of first-episode schizophrenia. *Br J Psychiatry* **193**(3): 203–209.

Cutajar MC, Mullen PE, Ogloff JRP, Thomas SD, Wells DL, Spataro J. (2010) Schizophrenia and other psychotic disorders in a cohort of sexually abused children. *Arch Gen Psychiatry* **67**(11): 1114–1119.

Lambert M, Conus P, Lubman DI, Wade D, Yuen H, Moritz S, Naber D, McGorry PD, Yung AR, Phillips LJ, Yuen HP, Francey S, Cosgrave EM,

Germano D, Bravin J, Mcdonald T, Blair A, Adlard S, Jackson H. (2002) Randomized controlled trial of interventions designed to reduce the risk of progression to first-episode psychosis in a clinical sample with subthreshold symptoms. *Arch Gen Psychiatry* **59**(10): 921–928.

Pekkala T, Merinder BL, (2010) Psychoeducation for schizophrenia: Cochrane database of systematic Reviews 2010.

Poulton R, Caspi A, Moffitt TE, Cannon M, Murray R, Harrington H. (2000) Children's self-reported psychotic symptoms and adult schizophreniform disorder: A 15-year longitudinal study. *Arch Gen Psychiatry* **57**(11): 1053–1058.

Starling J, Dossetor D. (2009) Pervasive developmental disorders and psychosis. *Curr Psychiatry Rep* **11**(3): 190–196.

Tiffin PA. (2007) Managing psychotic illness in young people: A practical overview. *Child and Adolesc Ment Health* **12**(4): 173–186.

Yung AR, Buckby JA, Cotton SM, Cosgrave EM, Killackey EJ, Stanford C, Godfrey K, Mcgorry PD. (2006) Psychotic-like experiences in nonpsychotic help-seekers: Associations with distress, depression, and disability. *Schizophr Bull* **32**(2): 352–359.

Chapter 29

Suicide and Self-Harm

Philip Hazell

1. Introduction

Deliberate self-harm is an act with a non-fatal outcome in which an individual deliberately did one or more of the following:

- Initiated behaviour (for example, self-cutting, jumping from a height), which intended to cause self-harm.
- Ingested a substance in excess of the prescribed or generally recognised therapeutic dose.
- Ingested a recreational or illicit drug that was an act that the person regarded as self-harm.
- Ingested a non-ingestible substance or object.

Most DSH is of low lethality and most people who engage in DSH are not at increased risk for suicide, at least in the short term. While an assessment for suicide risk is mandatory in the clinical work up of patients who engage in DSH, this should not be the only focus of assessment. The patient will be much better helped if the clinician tries to understand the patient's predicament and assists them to find solutions. Self-injurious behaviour is a term reserved for the seemingly stereotypic self-harm associated with some forms of intellectual disability, such as Lesch–Nyan and Cornelia de Lange syndromes.

Suicide of a young person is rare, but has a devastating effect on families, peers, the community, and on any individual who has had prior clinical involvement with the deceased. A significant proportion of adolescent suicide deaths progress to coronial inquiry. While it is important to explore all factors that could have contributed to a death, the reality is that such investigations focus on that which can be admitted in evidence. This can lead to the spurious conclusion that good note taking and form filling will prevent suicide, whereas good clinical and communication skills are more relevant.

2. Deliberate Self-Harm

2.1. *Clinical Description*

The most common methods of DSH identified in a large multi-national study of 15–16 year olds by Madge *et al.* were self-cutting and overdosing. Self-battery, jumping, and hanging were less frequent. Females were more likely than males to report self-cutting only (59.5% compared with 44.3%) and overdose only (23.1% versus 19.5%), but less likely to have used another single method (6.4% compared with 26.0%). From a menu of options, the most commonly chosen motivations for DSH were related to internal states and included obtaining relief from a terrible state of mind, a wish to die, and desire to punish oneself. Less commonly chosen motivations to self-harm related to interaction with others. These included showing how desperate they were feeling, finding out if others loved them, revenge, to attract attention, and to frighten others. Three quarters of those who self-harmed reported that others knew of their behaviour. Nearly half (48%) of those who had self-harmed said they had decided to do so within an hour of the episode in question. Most DSH episodes (83.3%) occurred at home. Hawton's sub-group analysis of respondents from the UK found of those reporting self-harm in the previous year, approximately one in eight had presented to a general hospital for help. The main determinant of whether a person went to hospital was the severity of the injury arising from the self-harm.

2.2. *Epidemiology*

One-year prevalence of DSH in a recent multinational study of adolescents was 8.9% for females and 2.6% for males. An Australian community survey found the four-week prevalence of DSH was highest for females in the age band 15–24 years, while for males it was highest in the age band 10–19 years. A collaborative Australian–US study of over 3,000 12–15 year olds found DSH among adolescents increased with advancing pubertal stage, but conversely declined with advancing age. The findings suggest that young adolescents who are already advanced in their puberty (early maturers) may be at increased risk of DSH.

2.3. *Associated Factors*

About 20% of self-harm episodes among a multinational sample of adolescents occurred under the influence of alcohol, and 12.8% occurred under the influence of illegal drugs. An Australian population survey found that those who had recently engaged in DSH were more likely than others to have a history of excessive drinking and substance abuse. They were also more likely to have experienced childhood abuse or neglect, and were more likely to be impulsive. Suicidal ideation was higher in this group than in the general population.

2.4. *Assessment*

Objectives of assessment of the self-harming patient include: establishing the immediate risk of repetition or suicide completion, identification of contextual crises that may have precipitated the self-harm, identification and mobilisation of any support systems that may be available to the patient, recognition and treatment where indicated of co-existing psychopathology. A practical approach to assessment is outlined in Table 1.

2.5. *Management*

It is standard practice for young people who have self-harmed to be referred to specialist mental health services for aftercare involving counselling and treatment directed to associated psychiatric conditions. Such aftercare is, however, poorly attended by young people and is of no proven benefit in reducing the repetition of self-harming behaviour.

Table 1:   Approach to the psychiatric assessment of the adolescent who has self-harmed.

- Attend to the adolescent's immediate discomfort and distress (may include strategies such as advocating to move the patient to a quieter area of the emergency department, and even arranging for fluids or a snack when there are no medical contraindications).
- Whenever possible first speak with the adolescent alone (promotes therapeutic alliance).
- Obtain corroborative information about the circumstances of the self-harm from accompanying relatives or friends after interviewing the adolescent, preferably with the adolescent's consent.
- Assess risk of repetition or completed suicide:

  Level of suicidal intent.
  Lethality of the attempt as perceived by the adolescent.
  Intensity of the precipitating crisis.
  Motivation.
  Previous self-harming.
  Concurrent mental disorder or substance abuse.
  Access to lethal means (especially firearms).

- Screen for psychopathology with specific attention to:

  Depression.
  Conduct problems.
  Personality disorder.
  Substance abuse.
  Anxiety.
  Less common conditions with a high risk of suicide such as psychosis and bipolar disorder.

- Mental state assessment with specific attention to continued intoxication and delirium (if either is suspected the clinician should delay decisions about disposition until the patient's sensorium is clear).
- Degree of hopelessness, impulsivity, and aggression displayed by the patient, since all have been associated with increased suicide risk.
- Assess stresses preceding the self-harm.
- Assess the motivation parents may have to assist the teenager in attending follow up appointments.
- Assess other support systems available to the adolescent (may include members of the extended family, peers, school welfare staff, and community youth support workers).

As a consequence, several centres have sought to develop specialised interventions to treat self-harmers. Such interventions include home-based family therapy, facilitation of follow up treatment through the use of an emergency card, rapid response outpatient treatment, inpatient dialectical behaviour therapy, and developmental group psychotherapy. For none of these interventions is there yet convincing evidence of superiority over treatment as usual for reducing repetition, although in some instances there are improvements in other markers of well-being. One non-randomised trial found higher rates of self-harm repetition in depressed adolescents receiving combined pharmacotherapy and cognitive behaviour therapy than in adolescents receiving one treatment modality alone, but the difference was statistically non-significant when analyses were adjusted for baseline characteristics. Dialectical behaviour therapy and mindfulness training are both used with adolescents who self-harm, but neither has been subjected to a controlled trial evaluation. Hospitalisation does not have an impact on rates of repetition of self-harm, and therefore should be reserved for patients deemed at imminent risk of completed suicide (see below), where there are child protection concerns, or where inpatient observation is required to clarify diagnosis. The status quo therefore is that there is no gold standard treatment for adolescents who self-harm. Treatment tends to be designed around the perceived needs of the patient, and the available skills within the treatment team.

2.6. *Outcome*

There is repetition of self-harm following the index episode in about half of cases, with recurrence most likely within the following four weeks. Multiple repetition is common, but within a year the behaviour will have attenuated in about one half of cases (Hazell, unpublished). A small number of individuals have very high recurrence rates of self-harm, presenting to hospital upward of 40 times per year. It is estimated that about 3% of people who self-harm with suicide intent will eventually die from suicide.

3. Suicide

3.1. *Clinical Description*

Among people of all ages, including adolescents and young adults, the most common methods of suicide in males are hanging and the use of firearms, while in females the most common method is self-poisoning. A high proportion of people who die from suicide have seen a medical practitioner within a month of death. A quarter to a half of completed suicides is known to be preceded by suicide attempts, but this is likely an underestimate. These attempts can be of escalating medical lethality. Some suicide deaths occur soon after the initiation of antidepressant treatment, raising the question as to whether it is an adverse effect of treatment, or whether the antidepressant reverses psychomotor retardation before it reduces motivation to suicide. That said, many of those patients prescribed anti-depressant treatment are not taking the medication at the time of their death.

3.2. *Epidemiology*

In most developed countries suicide is a leading cause of death among young people aged 15–25 years. In contrast to self-harm, death from suicide is more common in males (14 per 100,000) than females (4 per 100,000). This is largely because males choose methods that are of higher lethality. Suicide rates among young people peaked in most countries in the 1990s and have since declined. A psychological autopsy of 53 suicide deaths among 13–19 year olds found evidence of mental illness in more than 90%. Mood disorders were most common, affecting about half the sample, but substance misuse and conduct problems also affected about a quarter of the sample each. There is high risk of eventual suicide with certain conditions such as bipolar disorder, schizophrenia, and anorexia nervosa but the absolute numbers are low.

3.3. *Prevention*

Clinical strategies most likely to assist in reducing suicides among young people include accurate detection and treatment of mood disorder and substance abuse. Despite controversy, antidepressant medication should be prescribed to young people whose depression is moderate to severe as there is evidence it lowers suicide rates in this population. Keeping suicide risk in mind is important and should trigger the clinician to enquire about access to means such as firearms. Population-based strategies of merit include the provision of student support to counter bullying and victimisation within schools and other institutions. School-based suicide prevention curricula have been found to be unhelpful and possibly harmful, and have been superseded by more generic school programs that promote mental health and well-being. Internet-based self-help programs are the way of the future, although their impact on suicide rates has yet to be demonstrated.

3.4. *Managing the Aftermath of a Suicide*

The suicide death of an adolescent has a devastating effect on family, peers, and the community. The morale of schools where there has been a suicide death can be adversely affected for years. Systematic approaches to the aftermath of an adolescent suicide are well documented. The family usually receive immediate support from primary care, but may be referred on later for focussed bereavement counselling. An approach to the community response to an adolescent suicide is summarised in Table 2.

Table 2: Elements common to the management of the aftermath of an adolescent suicide.

1. Response plan:

- Developed by senior members of community.
- Discussed widely amongst the community.
- Some individuals become expert in the content and implementation of the plan.
- Criteria established for determining when plan should be initiated.

2. Information:

- Following a suicide, steps are taken to obtain accurate information regarding circumstances of the death.
- The death is acknowledged publicly as soon as practicable, in a manner that avoids sensationalism.
- Accurate and appropriate information is provided to the media by a designated media liaison person, who will emphasise the positive steps taken by the community to cope with the tragedy.

(Continued)

Table 2:   *(Continued)*

---

3. Risk assessment:

- Steps are taken to identify and counsel individuals considered to be at high risk of imitation (close friends of the deceased, adolescents with a known history of depression or suicidality).
- Adequate follow-up is arranged in consultation with parents or guardians.

4. Promotion of healthy recovery of the community:

- Input is provided to individuals less directly involved with the deceased by way of teaching sessions which focuses on the normal response to grief.

5. Prevention:

- Input is provided to individuals who focus on means of suicide prevention, such as early recognition of adolescents at risk, and the teaching of problem solving strategies as an alternative to suicidal behaviour.

References

Brent DA, Greenhill LL, Compton S, Emslie G, Wells K, Walkup JT, Vitiello B, Bukstein O, Stanley B, Posner K, Kennard BD, Cwik MF, Wagner A, Coffey B, March JS, Riddle M, Goldstein T, Curry J, Barnett S, Capasso L, Zelazny J, Hughes J, Shen S, Gugga SS, Turner JB. (2009) The treatment of adolescent suicide attempters study (TASA): Predictors of suicidal events in an open treatment trial. *J Am Acad Child Adolesc Psychiatry* **48**(10): 987–996.

Garland A, Shaffer D, Whittle B. (1989) A national survey of school-based, adolescent suicide prevention programs. *J Am Acad Child Adolesc Psychiatry* **28**(6): 931–934.

Hawton K, Rodham K, Evans E, Harriss L. (2009) Adolescents who self harm: A comparison of those who go to hospital and those who do not. *Child Adolesc Ment Health* **14**(1): 24–30.

Hazell P. (1993) Adolescent suicide clusters: Evidence, mechanisms and prevention. *Aust N Z J Psychiatry* **27**(4): 653–665.

Hazell PL, Martin G, Mcgill K, Kay T, Wood A, Trainor G, Harrington R. (2009) Group therapy for repeated deliberate self-harm in adolescents: Failure of replication of a randomized trial. *J Am Acad Child Adolesc Psychiatry* **48**(6): 662–670.

Madge N, Hewitt A, Hawton K, De Wilde EJ, Corcoran P, Fekete S, Van Heeringen K, De Leo D, Ystgaard M. (2008) Deliberate self-harm within an international community sample of young people: Comparative findings from the Child & Adolescent Self-harm in Europe (CASE) study. *J Child Psychol Psychiatry* **49**(6): 667–677.

Martin G, Hazell P, Harrison J, Taylor A, Swannell S, Page A. (2008) *Appendix to the final report for the research project Australian National Epidemiological Study of Self Injury (ANESSI)*. Report for University of Queensland, Brisbane.

Martin G, Swannell SV, Hazell PL, Harrison JE, Taylor AW. (2010) Self-injury in Australia: A community survey. *Med J Aust* **193**(9): 506–510.

Marttunen MJ, Aro HM, Henriksson MM, Lonnqvist JK. (1991) Mental disorders in adolescent suicide. DSM-III-R axes I and II diagnoses in suicides among 13- to 19-year-olds in Finland. *Arch Gen Psychiatry* **48**(9): 834–839.

Olfson M, Shaffer D, Marcus SC, Greenberg T. (2003) Relationship between anti-depressant medication treatment and suicide in adolescents. *Arch Gen Psychiatry* **60**(10): 978–982.

Patton GC, Hemphill SA, Beyers JM, Bond L, Toumbourou JW, Mcmorris BJ, Catalano RF. (2007) Pubertal stage and deliberate self-harm in adolescents. *J Am Acad Child Adolesc Psychiatry* **46**(4): 508–514.

Piacentini J, Rotheram-Borus MJ, Gillis JR, Graae F, Trautman P, Cantwell C, Garcia-Leeds C, Shaffer D. (1995) Demographic predictors of treatment attendance among adolescent suicide attempters. *J Consult Clinl Psychol* **63**(3): 469–473.

Chapter 30

Mental Health in Young People with Intellectual Disability and Autism

David Dossetor and Rameswaran Vannitamby

1. Introduction

Young people with intellectual disability (learning disability in the UK; mental retardation in the US) have levels of health problems as high as the most disadvantaged in our community, and similar problems of equity of access to services. Their emotional and behavioural problems are affected by developmental factors more akin to those of a much younger chrono-logical age, yet they are subject to the same bio–psychosocial problems as any other young adult person. Young people with ID strive for independ-ence as other young people do, but are likely to be more highly dependent on carers and family than other teenagers. There is a lack of specialist and coordinated services whether this is for primary health care, access to sec-ondary services or complex tertiary care, possibly because of their minority status and problems of communication and political participation. With the achievement of school leaving and young adult status, the availability of specialist services declines yet further.

2. Stigmatisation

Teenagers and young adults with ID may never fully participate in expected social roles, yet small but significant gains in health and function can have huge impacts. Legally, as a special need population, they have an entitlement to participation, recognition, and a quality of life like any other young person. Institutional care has been progressively dismantled. Teenagers and young adults with ID are subject to community ignorance, fear, and avoidance that constitute the stigma which minority groups experience. With the concomitant rights to 'normalisation' and community care, mainstream services have needed to change and to understand and be educated about the special needs of people with ID. Improving physical and mental health care of people with ID should be a priority for all health professionals. Health reform is needed around personal and sexual relationships, accommodation, occupation, and access to appropriately skilled community health and mental health services.

3. Prevalence of Intellectual Disability and Autism

Moderate, severe and profound ID (IQ 35–50; 20–35; <20 respectively) occur in 1% of any population, and mild ID (IQ 50–70) occurs in 2%–3% of any population.

ID is defined by three criteria:

- An IQ below 70 or two standard deviations below average.
- Significant limitations in two or more areas of adaptive behaviour, including communication, self-help skills, interpersonal skills.
- Evidence that the limitations were apparent before the age of 18.

ID is formally diagnosed by professional assessment of intelligence, such as the Wechsler Intelligence Scale for Children and adaptive behaviour assessment, such as the Adaptive Behaviour Assessment System - Second Edition. In order to move away from judging people by an IQ or their deficits, there are moves to focus more on the levels of support that define individual needs.

Over half of those with Autism and Autistic Spectrum Disorder have an ID, with an IQ <70. However most others have special needs with problems of adaptability and needs for special support and have similar mental health management issues to those with ID. Conversely, about one third of those with ID have ASD.

4. Aetiology

Those with moderate, severe and profound ID are generally found to have an abnormality of brain and neurological development. Over 90% have genetic conditions, prematurity, or other recognisable syndromes. The aetiology of mild ID may be viewed as being caused by the interaction of polygenic–socio–cultural factors. This is well illustrated by foetal alcohol spectrum disorder. Those with borderline intelligence (IQ 70–85) also present with a range of problems of chronic health and behaviour difficulties. UK epidemiological data have shown that despite being a small proportion of the population, young people with ID constitute close to 15% of the mental health needs of the population.

5. ID and Mental Health

5.1. *Associated Physical Health Needs*

Significant emotional behaviour problems, particularly with self injurious behaviour, in someone with limited communication skills requires a thorough medical assessment and active investigation, as physical health problems may masquerade as mental health issues. Routine annual health assessment has been recommended for those with ID. Young adults with ID have on average four physical health problems. These include constipation, oesophageal reflux and indigestion, problems of mobility/walking, poor dental health, seizures, sleep disorders, and visual, aural, cardiac, and renal disorders. Many of these conditions may involve pain that cannot be easily communicated.

5.2. *Communication and Problem Solving Skills and Mental Health*

Lack of such skills may lead to mental health problems, as well as limiting access to normal social roles and valuation which are important for quality of life. Limited communication and problem solving skills lead to difficulties in understanding and expressing one's internal subjective state, comparing it to past experience and rating it against social norms. Much can be done to aid understanding, including simplifying the discussion, and using visual and other communication aids. Regardless of age, information is required from additional sources to that of the patient.

A range of other competencies need to be taken into account in communicating with someone with ID, such as motor development, attention, and executive function, memory, theory of mind, social and emotional understanding, and insight. Many of these elements may be specifically delayed in those with ID or ASD. Indeed these qualities may be more important than the simple measure of intelligence, and reminds us why people with ASD also have problems with adaptation to their environment.

5.3. *Challenging Behaviour Versus Mental Health Disorder*

Adolescent mental health defines a psychiatric disorder as any emotions or behaviour that cause additional developmental impairment or persisting handicap to self or others, whereas adult mental health restricts mental disorder to a recognisable mental illness. Challenging behaviour is predicated on the notion that behaviour is related to the environment and therefore treatable by identifying the antecedents and consequences of the behaviour, and designing an intervention that will change the behaviour. A mental illness is predicated on the notion that the problem is caused by an illness process of the mind that will require specific treatment often with medication. In ID this dichotomous thinking often underlies the boundary battles between services and emphasises the need for a continuum in ID mental health services from child to adult. Overall studies propose that about 50% of those with behavioural problems also have significant mental ill-health disorders. The more severe the challenging behaviour, whether this is aggressive or self-injurious behaviour, the stronger is the association with mental ill-health.

5.4. *Diagnosis*

The Mini Psychiatric Assessment Schedule for Adults with Developmental Disability is a widely used screening instrument to enable those not specially trained in the psychiatry of intellectual disability to be able to make reliable diagnoses of anxiety disorder, depression, obsessional compulsive disorder, bipolar disorder, schizophrenia, autism, and dementia. The Child and Adolescent Psychiatric Assessment Schedule also includes attention deficit hyperactivity disorder and conduct disorder.

5.5. *Prevalence of Mental Disorders in Adolescents and Young Adults with ID and Transition Issues*

There are increased rates of anxiety disorder (15%), ADHD (30%), oppositional defiant disorder (10%), disruptive behaviour disorder, and ASD. Substance abuse is less frequent. Prevalence of depression is controversial because of the difficulties of diagnostic reliability, with studies suggesting a 10% prevalence. Self-injurious behaviour occurs in 10% and psychosis in 1%. ADHD and ASD are seldom diagnosed in adult mental health practice possibly reflecting the view that these are developmental disorders, not psychiatric illnesses. Although these conditions are often recognised to persist into adulthood, many improve. Adults with ID and ASD have higher rates of hospital admission, psychotropic medication use, and behaviour problems, and a higher rate of schizophrenia compared with those with ID without ASD. ADHD prevalence rises in adult with ID with increasing impairment of ID from 3% in borderline, 12% in mild, 25% in moderate and 35% in severe, with an overall prevalence of approximately 20%. Often adult and adolescent mental health services consider disruptive behaviour disorders to be outside their remit, and the criminal justice system is the default service.

5.6. *Specific Mental Health Diagnoses in ID*

5.6.1. *Depression*

The challenge is eliciting the classic features of persisting low mood, loss of energy, anhedonia, social withdrawal, reduced memory and concentration, and altered sleep and appetite. Those with ID are unlikely to complain of depressed thoughts, but often a close friend or relative can confirm an impression of persistent mood change. If there is a change of social and functional trajectory, it is quite reasonable to test a hypothesis of depression with a trial of pharmacotherapy.

5.6.2. *Anxiety disorders*

Anxiety disorders, including post traumatic stress disorder, are often the result of abuse (including sexual abuse) and other experiences of stigma and prejudice. Again the diagnosis and disclosure of associated abuse may be difficult. The first line treatment for both depression and anxiety is CBT or IPT. In those with ID, CBT or IPT may need modification, and will require special psychological skills and experience. Therapy may require both a greater level of prompting in problem solving approaches and a greater emphasis on the behavioural component. Therapy may also need a more directive educative approach to emotional recognition, theory of mind, and problem solving.

5.6.3. *Psychoses*

The diagnosis and treatment of psychotic illnesses are presented in Chapter 28. The characteristic features of hallucinations and delusions are often difficult to elucidate in the context of ID, ASD, and limited communication skills. Whereas there are reliable observations of depression and mania, sometimes behavioural features of schizophrenia are indicated by a consistent change in patterns of behaviour and social coherence, with other difficult to define or bizarre symptoms. Additional features can include thought disorder, disorganised behaviour, and negative features of blunted affect (lack or decline in emotional response), alogia (lack or decline in speech), or avolition (lack or decline in motivation). Catatonia is the motor presentation of schizophrenia, but features of catatonia also occur in autism and a range of neurological conditions. Lorazepam can improve symptoms.

Acute confusional states are a cause of psychotic phenomena, and a loss of orientation in time, place and person, is indicative of a medical aetiology which needs thorough investigation. Furthermore, ASD and ID increase the presence of normal developmental phenomena such as pretend friends, and stereotypic or concrete thinking which can easily be misattributed as psychotic phenomena. Often the presentation of schizophrenia in ID is more difficult to treat, with slow or atypical response to anti-psychotics. The presence of ID and abnormal brain biology increase the risk of adverse effects of therapy. The utility of non-pharmacological therapies is often also diminished. It is in this context that admission to a mental health unit with a rehabilitation program may be indicated.

5.6.4. *Impulse control disorders*

These are a group of psychiatric disorders that include:

- Intermittent explosive disorder (hot-headedness).
- Kleptomania (stealing).
- Pathological gambling.
- Pyromania (fire-starting).
- Trichotillomania (a compulsion to pull one's hair out).
- Onychophagia (compulsive nail biting).
- Dermatillomania (compulsive skin picking).

The onset of these disorders usually occurs between the ages of 7 and 15 years. Impulsivity, the key feature of these disorders, can be thought of as seeking a small, short term gain at the expense of a large, long term loss. Those with the disorders repeatedly demonstrate failure to resist their behaviour and the impulsive behaviour act is felt to be a compulsion beyond the personal control of the individual, despite the irrationality of the behaviours. Terms used to describe impulsive behaviour denote an absence of executive function, and suggest loss of or failure to attain inhibition control. A number of factors make people with ID more prone to impulse disorders, including their delayed development and neurobiological factors, and these factors may be reinforced by the social environment. Treatment involves behavioural, cognitive behavioural and drug treatments which all help to manage and improve the processing of excessive arousal.

5.6.5. *Organic mental disorders*

These describe a range of acute or chronic symptoms of impaired cognitive function due to brain abnormalities such as abnormal physiology, injury, or disease affecting brain tissues, chemical or hormonal abnormalities, exposure to toxic materials, neurological impairment, or abnormal changes associated with premature ageing in ID. ASD and impulse control disorders are often present. Treatment usually involves both psychological and pharmacological approaches.

6. Barriers To Mental Health Care in ID and How to Overcome These

Entry into mental health services requires referral and triage processes which are appreciative of the complex needs of people with a dual diagnosis of mental health disorder and ID. Due to the intrinsic nature of ID, people with ID are not able to express their distress or carers fail to identify mental health problems. There may be difficulty identifying to whom to refer the patient. Conceptual and operational difficulties between disability and mental health services may also provide challenges to the provision of quality care. Mental health services adopt a medical model of care, which in contrast to disability services, can be focused on the individual rather than encompassing carers and community needs. Inter-agency cooperation, communication, and commitment are all required for care of people with ID and mental health problems. Advocacy for people with ID from professionals, services and government, and training of nurses, psychologists, occupational therapists, speech therapists, and medical professionals in ID are all areas of need.

7. Models of Care

Models of care need to take account of geography, with a tiered structure, whereby more complex problems access greater and more specialised multidisciplinary expertise. This structure includes:

1. Primary health/mental health care, including general practitioners/ family physicians and community health services who co-ordinate and provide day to day health care.
2. Secondary health, disability services and generic mental health care services provide the next layer of care if required. Referral pathways may need to enable cross agency and multidisciplinary collaboration.

3. Specialist mental health services for ID in partnership with disability services.
4. Specialist specific programs for mental health and ID.
5. The fifth tier is government supported networks to provide clinical leadership and advice to government on cost effective essential service development, linked to advancing knowledge from a network of academics in ID and mental health.

Access to and use of generic services is greater, but evidence would suggest that specialist services by provision of longer and more focussed care are associated with better carer satisfaction and improved clinical outcomes. A mixed model which has an up-skilled generic mental health service and which is guided by a specialist mental health ID service is likely to be the most successful and the most resource attractive.

8. Conclusions

Working with people with ID and mental health problems requires a greater range of multidisciplinary skills both from disability services and for the modification of mental health interventions. Involvement with medical practitioners and psychiatrists is more likely to be needed where the ID is more severe, behavioural interventions have failed, treatment of developmental disorders require complex psychopharmacology and if mental health problems are suspected. Despite the emphasis of holistic multidisciplinary approaches to community based treatment in those with ID, those with more severe disturbance are also likely to need empirical interventions with psychopharmacology, whether disturbances are due to challenging behaviour, developmental disorders, or severe mental illness.

References

Bouras N, Holt G. eds. (2007) *Psychiatric and behavioural disorders in intellectual and developmental disabilities*, 2nd ed. Cambridge University Press, UK.

Bradley EA, Summers JA, Wood HL, Bryson SE. (2004) Comparing rates of psychiatric and behavior disorders in adolescents and young adults with severe intellectual disability with and without autism. *J Autism Dev Disord* **34**(2): 151–161.

Chaplin E, Paschos D, O'Hara J, McCarthy J, Holt G, Bouras N, Tsakanikos E. (2010) Mental ill-health and care pathways in adults with intellectual disability across different residential types. *Res Dev Disabil* **31**(2): 458–463.

Dossetor D, White D, Whatson L. (2011) *Mental Health for Children and Adolescents with Intellectual Disability*. IP Communication, Melbourne.

Emerson E, Einfeld S. (2011) *Challenging behaviour*, 3rd ed. Cambridge University Press, UK.

Hurley AD. (2008) Depression in adults with intellectual disability: Symptoms and challenging behaviour. *J Intellect Disabil Res* **52**(11): 905–916.

Matson JL, Shoemaker M. (2009) Intellectual disability and its relationship to autism spectrum disorders. *Res Dev Disabil* **30**(6): 1107–1114.

Mccarthy J, Hemmings C, Kravariti E, Dworzynski K, Holt G, Bouras N, Tsakanikos E. (2010) Challenging behavior and co-morbid psychopathology in adults with intellectual disability and autism spectrum disorders. *Res Dev Disabil* **31**(2): 362–366.

Torr J, Iacono T, Graham MJ, Galea J. (2008) Checklists for general practitioner diagnosis of depression in adults with intellectual disability. *J Intellect Disabil Res* **52**(11): 930–941.

Underwood L, McCarthy J, Tsakanikos E. (2010) Mental health of adults with autism spectrum disorders and intellectual disability. *Curr Opin Psychiatry* **23**(5): 421–426.

Chapter 31

Sleep and Sleep Disorders in Adolescents

Karen Waters

1. Introduction

Sleep disorders compromise daytime performance, quality of life, and health, but with appropriate identification and treatment, many sleep disorders can be effectively treated. A number of physiological and social factors during and around puberty affect sleep patterns with a tendency to later sleep onset, later awakening, and shorter sleep time. A number of specific sleep disorders that cause either excessive sleepiness or poor sleep quality, have their onset around the time of puberty and their concurrent onset with the normal adolescent changes may result in delayed diagnosis. It is extremely important to be aware of and to distinguish these abnormal phenomena in order to provide appropriate treatment for affected individuals in a timely manner.

2. Normal Changes in Sleep with Puberty and Adolescence

Changes during adolescence exist worldwide and include a *delayed sleep phase* with a marked tendency for later bedtimes and later rise times. There is also a *reduction in sleep quality* with more awakenings, and *lower sleep efficiency* (percent of the time in bed spent asleep). The major changes in sleep timing and sleep quality appear in the early stages of puberty. There is also *shorter sleep time* that tends to be associated with *increased daytime sleepiness* although there is greater tolerance for sleep deprivation or extended wakefulness as puberty progresses.

The quality of the sleep EEG also changes, and there is a steep decrease in delta non-REM sleep, that is also linked to increased sleepiness. Hormonal changes during this period of development include reduction in melatonin levels that fall mainly between Tanner Stages I and II. There are no longitudinal studies on puberty hormones and sleep.

Social factors mean that these normal sleep changes frequently coincide with a tendency to irregular sleep patterns, particularly sleeping less during weekdays, and accumulating sleep debt, and then sleeping for longer during weekends as partial compensation.

2.1. *Circadian Rhythm*

Adolescent shifts between week and weekend sleep times interact with circadian physiology wherein the trend to the later sleep times of the weekend is relatively easy. However, the shift to an earlier sleep onset and wake time during the week days takes most of the week to occur, since it is a difficult adaptation for the body's circadian pacemaker to make.

Over a number of studies, it has been demonstrated worldwide that the trend is for a shift of two hours or more between week and weekend sleep times. Asian adolescents have the most restricted sleep and suffer more daytime sleepiness than European and North American groups.

2.2. *Psychosocial Factors*

Psychosocial factors that contribute to the sleep phase delay include academic demands, social activities, after-school employment, TV, computer and internet attractions. There is increasing evidence that many adolescents obtain insufficient sleep, resulting in chronic sleep deprivation that can reduce control of behaviour, emotions and attention. Health consequences include high risk behaviours associated with substance abuse and car accidents, along with increased risk for mental illness.

2.3. *Week Day and Weekend Sleep*

The most common problem with adolescent sleep is the shift that occurs between weekend and week day sleep times. Poor sleep affects cognitive performance and is associated with poor emotional and physical health, behaviour problems and substance abuse.

2.4. *Sleep Hygiene*

Sleep hygiene relates to the habits surrounding sleep and optimising those habits to achieve regular and restful sleep. The first step in optimising sleep in adolescents is to narrow the gap between weekend and week day bedtimes and sleep opportunities. Given the limits of their social parameters, this can be hard to achieve. However, narrowing the gap may be essential in those who present with sleep difficulties in order to make progress with the diagnosis and management of any pathological sleep problems.

3. Sleep Disordered Breathing

The most common sleep disorder at all ages is obstructive sleep apnoea. Amongst adolescents with sleepiness, sleep disordered breathing may well be the most common diagnosis. The predominant symptom of the disorder is regular or frequent snoring, but with adolescents frequently sleeping alone, this history may not be reliable unless there is recent occurrence of shared sleep quarters. Daytime consequences include:

- Excessive daytime sleepiness.
- Impaired school performance.
- Depression.
- Behavioural problems resembling ADHD.

The prevalence of OSA is around 3% in children, increasing to 6% during teenage years. Factors increasing the risk for OSA include obesity, chronic rhinitis, passive second-hand cigarette smoking, a positive family history for the disorder, ethnicity with higher prevalence in African-American and some Asian races, and any underlying disorder that affects craniofacial growth. It is important to note that the features of daytime sleepiness as a symptom of OSA and a male predominance of OSA both emerge during adolescence.

3.1. *Diagnosis*

Diagnosis is made on an overnight sleep study (polysomnography), usually in a sleep laboratory, to determine the frequency of obstructive respiratory events and associated changes in gas exchange including oxygen desaturations and CO_2 retention.

3.2. *Treatment*

Where possible, adenotonsillectomy is undertaken. As the adenoids and tonsils are less frequently the underlying pathology in adolescents, the use of nasal mask continuous positive airway pressure is the treatment of choice. Other management strategies may include surgical options such as clearance of nasal passages where these are restricted, and rapid maxillary (palatal) expansion to broaden lateral airway dimensions. Weight loss should be encouraged in the overwight adolescent.

4. Hypersomnolence

Disorders of excessive sleepiness that lead to daytime dysfunction and interfere with social activities are termed hypersomnolence. The known disorders of hypersomnolence often have their onset during adolescence and without proper identification and treatment can lead to long term disability. To confirm these diagnoses, it is important to ensure that any daytime sleepiness is not simply caused by lack of sufficient sleep. The most accurate way to assess this is by monitoring sleep times, for example by actigraphy (a sensor which measures gross motor activity) over a period of two or three weeks.

5. Delayed Sleep Phase Syndrome

5.1. *Diagnosis*

In this disorder sleep episodes occur later than desired, and this is associated with difficulty falling asleep, problems awakening on time (for example to meet work or school obligations) and daytime sleepiness. Sleep is otherwise normal. In this group, preferred later sleep times are between 2:00 am and 6:00 am, and preferred later wake times are 10:00 am to 1:00 pm. The reported prevalence of DSPS varies between 0.1% and 3.1% of the population, and tends to be higher in adolescents than adults. Circadian rhythm sleep disorders arise from a desynchronised biological clock, account for around 10% of chronic insomnia patients, and often co-exist in the presence of psychiatric comorbidities including personality disorders and depression.

5.2. *Treatment*

Treatment for DSPS is designed to resynchronise the circadian system, but it is imperative that a rigid sleep/wake schedule be maintained for persisting improvement. This can be achieved by progressively further delaying sleep times until the desired sleep time is reached, or by bright light exposure with regular morning awakening. These patients may also benefit from the sedative effects of melatonin administered a few hours before their natural melatonin secretion (when circulating melatonin levels are low) while they attempt to advance their circadian timing. Whether DSPS is an extreme expression of the adolescent pattern of sleep or the true expression of the disorder when seen in adolescents, the approach to treatment remains the same. If adolescents are provided with the skills to modify their sleep habits, it may help circumvent chronic disability in adulthood due to an established circadian rhythm sleep disorder.

6. Narcolepsy

Narcolepsy is a life-long but non-progressive disease characterised by abnormal regulation of the sleep–wake cycle and increased penetration of rapid eye movement sleep so that features of REM sleep, such as motor paralysis and dreaming, intrude into wakefulness. The specific pathology is a mutation of the hypocretin receptor-2 or sporadic hypocretin deficiency due to a neurodegenerative process affecting hypocretin/orexin neurons in the lateral hypothalamus. Narcolepsy occurs in approximately 1:2,000 in the general population. More specifically, the estimated prevalence of narcolepsy with cataplexy (sudden physical collapse triggered by strong emotion) is 36 per 100,000, and for narcolepsy without cataplexy is 32 per 100,000 in males and 12 per 100,000 in females.

6.1. *Diagnostic Criteria*

Diagnostic criteria for narcolepsy (Table 1) include documentation of hypersomnolence. Mean daytime sleep latency for narcoleptics is very short at 3.1 ± 2.9 minutes. The study to document narcolepsy should be undertaken after documentation of adequate sleep, by diary or preferably by actigraphy for a period of two weeks. After an overnight sleep study, in order to demonstrate an adequate night of sleep (defined as at least six hours of polysomnographically defined sleep), a daytime Mean Sleep Latency Test is performed. The MSLT includes a drug screen to confirm that the patient is free of drugs that influence sleep. The mean sleep latency over the course of five daytime nap opportunities should be less than eight minutes to define excessive sleepiness, since 90% of narcoleptic patients have sleep latency below this level.

Table 1: Diagnostic criteria for narcolepsy — International Classification of Sleep Disorders-2.

Current Definition

A. The patient has a complaint of excessive daytime sleepiness occurring almost daily for at least three months.

B. A definite history of cataplexy, defined as sudden and transient episodes of loss of motor tone triggered by emotions, is present.

C. The diagnosis of narcolepsy with cataplexy should, whenever possible, be confirmed by nocturnal polysomnography followed by a MSLT; the mean sleep latency on MSLT is less than or equal to eight minutes and two or more sleep onset REM periods are observed following sufficient nocturnal sleep (minimum six hours) during the night prior to the test. Alternatively, hypocretin-1 levels in the CSF are less than or equal to 110 pg/ml or one-third of mean normal values.

D. The hypersomnia is not better explained by another sleep disorder or neurological disorder, mental disorder, medication use, or substance use disorder.

6.2. *Treatment*

Treatment of sleepiness involves the use of stimulants, typically amphetamines, to maintain wakefulness. Modafinil is a dopamine reuptake inhibitor that aids in the maintenance of wakefulness, but is a low potency compound. Treatment of cataplexy involves use of tricyclic anti-depressants, serotonin reuptake blockers, or venlafaxine which is a serotonin and noradrenaline reuptake inhibitor (serotonin $\geq$ noradrenaline). Other therapies are experimental at this stage, including immune modulation near the time of disease onset and ongoing research into replacement or boosting of hypocretin levels.

Idiopathic hypersomnolence also occurs, and management follows essentially the same strategies as for narcolepsy, ensuring that other causes for the hypersomnolence have been excluded.

7. Periodic Hypersomnolence: Including Kleine–Levin Syndrome and Menstrual-Related Hypersomnolence

7.1. *Diagnosis*

Subjective hypersomnolence occurs in around 5% of the population. The diagnosis of hypersomnolence disorders requires the exclusion of other sleep problems, such as OSA or circadian rhythm disorders. The ICSD-2 definition includes:

- Recurrent episodes of excessive sleepiness of two days to four weeks duration.
- Episodes recur at least once a year.
- Normal alertness, cognitive functioning, and behaviour between attacks.
- The hypersomnia is not better explained by another sleep or medical disorder, or caused by substance use.

There are hypersomnia syndromes with characteristic features.

7.2. *Presentation and Treatment*

The *Kleine–Levin Syndrome* is rare and mainly affects adolescents (median age 15 years, 80% male). It involves recurrent episodes of hypersomnia (median recurrence interval 3.5 months), usually accompanied by hyperphagia (66%–80%), cognitive and mood disturbances, with abnormal behaviour like hypersexuality (43%–53%), and signs of dysautonomia. It can occur secondary to infection or head trauma. The majority of patients outgrow these symptoms.

Menstrual-related hypersomnia also involves recurrent episodes of hypersomnia that are clearly associated with menstruation and/or puerperium, and may include other symptoms of Kleine Levin Syndrome. Whereas there have been no consistent therapeutic successes with treatment of Kleine Levin Syndrome, the menstrual-related hypersomnia responds to treatment with oral contraceptives.

8. Insomnia

8.1. *Definition*

Insomnia is repeated difficulty with sleep initiation, duration, consolidation or quality, despite age-appropriate time and opportunity for sleep. It should also result in daytime dysfunction. The prevalence of insomnia is estimated to be 1%–6% in those ≤ 17 years with much higher prevalence (10%–30%) if the definition includes bedtime refusal and night awakenings. These sleep problems have a higher prevalence in adolescents with other neuro-developmental or psychiatric problems.

8.2. *Contributing factors*

A large epidemiological survey of adolescents in the US found that the median age of onset of insomnia was 11 years. Of those adolescents with insomnia, 53% also had a psychiatric disorder. The major factor associated with increased risk for insomnia is the onset of menses, when the risk for insomnia is increased 28-fold. There is no developmental change in the prevalence of insomnia for boys. Amongst those adolescents with insomnia, half of them had primary insomnia, 27% had insomnia related to a psychiatric disorder, 12% had insomnia related to substance use, and 7% had insomnia related to a medical condition. The population prevalence estimate for primary insomnia is 2.2%, for insomnia linked to a psychiatric condition 1.1%, for substance abuse 0.5%, and for insomnia linked to a medical condition 0.3%.

8.3. *Management of Sleep Disorders*

Adolescents comprise a large proportion of those attending paediatricians or psychiatrists for sleep problems and of those who are likely to have medication prescribed if they complain of insomnia.

8.3.1. *Optimisation of sleep hygiene*

Optimisation of sleep hygiene should always be the first priority in managing insomnia in adolescents, especially because of the above mentioned trends in sleep patterns that are common for this age group. As part of sleep hygiene, it is important to elucidate any current use of nicotine, alcohol, or other drugs as well as evaluating caffeine intake (through soft drinks and energy drinks as well as coffee). The use of technology in the bedroom (TV, computers, mobile phones) is also important since increased media use is related to decreased sleep time and the stimulation associated with various media can also affect sleep quality.

8.3.2. *The primary behavioural management principle*

The primary behavioural management principle after optimisation of sleep hygiene is that the bed should only be used for sleep, although this may extend to the bedroom to optimise sleep conditions. If the basis of the sleep problems is behavioural, or due to media activities in the bedroom, then appropriate management requires that these issues are addressed. Both behavioural and medication therapies may be appropriate and tend to be prescribed.

8.3.3. *Medication*

There is agreement that medication use should, wherever possible, be only short term. Varieties of medications in use include melatonin, antihistamines, and benzodiazepines as well as non-benzodiazepine hypnotics.

9. Sleep in Other Disorders

Adolescents with other chronic medical, psychiatric, and developmental disorders appear likely to have an increased frequency of concurrent sleep disorders. In some medical conditions, this will relate to medications, while in others to associated physical problems, for example nasal polyps in cystic fibrosis.

9.1. *Intellectual Disability*

The most evidence exists for sleep problems in the presence of intellectual disability. Prevalence is lower in adolescent and adult populations than in children, where estimates of the frequency of sleep problems in ID vary from 15%–80%. These observations suggest that the prevalence of sleep problems reduces with age. Nonetheless, more severe sleep problems tend to occur in those with more severe ID, epilepsy, and cerebral palsy. EEG abnormalities have been linked to abnormal sleep in the presence of ID, including specific problems such as increased light (Stage 1) sleep, reduced slow wave sleep, and decreased sleep time.

9.2. *Change at Adolescence*

During adolescence, concurrent morbidities such as obesity or mental health problems such as anxiety or depression can predispose to new sleep problems. The link between sleep problems and mental illness needs close scrutiny, as it has been repeatedly demonstrated that prescriptions of psychotropic medications are common in adolescents and adults without a clear evidence base. Sleep problems, particularly poor quality sleep, are associated with daytime problem behaviours, respiratory illness, and anti-convulsant medications.

9.3. *Specific Syndromes*

Specific syndromes are commonly associated with sleep problems, such that it seems likely that some genetic abnormalities also disrupt sleep functions. Examples include Angelman syndrome, Prader–Willi syndrome, tuberous sclerosis, Sanfilippo syndrome, and Smith–Magenis syndrome. Some of these disorders may be specifically associated with abnormalities of the hypothalamus, and include alteration in circadian regulation, and/or lower sleep requirements. Those with autistic spectrum disorders appear to be specifically vulnerable to insomnia. It has been postulated that ASD is associated with abnormal melatonin secretion which accounts for why long term therapy with melatonin appears to be effective and safe, although controversy remains, since the presence of ID *per se* is often associated with circadian rhythm disturbances.

9.4. *Treatment*

Improving sleep hygiene is an important general management strategy. Melatonin reduces sleep latency in a broad range of developmental disabilities, being more effective with the more severe sleep disruptions. However, there is very little evidence of any effect on sleep maintenance or sleep duration, although melatonin appears to improve both sleep and daytime function in adults with ID. Concurrent anxiety and mood disorders can also contribute to the presence of sleep dysregulation and should be addressed in the course of any treatment. A better understanding of the association between sleep disorders and daytime behavioural dysfunction in sleep disorders of specific syndromes is needed.

10. Conclusion

Adolescence is a time when sleep patterns frequently become disorganised, to the extent that this can affect daytime function. It is tempting to assume that the major factors associated with resolution of these disrupted sleep patterns are socially-driven, but further research is required to identify what physical and physiological factors stabilise during adulthood. Some individuals will be more susceptible to the dysfunction that disruption of sleep patterns induces, either because they have greater sleep needs, or because they have greater susceptibility to sleep deprivation. At any age, sleep-disordered breathing is the most common sleep problem to be identified and should be investigated and treated due to the immediate and long term medical and psychosocial consequences. Chronic sleep disorders may have their onset around the time of puberty, and it is important to identify those associated with pathological hypersomnolence. Insomnia may also begin during this developmental period, and it is a common association with ID. Early identification and treatment of these disorders is important to avoid long term social and physical disability.

References

Aran A, Einen M, Lin L, Plazzi G, Nishino S, Mignot E. (2010) Clinical and therapeutic aspects of childhood narcolepsy-cataplexy: A retrospective study of 51 children. *Sleep* **33**(11): 1457–1464.

Arnulf I, Zeitzer JM, File J, Farber N, Mignot E. (2005) Kleine-Levin syndrome: A systematic review of 186 cases in the literature. *Brain* **128**(12): 2763–2776.

Billiard M, Jaussent I, Dauvilliers Y, Besset A. (2011) Recurrent hypersomnia: A review of 339 cases. *Sleep Medicine Reviews* **15**(4): 247–257.

Cortesi F, Giannotti F, Ivanenko A, Johnson K. (2010) Sleep in children with autistic spectrum disorder. *Sleep Medicine* **11**(7): 659–664.

Crowley SJ, Acebo C, Carskadon MA. (2007) Sleep, circadian rhythms, and delayed phase in adolescence. *Sleep Medicine* **8**(6): 602–612.

Didden R, Korzilius H, Van Aperlo B, Van Overloop C, De Vries M. (2002) Sleep problems and daytime problem behaviours in children with intellectual disability. *J Intellect Disabil Res* **46**(7): 537–547.

Fuentes-Pradera MA, Sanchez-Armengol A, Capote-Gil F, Quintana-Gallego E, Carmona-Bernal C, Polo J, Delgado-Moreno F, Castillo-Gomez J. (2004) Effects of sex on sleep-disordered breathing in adolescents. *European Respiratory Journal* **23**(2): 250–254.

Johnson EO, Roth T, Schultz L, Breslau N. (2006) Epidemiology of DSM-IV insomnia in adolescence: Lifetime prevalence, chronicity, and an emergent gender difference. *Pediatrics* **117**(2): e247–256.

Mindell JA, Emslie G, Blumer J, Genel M, Glaze D, Ivanenko A, Johnson K, Rosen C, Steinberg F, Roth T, Banas B. (2006) Pharmacologic management of insomnia in children and adolescents: Consensus statement. *Pediatrics* **117**(6): e122332.

Sass AE, Kaplan DW. eds. (2010). *Sleep and Sleep Disorders in Adolescence* Adolescent Medicine: State of the Art Reviews. American Academy of Pediatrics.

Chapter 32

Attention Deficit Hyperactivity Disorder

Michael R Kohn and Deborah Erickson

1. Introduction

Attention deficit hyperactivity disorder is the most common neuro-behavioural disorder in childhood. It is characterised by the inability to attend to salient stimuli, ignore irrelevant stimuli and exhibit developmentally appropriate self-regulatory behaviours. All are key components in the development of brain function. Diminished executive function and diminished ability to organise, plan and anticipate underpin the behaviours required for the clinical diagnosis of ADHD as per the Diagnostic and Statistical Manual for Mental Disorders. While commonly viewed as a childhood disorder, ADHD is recognised as persisting into adolescence and adulthood.

The diagnosis and management of ADHD remains controversial. The lack of accepted biological markers results in the diagnosis being made from subjective observations of behaviours that change with development. Standardised psychometric measures help determine specific strengths and weaknesses in cognitive processing, but there is limited scientific evidence that such measures correlate with sub-types or treatment response. Controversy is heightened by the lack of evidence to support many of the currently used treatment regimens.

ADHD impacts all aspects of the adolescent's health and well-being. Young persons with ADHD experience under-achievement, low self esteem, chronic employment challenges in the workplace, difficulty in social relationships and have a greater frequency of motor vehicle accidents, substance abuse and difficulty with the law.

2. What is ADHD?

ADHD is diagnosed by a persistent pattern of inattention and/or hyperactive and impulsive behaviour that is more frequent and more severe than is typically seen at a given stage of development. Symptoms are usually present from early childhood, and tend to become particularly troublesome when the child starts school. Up to 65% of children diagnosed with ADHD have difficulties that persist through adolescence and across the life span. Most individuals with ADHD have problems in areas including language, learning, mood, emotional regulation, and motor control.

2.1. *Aetiology*

ADHD is thought to result from impaired frontal lobe function, attention, orientation, and executive function. Current modelling proposes the following:

- primary impairment of frontal lobe function.
- secondary effects on frontal lobe function from ascending subcortical pathways.

Much research is focused on genetic markers. Neuroimaging techniques such as MRI, functional MRI, DTI, PET and SPECT have also been used to assess differences in brain structure and function. To date, research using these imaging techniques has not added substantially to information gained from clinical assessment and standardised psychometric measures. Imaging data have shown group differences, though the capacity to discriminate individual information is yet to be shown.

A measurable impact of environmental factors on the severity of ADHD has been shown although the relative contribution of these risk factors remains unclear. Antenatal influences, psychological trauma, and acquired or traumatic brain injury all occur with more frequency in adolescents diagnosed with ADHD.

2.2. *Epidemiology*

ADHD occurs in all ethnic groups and social classes. The childhood community prevalence of 6.8% found in Australia is similar to that reported in other countries, 7.4% in the UK and between 3%–7% in the US. The male:female ratio varies, but is typically reported to be greater than 4:1.

3. Diagnosis and Assessment

The two diagnostic schedules for ADHD most commonly used in both clinical practice and research are the DSM-IV-TR, published by the American Psychiatric Association, and the ICD published by the World Health Organization. Symptoms must be present by the age of seven years.

3.1. *DSM-IV-TR*

The DSM-IV-TR requires that six inattentive and/or hyperactive/impulsive criteria must be met to make the diagnosis of ADHD. Formal diagnosis is predicated upon a comprehensive clinical assessment with subjective information from family members and teachers. Psycho-educational assessment is also used.

3.2. *ICD-10*

ICD-10 diagnosis requires the presence of at least six inattentive symptoms, at least three hyperactive symptoms and at least one impulsive symptom. ICD-10 criteria for hyperkinetic disorder require the presence of symptoms 'excessive for the age and IQ of the child' and exclusion of certain other psychiatric disorders.

3.3. *Other Diagnostic Tools*

Specific neuro-psychological tests have been proposed for the diagnosis of ADHD, and which focus on executive function and working memory. Tests such as the Conners and Tests of Variables Attention asssess continuous performance. EEG studies in ADHD show sensitivity and specificity for diagnosis compared to clinician rating of ADHD to be around 90%. Diagnostic approaches have *not* been shown to predict comorbidity or treatment response. Despite their appeal to consumers, careful consideration must be given to how results from these investigations are clinically interpreted and used.

3.4. *Differential Diagnoses*

Symptoms must persist across a range of environments — home, school, and social. Differential diagnoses include learning difficulties, sleep deprivation, hearing impairment, substance abuse, and affective disorders such as anxiety and depression. Family conflict, bullying, and child abuse can also lead to presentation with ADHD-like symptoms.

4. Comorbidities

4.1. *Psychiatric Disorders*

Oppositional defiant disorder and conduct disorder are the most common comorbid psychiatric disorders. Somewhere between 45%–84% of children and adolescents with ADHD meet diagnostic criteria for either of these conditions. There is evidence that adolescents with ADHD are especially at increased risk for major depressive disorder or dysthymic disorder. Adolescents with ADHD are more likely than their peers to meet criteria for anxiety disorder. In Bird *et al.*'s study of 9–16 year olds with ADHD, 48% had comorbid depression or a dysthymic disorder, 36% had comorbid ODD/CD and 36% had comorbid anxiety disorder. Data from the Australian Twin ADHD Project suggest higher rates of ODD and CD occur in males and higher rates of anxiety disorder in females.

4.2. *Learning and Development*

Individuals with ADHD experience lower levels of intellectual performance, higher rates of learning disorders, and problems with academic performance. They display movement difficulties consistent with developmental coordination disorder. Fine motor difficulties are present in the inattentive subtype of ADHD, while those with the combined impulsive/inattentive subtype display greater difficulty with gross motor skills. These findings are consistent with the observation that adolescents with ADHD are at greater risk for accidents, findings which extend to increased motor vehicle accidents and traffic violations in older individuals.

4.3. *Other Assessments*

Medical review is required for potential contraindications to medication (such as pre-existing cardiac problems). Speech or language difficulties may need allied health assessment. Formal psycho-educational assessment should be undertaken in the presence of academic difficulties. Evaluation of family and social issues, such as behavioural management strategies, must be undertaken at the time of initial assessment and repeated at times of apparent deterioration.

5. Management

5.1. *Introduction*

There are marked differences in the medical approaches in the treatment of ADHD, but a multimodal approach is always recommended. These interventions are designed to help overcome reinforcing factors for the ADHD pattern of behaviour. Effective multidisciplinary care requires cooperation amongst health professionals, as well as effective liaison with families, schools, and community support services. This approach also enables planning for psycho-educational interventions and/or transition of adolescents into adult services for those requiring ongoing care. The American National Initiative for Children's Healthcare Quality has proposed that communities support those with ADHD, including teens and young adults, by using a 'chronic care model' to assure a seamless transition between support services given to children, and those given to adolescents and adults.

The individual management plan addresses behavioural, relationship, and psychosocial issues, including associated learning difficulties, peer relationships, low self-esteem, and family function. Families and carers should be provided with information about ADHD and the advantages and disadvantages of potential treatment strategies. Presenting the treatment alternatives and engaging the adolescent and their family in selecting a treatment option improves the doctor–patient relationship and adherence. Local ADHD support groups may also have a role to play, if they provide good quality information.

5.2. *Medication*

A majority of adolescents with ADHD have a positive response to medication. Medication has the capacity to modify behaviour sufficiently to permit participation in main-stream educational and social activity. Learning and social experience then enable the individual to develop alternative coping strategies to improve function. The need for support from medication in the performance of daily activities will reduce over time in conjunction with further developmental brain maturation.

5.2.1. *Stimulants*

Stimulant medications, such as methylphenidate and dexamphetamine, are available in various formulations. The short acting formulations have an immediate release with effects evident for 4–6 hours and 2–3 daily doses required. Extended release formulations of methylphenidate need only be taken once daily. Typically, lower doses are required to manage attention and higher doses for management of behaviour. Extended release medications assist in decreasing the stigma and inconvenience of taking medication at school. In comparison with immediate release preparations these are better tolerated with decreased side effects of appetite suppression and mood lability. Immediate release stimulants, in higher doses, are more likely to be associated with headache, loss of appetite, stomach ache, and insomnia. These adverse effects can also occur with extended release preparations. In the younger adolescent, decreased growth velocity appears related to change in weight, underscoring the importance of regular medication review with physical examination. Stimulants have the potential to be abused, and care should be taken that adolescents are not 'on-selling' or trading their prescription medication.

The largest study to examine the effects of medication and psychosocial treatment is the Multimodal Treatment of ADHD study. Key findings were:

- Both methylphenidate and psychosocial treatments were effective in reducing ADHD symptoms, but psychosocial treatments alone had smaller effect sizes than either methylphenidate or combined treatment.
- For ODD symptoms both psychosocial interventions and methylphenidate generated significant improvements; however, the latter was significantly more effective.
- For social behaviour, the psychosocial, methylphenidate and combined interventions were equally effective.
- Academic function did not improve with any treatment.

5.2.2. Atomoxetine

Atomoxetine is a non-stimulant pharmacological agent for ADHD. Atomoxetine is primarily a noradrenaline reuptake inhibitor. Studies using atomoxetine at a dose of between 1.0 and 1.5 mg per kg per day demonstrate improvement in ADHD symptoms and comorbid symptoms. It is given as a once daily dose though side effects may be diminished by splitting the dose. Compared to stimulants, atomoxetine is generally superior in decreasing comorbid mood symptoms and has a lesser impact on appetite and sleep. Adverse effects include headache, nausea, and abdominal pain.

5.2.3. Other medications

In some countries use of medications may be off label.

Clonidine is an alpha-adrenergic agonist, used in the treatment of ADHD, both because of its capacity to decrease core symptoms and its positive effect on stimulant side effects. A dose of 100–200 mcg is usually prescribed to be taken at night. Clonidine may also be of benefit where there has been an unsatisfactory clinical response to stimulants and atomoxetine.

Though *modafinil* functions as a stimulant it is chemically different to both methylphenidate and dexamphetamine. Erythema multiforme major and Stevens–Johnson syndrome have been associated with its use. Like stimulants this medication is subject to abuse potential.

Though current research suggest that *nicotine patches* are of limited or no benefit in treating ADHD in adolescents, they are increasingly used to support smoking cessation in this age group.

Other medications such as *selegiline, bupropion,* and *guanefacine* remain specialist and research agents and should only be used in clinical research services.

5.3. *Psychosocial Management*

Relatively little quality research has been conducted examining psychosocial treatments for adolescents with ADHD. Psychosocial interventions include cognitive behavioural therapy, behavioural modification, social skills training, and educational strategies. As well as addressing core ADHD symptoms, psychosocial interventions need to focus on improving day to day function at home and at school, and further education and employment. An integrative, cognitive–behavioural, systemic approach in the school setting with students with ADHD has proven to be effective. Programs are especially effective in combination with medication, but the effectiveness does not always translate to settings not included in the intervention. Parenting programs and family therapy interventions require strong parental commitment. Continuing to reinforce stronger parent–child relationships into adolescence and good parenting skills give adolescents more opportunities for development and practice of social skills within the family setting. Behavioural modification and contingency management systems use a combination of strategies such as structured reward systems and disciplinary techniques to encourage behavioural change. While there is a significant overlap between ADHD and academic underachievement, limited systematic research has been conducted on psychosocial strategies to assist students in the educational arena. Research which addresses non-medical intervention strategies for academic success, has examined behavioural approaches for time management, note-taking, and study skills. However, very few conclusions can be drawn about any effective educational interventions, particularly in secondary and tertiary settings.

5.4. *Complementary and Alternative Treatments*

Approximately two-thirds of Australian families with an adolescent with ADHD report using CAMs, although usually in conjunction with medication or behavioural strategies. The expense of many CAM approaches in conjunction with the lack of an evidence base to support their use necessitates caution in their recommendation. It is important that health professionals inquire about their patient's use of such treatment approaches and openly discuss these with patients and their families.

Elimination diets and *dietary supplements* remain popular. Food colouring and sugar are commonly described triggers for ADHD behaviour. Provocation studies rather than well designed treatment studies are the main evidence for restrictive dietary approaches. Omega-3 fatty acid dietary supplements are the most researched. Their use as a dietary supplement however is only supported by parallel research on brain development, and not by specific treatment studies. *Behavioural optometry* uses visual training techniques to improve coordination and sequencing, but has not been examined in controlled studies. Neither has the use of *coloured (Irlen) lenses*. In *neuro-feedback*, individuals are trained to self-regulate their brain activity. Unlike many other CAMs, neuro-feedback has been compared to medication in clinical trials and shows promise in the treatment of ADHD. The benefit of *chiropractic* and other kinaesthetic interventions is yet to be examined in the treatment of ADHD.

5.5. *Review and Ongoing Management*

An initial review during the first month after medication is initated assists in establishing the optimal dosing required. Patients receiving treatment for ADHD should be reviewed each school term by their general practitioner/family physician and have, at a minimum, a six monthly specialist review to ensure that the management strategies remain appropriate and effective. Clinical review covers medication and other interventions, educational progress and behaviour in the home and other settings, and should occur more frequently in younger adolescents. Progress information should be sought from multiple sources, including parents and other significant care givers and teachers. Follow up is also required to assess the impact of treatment side effects, particularly for growth and development in the younger adolescent on stimulant medication.

The primary care physician is well placed to monitor treatment adherence, treatment efficacy, and side effects and will also be aware of local services to support educational, psychosocial, and family interventions.

5.6. *Transition*

Three areas of transition are important to consider as the adolescent enters young adulthood. Some will move into a university setting, others into a vocational career. All will need assistance negotiating the health care system as an adult.

5.6.1. *College and tertiary education*

Students in the US and elsewhere are entitled to educational support services and an increasing number of college age students with ADHD are requesting the special accommodations allowed. Upwards of 9% of college students are now disclosing their history as children and adolescents with ADHD. This phenomenon places the onus on educational institutions to decide what support strategies they need to put in place, in order to achieve optimal outcomes for individual students. Strategies such as technology for note-taking, time management workshops, individual tutoring sessions, and extra study sessions and examination time are just some of the support needed for college students with ADHD. While there is limited research in academic achievement in college students with ADHD, there is evidence of risk for lower grades, challenging social interactions, and overall difficulty adjusting to college life. Students who self report ADHD had greater concerns about their academic performance and exhibited more depressive symptoms during the transition to college as compared to other college students.

5.6.2. *Workplace*

As adolescents and young adults with ADHD develop, evidence of hyperactivity decreases but problems with inattention, distractibility, and executive function may remain. These limitations have a direct effect on workplace success. The combination of poor time management skills leading to missed deadlines and misplaced work, along with difficulty prioritising tasks, lack of self-regulation, and social skills deficits make it challenging for the adult with ADHD to work independently and complete multistep tasks. It is essential that young adults obtain career guidance to examine which careers are most appropriate for them as individuals. Guidance regarding the degree of job match with the individual's strengths and weaknesses along with an analysis of the job expectations and supervisory styles should occur. In addition, education about potential strategies to negotiate the complex issues in a work environment enables the person with ADHD to be ready for challenges that might occur on the job.

5.6.3. *Independence from family*

Young adults with ADHD will also need individual guidance to access services for continued success living with ADHD. Negotiating different insurance and medical care plans, finding community support services and choosing medical treatments become their responsibility as adults. A study in the UK indicated that three quarters of young people with ADHD reaching adulthood required continued services in some form.

6. Conclusions

ADHD, the most common behavioural disorder of childhood, is now known to continue into adolescence and adulthood in over 65% of childhood diagnoses. While most have less hyperactivity as they mature, they still demonstrate challenges in attention, self-regulation, and learning. Other comorbid conditions present with age, such as CD/ ODD, depression, and anxiety. Clinical diagnosis, using standardised subjective rating of behaviour remains the current gold standard over objective measures of brain function such as imaging or EEG. Medication provides an effective strategy to improve attention and decrease impulsivity. Educational, psychosocial, and family support are all important components of a treatment plan for adolescents with ADHD. CAMs require further investigation before these can be recommended in routine clinical care for adolescents with ADHD. The most important treatment process is a systematic assessment of each individual's needs and the creation of an individualised intervention plan.

Case History

Peter has been managed for ADHD for 10 years and has progressed from being oppositional, hyperactive, and constantly in trouble at school to being a young man whose ADHD symptoms are reasonably well controlled on dexamphetamine. He was changed to dexamphetamine because of adverse effects. At 18, Peter wonders if he will need to continue to use medication as an adult. At this stage he has taken himself off dexamphetamine, however is somewhat ambivalent about stopping the medication. Although he feels that he copes well without it, there are times when he knows he needs to concentrate. He recently got a job and admits there has been quite a difference between being on the medication and off it. His boss said he noticed that Peter was far more focused and a better worker when on the medication. Peter wants to know whether it is appropriate to continue medication both for his job and further education. Dexamphetamine at a lower dose than in adolescence is effective. Peter can be reassured that he can continue to take the medication and that he may have a trial off stimulants when he finishes further education. One third of patients need medication for life. In many countries there may be a limited choice of stimulant prescribers in adulthood.

References

American Psychiatric Association (2000) *Diagnostic and statistical manual of mental disorders Text Revision (DSM-IV-TR)*, 4th edn. American Psychiatric Publication, Washington, DC.

Bird HR, Gould MS, Staghezza BM. (1993) Patterns of diagnostic comorbidity in a community sample of children aged 9 through 16 years. *J Am Acad Child Adolesc Psychiatry* **32**(2): 361–368.

Clarke S, Heussler H, Kohn MR. (2005) Attention deficit disorder: Not just for children. *Intern Med J* **35**(12): 721–725.

MTA Cooperative Group (2004) National Institute of Mental Health Multimodal Treatment study of ADHD follow-up: 24-month outcomes of treatment strategies for attention-deficit/hyperactivity disorder. *Pediatrics* **113**(4): 754–761.

Hinshaw SP. (2007) Moderators and mediators of treatment outcome for youth with ADHD: Understanding for whom and how interventions work. *J Pediatr Psychol* **32**(6): 664–675.

Huang Y-S, Tsai M-H. (2011) Long-term outcomes with medications for attention-deficit hyperactivity disorder: Current status of knowledge. *CNS Drugs* **25**(7): 539–554.

Lara C, Fayyad J, De Graaf R, Kessler RC, Aguilar-Gaxiola S, Angermeyer M, Demytteneare K, De Girolamo G, Haro JM, Jin R, Karam EG, Lepine J-P, Mora MEM, Ormel J, Posada-Villa J, Sampson N. (2009) Childhood predictors of adult attention-deficit/hyperactivity disorder: Results from the World Health Organization World Mental Health Survey initiative. *Biol Psychiatry* **65**(1): 46–54.

Loe IM, Feldman HM. (2007) Academic and educational outcomes of children with ADHD. *J Pediatr Psychol* **32**(6): 643–654.

Nigg JT. (2005) Neuropsychologic theory and findings in attention-deficit/hyperactivity disorder: The state of the field and salient challenges for the coming decade. *Biol Psychiatry* **57**(11): 1424–1435.

Nutt DJ, Fone K, Asherson P, Bramble D, Hill P, Matthews K, Morris KA, Santosh P, Sonuga-Barke E, Taylor E, Weiss M, Young S. (2007) Evidence-based guidelines for management of attention-deficit/hyperactivity disorder in adolescents in transition to adult services and in adults: Recommendations from the British Association for psychopharmacology (guidelines). *J Psychopharmacol* **21**(1): 10(32).

Swanson JM, Kinsbourne M, Nigg J, Lanphear B, Stefanatos GA, Volkow N, Taylor E, Casey BJ, Castellanos FX, Wadhwa PD. (2007) Etiologic subtypes of attention-deficit/hyperactivity disorder: Brain imaging, molecular genetic and environmental factors and the dopamine hypothesis. *Neuropsychol Rev* **17**(1): 39–59.

Wolraich ML, Wibbelsman CJ, Brown TE, Evans SW, Gotlieb EM, Knight JR, Ross EC, Shubiner HH, Wender EH, Wilens T. (2005) Attention-deficit/ hyperactivity disorder among adolescents: A review of the diagnosis, treatment, and clinical implications. *Pediatrics* **115**(6): 1734–1746.

Chapter 33

Immunisation and Infectious Diseases

Melina Georgousakis, Alexa Deirig
and Robert Booy

1. Introduction

Historically, the clinical focus of vaccination has been largely restricted to children and the elderly due to the high morbidity and mortality from the vaccine preventable diseases seen in these age groups. However, over the past decade, vaccination of adolescents has become a priority. Pertussis, meningococcal disease, and human papilloma virus have high incidence rates in adolescents and young adults due to age specific behaviours including school attendance, social activities, and sexual debut. In addition, sporadic epidemics of diseases for which vaccinations are delivered during childhood (such as measles) still occur among adolescents because of incomplete or missed childhood vaccinations. Thus, timely vaccine delivery during adolescence is not only crucial to introduce protection against new diseases relevant to adult life but also to maintain protection gained through childhood into adulthood.

In recent years the number of vaccines recommended specifically for adolescents has increased. In general, routine adolescent vaccinations include booster doses for diphtheria, tetanus, and pertussis, as well as the complete primary schedule against HPV. There are also circumstances that can put adolescents in need of additional vaccinations, including catch-up schedules, and medical and lifestyle risk factors. However, there are a number of challenges that affect the timely delivery of these vaccinations including adolescent rebelliousness, lack of parental education, and deficiencies in funding or delivery systems.

2. General Immunisation Guidelines

Before deciding on necessary vaccinations, one should take into account current personal circumstances of the adolescent. To initiate discussions on vaccination, several points should be considered:

- Is the individual suffering from an acute illness or a chronic disease?
- What is their country of origin and their country of residence?
- Is the individual living with chronically ill family members?

Once the required vaccinations are established, it is important to:

- Check for any contraindications.
- Provide information on, and discuss disease risk and the benefit of vaccination, as well as any expected adverse events following immunisation.
- Be prepared to manage anaphylactic reactions.
- Record any vaccinations administered and any future doses or new vaccinations required.

3. Vaccinations Recommended for All Adolescents

3.1. *Primary Immunisations*

These provide protection against diseases that peak in adolescence and in early adult life. HPV is the only VPD for which delivery of the complete vaccination course is recommended during adolescence as standard practice. HPV is a sexually transmitted disease that is responsible for a number of benign and malignant lesions in women and men including respiratory papillomatosis, condylomata acuminate, and various cancers of the anogenital and upper-respiratory tracts. However, the primary goal of vaccination has been the prevention of cervical cancer in women, which has the highest rates of morbidity and mortality of all the HPV associated diseases.

Currently, two HPV vaccines are registered in many countries; Cervarix® (2-valent) and Gardasil® (4-valent). Both vaccines provide protection against HPV types 16 and 18 which are responsible for over 70% of cervical cancers. However Gardasil® also provides protection against an additional two HPV types, HPV 6 and 11, which are associated with 90% of cases of genital warts. Both vaccine formulations are delivered in a three dose schedule; Cervarix® on months 0, 2, and 6; and Gardasil® on months 0, 1, and 6. As applicable to all vaccines, an important contraindication for HPV vaccination is anaphylaxis following a previous dose of the vaccine or anaphylaxis following any component of the vaccine, in particular, the yeast (*Saccharomyces cerevisiae*) component of Gardasil®. HPV vaccines are based on virus like particles, hence they do not replicate in the host.

HPV vaccination is most effective when the recipient is naïve to the HPV types covered by the vaccine. More than three quarters of new HPV infections occur during adolescence and young adulthood hence vaccination is targeted to early adolescence prior to the onset of sexual activity. The recommended age for HPV vaccination, the funding arrangements, and delivery programs vary between countries and jurisdictions. Every effort should be made to identify adolescent and younger adult women who may not have been vaccinated against HPV and may benefit from vaccination. It is important to keep in mind that vaccine effectiveness will reduce with increased exposure to HPV as occurs with increasing age.

In 2010 Gardasil® was approved by the US Federal Drug Administration for use in males 9–26 years of age for the prevention of external genital lesions, including genital warts, and infection caused by the HPV types in the vaccine. Routine vaccination of males will start in Australia in 2013. Males who would like protection against HPV, or those at high risk of HPV infection such as men who have sex with men, may be able to access the vaccine through private prescription where it is not government funded. Gender neutral HPV vaccination programs are likely to expand.

3.2. *Booster Immunisations*

Booster doses are necessary to increase immunity against a specific vaccine antigen to at least the level achieved following primary immunisation. A routine adolescent booster dose using the combined diphtheria, tetanus and acellular pertussis vaccine has been added to the immunisation schedule of many countries including Australia and US. The booster dose is given between 9–18 years of age, depending on the country's schedule, using the adolescent/adult vaccine formulation (dTap). This combined vaccine has a good safety record, however local injection site reactions do occur with repeat vaccinations containing DT. To increase tolerability of this vaccine the adult formulation has reduced amounts of the diphtheria and pertussis vaccine components.

3.3. *Catch-Up Programs*

Any routine outpatient visit by an adolescent is an opportunity to review if they are up to date with all vaccinations required from birth. If childhood vaccinations have not been completed as per the recommended schedule, a catch-up program should be developed. The development of a catch-up program should be based on the local schedule.

3.3.1. *Measles, mumps, and rubella*

In many countries, it is recommended that all individuals born after 1960 receive two doses of MMR, at least four weeks apart, to induce optimal immunity against the three diseases. A large proportion of this age cohort would not have developed natural immunity to the viruses and may not have received two doses of MMR in childhood. This is particularly true for adolescents who may have missed the implementation of a routine second dose in their country. The MMR vaccine is a trivalent live attenuated vaccine. Monovalent vaccines are less often available and though licensed in some countries it is usually preferable to use the combined MMR vaccine. Pregnant women or individuals with impaired immunity should not receive live vaccines like MMR. Individuals with egg allergy can safely receive the vaccine as it contains only negligible amounts of egg protein.

3.3.2. *Polio*

Polio vaccination is part of the routine immunisation schedule in most countries which has resulted in its eradication from the developed world.

There are two highly effective vaccines available against polio; an inactivated poliovirus vaccine (IPV; "Salk"), given intramuscularly and a live-attenuated oral vaccine (OPV; "Sabin"). The Salk vaccine covers the three serotypes whereas the oral vaccine is available in several formulations of varying valency. Due to the risk with OPV of vaccine associated paralytic poliomyelitis and prolonged shedding of vaccine strains in individuals with impaired immunity, its routine use in developed countries (and some developing countries) was stopped in recent years and it was replaced with IPV. There are fewer safety concerns with IPV.

If no, or an incomplete, primary course was given in childhood, three doses, at least four weeks apart, of IPV are necessary.

3.3.3. *Hepatitis B*

The hepatitis B vaccine is usually given as a three dose primary series and is part of the routine childhood immunisation schedule in most developed and some developing countries. The World Health Organization estimates that approximately two billion people worldwide have been infected with the hepatitis B virus and about 350 million live with a chronic infection. The hepatitis B vaccine is a recombinant vaccine based on the hepatitis B surface antigen. Different formulations are available including combined antigen formulations. If an adolescent presents who has not been appropriately immunised in childhood, there are multiple options for the catch up schedule which depend on their age, the vaccine being used and their place of residence. In Australia, for example, if the young person is between 8 and 19 years of age, three doses of the paediatric dose of hepatitis B vaccine with a minimum interval of four weeks between the first and second dose and eight weeks between the second and third dose is recommended. For individuals aged 11–15 years, an alternative two dose catch up schedule is available using the adult formulation which contains double the amount of the HBsAg protein. A minimum interval of 4–6 months between doses is required.

In most countries, the completion of the childhood hepatitis B vaccination schedule is enough to provide long lasting protection against hepatitis B. For individuals with impaired immunity booster doses might be necessary, and serology should be taken to determine the anti-HBs levels following vaccination. The hepatitis B vaccine is well tolerated and most adverse events are minor and transient.

3.3.4. *Varicella*

Varicella vaccination has been introduced in the childhood immunisation schedule in a number of developed countries including Australia, Canada, Japan, Germany and the US. If an adolescent in a country where the vaccine is part of the routine immunisation program has either not received a previous varicella vaccination or has no history of natural varicella infection, a catch up vaccination should be administered. Depending on the country, one or two doses of the vaccine are required.

Varicella is a monovalent live attenuated vaccine and has the same contraindications as other live attenuated vaccines. In some countries a combined vaccine, consisting of MMR and varicella, is also available.

3.3.5. *Meningococcal C*

Meningococcal disease can occur at any age; however, a higher incidence is seen in young children with a second peak in adolescence. Several vaccines are available against meningococcal disease, which differ by the number of meningococcal serotypes they protect against and also their formulation and recommendations. A majority of countries in the developed world recommend the use of the conjugate meningococcal C vaccine (MenC), in their childhood immunisation schedule. However, in the US and Canada the tetravalent A, C, Y, W135 conjugate vaccine is licensed for use in children, teenagers, and adults. In the US, meningococcal vaccination of adolescents aged 11–12 years is routinely recommended followed by a booster dose at 16 years of age. Adolescents in countries where a meningococcal vaccine is part of the immunisation schedule but who have never been vaccinated should be offered the vaccine.

Although meningococcal vaccination is not a standard travel vaccination, health care providers caring for adolescents planning international travel or residency in an endemic country, should counsel them regarding the risk of different meningococcal serogroups. For example major meningococcal epidemics occur regularly in the sub-Saharan meningitis belt of Africa.

4. Immunisations for Adolescents at Risk

In addition to vaccinations routinely recommended during adolescence, others may be required due to life style or medical factors which increase the risk for particular VPDs. It is important for health care providers to implement strategies to identify adolescents who may have one or more of these risk factors so that the appropriate vaccinations are delivered.

4.1. *Underlying Medical Conditions*

4.1.1. *Influenza*

Persons of any age, including children and adolescents, with a serious or chronic medical condition have an increased risk of hospitalisation and morbidity following an influenza infection. The WHO recommends that seasonal influenza vaccinations are given yearly to any person who has an underlying medical condition that increases their risk of influenza associated complications. Medical conditions which increase a person's risk of serious influenza include, but are not limited to:

- Cardiac disease.
- Chronic respiratory conditions (including severe asthma).
- Chronic neurological and neuromuscular conditions.
- Chronic renal or liver disease.
- Diabetes mellitus.
- Morbid obesity.
- Impaired immunity (either through disease or treatment).

Identification and annual vaccination of adolescent patients who have one or more of these health conditions should be a primary focus of physicians.

While healthy children and adolescents are not at higher risk of influenza complications, their high attack rates of infection during influenza seasons mean they are a common source of transmission to those at increased risk. In the US, annual influenza vaccination is recommended for any child aged six months or more, independent of health status.

Two vaccine formulations are available against seasonal influenza; the trivalent inactivated influenza vaccine and the live attenuated influenza vaccine. Currently, LAIV is only registered for use in the US. Both vaccines should contain the strains of influenza virus that are recommended for that season's formulation by the WHO. In adolescents and young adults, a single intra-muscular dose of TIV is required to provide protection against influenza. Vaccination should occur yearly so that protection is gained against newly circulating strains. In clinical studies TIV has been shown to be safe and effective in persons with underlying medical conditions. However, LAIV is not registered for use in at-risk persons. Contraindications for influenza vaccination include any person who has anaphylactic sensitivity to egg or other components of the vaccine unless they have been de-sensitised.

4.1.2. *Pneumococcal vaccination*

Although the greatest disease burden due to invasive pneumococcal disease is in children <2 years of age and elderly persons >85 years, persons of any age with certain medical conditions can be at high risk of infection. This has resulted in pneumococcal vaccination recommendations specifically for these individuals in many countries. The indicated at-risk conditions include but are not limited to:

- Chronic medical conditions (including heart disease, lung disease, diabetes, cerebral spinal fluid leaks, and cochlear implants).
- Conditions that reduce immunity against infection (HIV or AIDS, organ transplant, various cancers, acute nephrotic syndrome, and asplenia).
- Therapy that reduces immunity against infection (long term steroids, certain cancer drugs, radiation therapy).
- Smoking.

Two types of pneumococcal vaccines are available. Conjugate vaccines, which combine between 10–13 pneumococcal polysaccharides with a protein carrier and pneumococcal polysaccharide vaccine, which contains 23 pneumococcal polysaccharides with no carrier (23vPPV). In most countries, the use of conjugate vaccines is limited to young children due to the incidence of disease and limited clinical data of their efficacy in adolescents and adults. 23vPPV can be given to children from two years of age, adolescents, and adults. The type of pneumococcal vaccine recommended varies between countries and jurisdictions; thus it is important to be familiar with local recommendations.

The effectiveness of 23vPPV may be lower in individuals with underlying medical conditions, in particular those conditions that affect immune function. A single re-vaccination with 23vPPV after 5 years is recommended in some countries to maintain immunity in individuals at high risk of invasive infection.

4.1.3. *Other medical conditions which may require additional vaccinations*

Patients with functional or anatomical asplenia have increased risk of infection with encapsulated bacteria including Pneumococcus, Meningococcus and *Haemophilus influenza*. If treating a patient prior to splenectomy or after unplanned splenectomy, specific local recommendations for each of these vaccinations should be followed. This is also the case when treating patients with other immune deficient conditions where alternate immunisation schedules are required, for example oncology patients, HIV infected individuals, and solid organ and bone marrow transplant recipients.

In addition, both hepatitis A and hepatitis B vaccination should be considered for patients with chronic liver disease of any cause, preferably early in the course of the disease.

4.2. *Immunisation in Pregnancy*

4.2.1. *During pregnancy*

Live attenuated vaccines are the only vaccines contraindicated for pregnant women because of the potential risk associated with the transfer of vaccine virus to the infant, albeit low. However, the use of vaccines in pregnancy, with the exception of inactivated seasonal influenza and pertussis, is avoided other than in situations where the benefits of protection following vaccination far outweigh the risks.

Seasonal TIV is routinely recommended during pregnancy due to the high risk of severe complications in the mother and also the foetus following an influenza infection. This risk is the highest in the third trimester so vaccination should still be considered at this later stage of pregnancy. Seasonal influenza vaccination has been shown to have a good safety profile in pregnant women when given in any trimester. The benefit of vaccination may also be extended to the new born child with recent evidence suggesting vaccination during pregnancy can also protect infants against influenza until up to six months of age.

4.2.2. *Planning or post pregnancy*

It is advisable to review the vaccination history of young women of child bearing age, in particular for immunity to rubella, pertussis, and varicella. Although rubella is usually a mild and self-limiting disease, rubella during early pregnancy can result in congenital rubella syndrome in infants. Immunity to rubella should be established prior to pregnancy, via serological screening and seronegative women are recommended to receive a dose of MMR. Seroconversion should be tested 6–8 weeks post vaccination, and women with low antibody levels should be revaccinated. MMR or monovalent rubella vaccines should not be given to a woman known to be pregnant. It is recommended that women who have received MMR should wait 28 days before becoming pregnant.

Varicella during pregnancy can result in increased maternal morbidity and mortality as well as congenital varicella syndrome or neonatal varicella. Varicella infection in early pregnancy has been associated with a 1% risk of congenital infection. Young women planning pregnancy who are non-immune to varicella are recommended to receive two doses of monovalent varicella vaccine at least four weeks apart to achieve maximum protection. Like MMR, VV is a live attenuated vaccine and should not be administered during pregnancy and women should wait for 28 days following vaccination before becoming pregnant.

Adults, in particular parents, are the main source of pertussis infection for infants. In a number of developed countries including the US,

Australia, Austria, and Germany, pertussis vaccination has been recommended for mothers, fathers, and carers of new-borns as a strategy to reduce transmission to infants, especially those who are too young to be vaccinated against the disease. Vaccination with dTpa can be given to women either when planning pregnancy, after 20 weeks of pregnancy or soon after the birth of the child. Although in many countries an adolescent booster dose of dTpa is recommended under national immunisation programs as described above, vaccination uptake is still lower than optimal, leaving a large proportion of adolescents and adults susceptible to infection. In the US in 2004 and 2005, more than 50% of pertussis cases were in those >11 years of age.

5. Travel Vaccinations

As adolescents become more independent, they often start to travel or work overseas where additional vaccinations might be needed in order to prevent disease. In addition to discussing specific travel vaccinations, international travel provides an opportunity to discuss and review an adolescent patient's vaccination history for routine vaccinations. Prior to recommending vaccinations, health care providers must acquire sufficient information on destination of travel, reason for travelling, planned activities and length of stay in order to provide each adolescent with appropriate and individual travel vaccine advice. It may be appropriate to direct adolescent patients to specialised travel vaccination clinics.

5.1. *Poliomyelitis*

Due to global eradication efforts infections with poliovirus have decreased by over 99% since 1988. Afghanistan, Nigeria, and Pakistan are the three remaining countries where polio is still endemic. If adolescent patients are planning to travel to these countries, their polio vaccination history should be reviewed. If they have not been vaccinated previously they should complete a primary schedule of polio vaccine. For patients who have previously completed a polio vaccination course, a single booster dose is recommended prior to travel to polio-endemic areas.

5.2. *Yellow Fever*

Yellow Fever is an acute viral haemorrhagic disease that occurs in sub-Saharan Africa and in tropical and sub-tropical Central and South America. Transmission of the virus is by mosquito bite. According to the WHO, more than 200,000 cases of YF, with approximately 30,000 deaths, occur each year. There is no treatment for the disease, so prevention with vaccination is crucial. There are several vaccine formulations on the market which are all live attenuated vaccines. The vaccine can only be administered by YF Vaccination Centres approved by the relevant health authorities and this should be recorded on an International Certificate of Vaccination against YF. For some areas, for example in South America, a proof of vaccination is required to enter the country. A single dose of the YF vaccine probably provides protection for at least 30 years, but in order to obtain a valid international vaccine certificate, revaccination is required after 10 years.

YF vaccine is usually considered to have only mild side effects, but in recent years some severe adverse events have been linked to the vaccine: vaccine-associated neurotropic disease and vaccine-associated viscerotropic disease. Therefore, it is important to ensure that young people have a good understanding of the side effects and are only vaccinated if their destination is clearly in the endemic YF zone. Contraindications are as for all live attenuated vaccines, but also include anaphylaxis to eggs, impaired immunity, and thymus disorders.

5.3. *Typhoid*

Typhoid fever, a systemic illness, caused by infection with *Salmonella typhi* (*S. enterica* serotype typhi), is known together with *S. paratyphi* A or *B* as enteric fever. Transmission usually occurs via the ingestion of faecally-contaminated food or water. It is estimated that 22 million cases of *S. typhi* occur annually incurring around 200,000 deaths with the highest incidence in Africa, Asia, and South America. In the developed world, the vast majority of typhoid fever is associated with travel. Typhoid can be treated with antibiotics, however, as more multidrug resistant strains are emerging, treatment is becoming more challenging.

For prevention of the disease, two different vaccines are currently available; a live attenuated oral vaccine and a capsular polysaccharide vaccine. These vaccines protect only against *S. typhi* and not *paratyphi*. Several doses of the oral, live attenuated vaccine are necessary for protection; the exact dosing schedule differs between countries. For example, Canada and the US use a four dose regimen with doses administered on alternate days, whereas a three dose regimen is followed in other countries. The oral vaccine is attractive to many travellers as it is given as a capsule. The capsule should be kept refrigerated, not be chewed and taken with cool liquid. On the other hand, the polysaccharide vaccine is inactivated and only one dose, given intramuscularly, is necessary. Travellers are advised to complete the schedule at least one week (for the oral vaccine) or two weeks (for the i.m. vaccine) prior to departure.

Booster doses are necessary for individuals with prolonged or repeat exposure. For the inactivated vaccine, it is recommended to revaccinate with one dose after three years. For the live attenuated vaccine, revaccination is recommended every three years with three doses if the three dose regimen was used, or every five years with four doses if the four dose schedule was used.

Both types of vaccines elicit few adverse events which are mostly mild. The oral live attenuated vaccine should not be given to pregnant women, to individuals with impaired immunity, and to individuals taking antibiotics. For adolescents requiring hepatitis A and typhoid vaccination a combined vaccine may be available.

5.4. *Hepatitis A*

Hepatitis A is an acute infection of the liver caused by the hepatitis A virus. It is spread via the faecal–oral route. It is more prevalent in developing countries and low socio-economic areas where lack of adequate sanitation and poor hygiene facilitate spread of the infection. The risk of hepatitis A is dependent on destination, the length of stay, the contact with the local population and both personal and local hygiene standards. There is no specific treatment for the disease, but vaccination is available. There are a number of different hepatitis A vaccine formulations; the majority are inactivated vaccines, however some countries, for example China, have a live attenuated vaccine. The different formulations have different hepatitis A virus antigen content, have different vaccination schedules, and can be licensed for different age groups. In most countries a two dose schedule is recommended with the second dose given 6–12 or 12–18 months after the first dose depending on the vaccine used.

Evidence suggests that high antibody response occurs after a single dose of the hepatitis A vaccine; however the second dose is expected to improve long-term protection. Those who do not have time to receive the two doses prior to departure may still benefit from receiving the first dose before travel and the second dose (to induce the anamnestic response) upon return. A second dose several years after the first has been shown to trigger an anamnestic response.

All hepatitis A vaccines are well tolerated with no severe adverse events recorded. Mild local and systemic reactions do occur. Prior to vaccinating with hepatitis A, health care providers should check if immunisation status for hepatitis B is up to date. In the case of an incomplete or even missing primary course of hepatitis B, there is the possibility to vaccinate with a combined hepatitis A and B vaccine.

5.5. *Rabies*

Rabies is a zoonotic viral disease which is one of the most deadly diseases known to mankind. Almost all individuals developing symptoms will die of the disease. Humans are at risk of infection through the transmission of the virus by close contact with an animal's saliva, via bites or scratches from infected animals (domestic and wild) and in rare cases through contact of infected material (usually saliva) with mucous membranes or fresh skin wounds.

There are several vaccines available for pre- and post-exposure prophylaxis which are highly effective. The vaccines are produced either from cell culture or embryonated eggs. Pre-exposure prophylaxis is not needed for most travellers, but recommended for anyone who is at increased risk of catching the disease due to travelling, or nature of occupation, or residence. Pre-exposure vaccination requires administration of three doses prior to travel (days 0, 7, and 21 or 28). A booster dose is not usually recommended unless individuals are expected to have ongoing exposure to rabies. If a non-immune traveller is exposed to rabies, post-exposure prophylaxis exists and should be administered. It consists of local treatment of the wound and, depending on the type of contact, vaccination (five doses at day 0, 3, 7, 14, and 28–30) and administration of rabies immunoglobulin (infiltration in and around the wounds, remainder of the dose intra-muscularly). Recently, the US reduced the recommended number of post-exposure rabies doses to four from the standard five dose schedule, which has also been recently considered in Australia.

The vaccines are in general well tolerated with few (and minor) systemic and local side effects. In the case of history of an anaphylactic sensitivity to eggs or to egg protein, the vaccine produced from cell culture should be used.

5.6. *Japanese Encephalitis*

Japanese encephalitis is a mosquito-borne viral infection caused by the JE virus, which belongs to the flavivirus family. The disease is endemic in parts of China and in Eastern, South and South-East Asia, and in Papua New Guinea. It has also emerged in Northern Australia and the Torres Strait Islands. The case fatality rate is high with approximately 10,000–15,000 deaths worldwide annually. No specific treatment for JE exists.

The risk of acquiring JE for travellers is low, but depends on time, duration and place of travel. The overall incidence is <1 per one million travellers. In expatriates and travellers staying for prolonged periods in rural areas, the risk is close to that of the local population.

According to the recommendations of the US Advisory Committee on Immunisation Practices, the following groups of people should be vaccinated against JE:

- Travellers who plan to spend a month or longer in endemic areas during transmission season.
- Recurrent travellers to JE endemic areas.
- Expatriates who are likely to visit rural or agricultural areas.

However, vaccination can be considered for short term travellers (<1 month) if they have increased risk of JE exposure, for example, travelling outside of an urban area or during a JE outbreak or if destination or activities are uncertain.

The currently available vaccine against JE for international travellers is the inactivated formulation IC51 vaccine (Ixiaro®). However, it is not licensed for individuals <18 years of age. Children and adolescents aged 1–17 can receive the inactivated mouse brain derived vaccine. However some countries may experience shortages in upcoming years due to discontinued production by the manufacturer. For adolescents, three doses administered on days 0, 7, and 28 are recommended. The mouse brain derived vaccine has been associated with serious, but rare, allergic and neurologic adverse events.

6. Future Vaccines for Adolescents

The number of vaccinations recommended during adolescence is expected to increase in the near future as new vaccines are developed, and also as changes are made to the schedule or the formulation of currently available vaccines. Vaccines against meningococcal B and herpes simplex virus, which are relatively common among adolescents, are in various stages of development. Although MenB is responsible for a majority of meningococcal disease in developed countries, the currently licensed vaccines only provide protection against meningococcal serotypes A, C, W135, and Y. The development of a vaccine that also protects against serotype B has been hindered by the genetic diversity of MenB strains circulating in the population. The most advanced MenB vaccine formulation is Bexsero® (Novartis) which was licensed in Europe in 2012. Other vaccines against MenB based on different strategies are in various stages of clinical development.

Various vaccine formulations against HSV have reached clinical trials however their success has been variable. The HSV viruses, HSV-1 and HSV-2, may lead to lifelong disease from genital ulcerations to skin and eye lesions. They are also the most common viral cause of encephalitis. The time period between clinical testing and availability of HSV vaccine for clinical use is hard to predict but the progression of multiple vaccine candidates into clinical trials is promising.

Next generation vaccines are being developed against a number of VPDs for which vaccines already exist with the aim of improving the current formulations, for example, using strategies to increase vaccine efficacy, reduce antigen content or increase compliance through less invasive delivery strategies.

7. Hurdles for Adolescent Vaccine Delivery

The recent introduction of a number of vaccinations during adolescence such as HPV, MenC, and dTpa booster has placed new emphasis on preventative health care among this age cohort. However, the delivery of adolescent vaccinations has been faced with a number of challenges which have reduced vaccine uptake when compared with programs in childhood.

In general, adolescents and their parents are often unaware of the need for vaccinations during this time of life. In many countries such as Australia, England, and provinces in Canada, delivery of adolescent vaccinations occurs through school based programs which are known to increase uptake. Other countries' vaccinations are delivered through general practitioners and other health services. In these instances, vaccine uptake relies on both patient recall and provider recommendation. Evidence suggests adolescents are less likely to seek preventative health care. For those who do visit a heath care provider, other challenges such as adequacy of adolescent consent interferes with uptake. The ability of an adolescent patient to consent to vaccination without a parent's consent varies between countries and even jurisdictions, and has become of increased importance in situations such as HPV vaccination, where parents' views may be more conservative than those of the adolescent.

The deficient health literacy of adolescents and the fact that they likely present for fewer preventative health care visits, means every opportunity should be taken by providers to discuss vaccination requirements with adolescents and their parents, and to plan the delivery of appropriate vaccines. Provider support has been cited as a major influence for vaccine acceptability by both parents and adolescents. However, in many developing countries, missed opportunities to vaccinate adolescents occur regularly, with physicians identifying barriers such as time constraints, lack of funding, and difficulties in obtaining consent.

References

Brabin L, Greenberg DP, Hessel L, Hyer R, Ivanoff B, Van Damme P. (2008) Current issues in adolescent immunization. *Vaccine* **26**(33): 4120–4134.

Centers for Disease Control and Prevention. (2010) Recommended immunization schedules for persons aged 0 through 18 years. Report for United States.

Dorell C, Stokley S, Yankey D, Cohn A, Markowitz L. (2010) National, state, and local area vaccination coverage among adolescents aged 13–17 years — United States, 2009. MMWR (Morbidity and Mortality Weekly Report).

Gruslin A, Steben M, Halperin S, Money DM, Yudin MH. (2009) Immunization in pregnancy: No. 220, December 2008. *Int J Gynaecol Obstet* **105**(2): 187–191.

Jelfs J, Rashid H, Booy R. (2010) Meningococcal vaccines. In: Zuckerman JN, Jong Ec (eds), *Travelers' vaccines*, 2nd ed. People's Medical Publishing House, USA, Shelton, CT.

Middleman AB, Rosenthal SL, Rickert VI, Neinstein L, Fishbein DB, D'angelo L, Society for Adolescent Medicine. (2006) Adolescent immunizations: A position paper of the society for adolescent medicine. *J Adolesc Health* **38**(3): 321–327.

Nakamura MM, Lee GM. (2008) Influenza vaccination in adolescents with high-risk conditions. *Pediatrics* **122**(5): 920–928.

Tan L, K, K, Carlone G, M, Borrow R. (2010) Advances in the development of vaccines against neisseria meningitidis. *N Engl J Med* **362**(16): 1511–20.

Chapter 34

Respiratory Disorders in Adolescence

Donald Payne and Siobhain Mulrennan

1. Introduction

Respiratory problems are common in the adolescent and young adult population. These include acute illnesses such as bacterial pneumonia and viral respiratory tract infections, as well as chronic illnesses such as asthma and cystic fibrosis. There is also an increasingly large cohort of adolescents and young adults growing up with childhood respiratory disorders, including chronic lung disease associated with extreme prematurity and neuromuscular disorders requiring respiratory support, conditions for which adult health professionals may have had little or no experience or training. These young adults often have associated comorbidities, such as significant neurological disease or cognitive impairment, which present an additional challenge to management.

2. Asthma

Asthma is a common condition characterised by intermittent episodes of difficulty in breathing associated with wheezing, with or without cough. Symptoms respond acutely to inhaled bronchodilator therapy. Objective evidence of reversible airways obstruction can be sought using spirometry before and after inhaled bronchodilator. The evidence suggests that prevalence rates of asthma remain high in adolescents and young adults. In Australia, the asthma prevalence rate in 2003 was 14% for those aged

12–14 years and 12% each for those aged 15–19 years and 20–24 years. In the same year, asthma was ranked second (behind anxiety and depression) in a list of the leading causes of the burden of disease among young Australian women aged 15–24 years. Asthma did not make the top ten in the corresponding list for young men, which was dominated by injuries, mental health problems, and drug use. During childhood, asthma is more common in boys than girls. However, during adolescence the balance shifts, with asthma becoming more common among women in young adulthood. Although rare, deaths from asthma still occur in young people, and more commonly than in younger children.

2.1. *The Diagnosis of Asthma*

The diagnosis of asthma should be relatively easy to make in adolescents and young adults, given their ability to perform simple lung function tests to assess airway obstruction and bronchodilator reversibility (an increase in FEV_1 following bronchodilator of >12% of the baseline value or >200 ml). However, under-diagnosis still occurs. Clinicians should therefore be alert to the possibility of diagnosing asthma for the first time in an adolescent or young adult.

Conversely, over-diagnosis is also a potential problem. There are a number of conditions in adolescence which may mimic asthma and which should be considered, particularly when conventional doses of asthma treatment fail to result in adequate asthma control. These include external airway compression due to a vascular ring or a mediastinal mass, tracheo/bronchomalacia, cystic fibrosis, dysfunctional breathing such as hyperventilation or vocal cord dysfunction, gastro–oesophageal reflux disease, immune deficiency, and primary ciliary dyskinesia. Simple tests, such as a chest X-ray, spirometry with inspiratory and expiratory flow-volume loops before and after bronchodilator, and an exercise-induced asthma test can help to establish the correct diagnosis.

2.2. *Treatment*

Current recommendations for the pharmacological treatment of asthma are similar in adolescents and adults. The most recent Australian guidelines for treatment are summarised in the Asthma Management Handbook (www.nationalasthma.org.au). In the UK, there are asthma guidelines developed by the British Thoracic Society and the Scottish Intercollegiate Guidelines Network. The areas of self-management and adherence to treatment are key factors in the management of asthma in adolescence (Chapter 11). Open discussions with adolescents around treatment adherence can be facilitated if they are seen alone and given some assurance of confidentiality. Other ways to optimise adherence include keeping the treatment regimen as simple as possible and explaining the reasons for taking treatment in language that adolescents are able to understand. For those with asthma severe enough to require the use of both inhaled corticosteroids and long-acting bronchodilator, use of budesonide/formoterol in a combination inhaler, for both preventer and reliever treatment, may improve adherence to treatment.

2.3. *Collaboration with High Schools and Transition from Paediatric to Adult Health Care*

Collaboration with schools should be an integral part of the health professional's role. This should include working with schools to promote asthma friendly practice and providing school staff with a copy of each student's asthma action plan. Another possible avenue includes peer-led asthma education programs, which have been demonstrated to have a positive impact on quality of life, school absence and asthma exacerbations in adolescents with asthma.

Transition can be a risky time and failure to link with an appropriate adult health care provider can result in missed appointments, loss to follow up and poor health outcomes over time. In addition to identifying a designated health professional to coordinate care, preparation should focus on the features of self-management, such as how to make an appointment, how to obtain new prescriptions and whom to contact in the event of a deterioration in their condition.

3. Cystic Fibrosis

Cystic fibrosis is an autosomal recessive genetic disorder that affects one in 2,500 Caucasians. The defect lies on chromosome 7 and leads to an abnormality in the CF transmembrane regulator protein which regulates chloride secretion. Defective chloride secretion leads to thick, dehydrated mucus within the lungs, pancreas, liver and bowel, and defective mucociliary clearance within the lungs. Newborn screening now identifies the majority of affected individuals in childhood, but prior to the introduction of newborn screening, people could and did present at any age. The diagnosis is made via a combination of clinical features plus identification of two CF mutations or a positive sweat test. Morbidity is usually related to recurrent respiratory infection and malnutrition, secondary to pancreatic insufficiency. The multisystem manifestations of CF are detailed in Table 1. Effective treatment is provided via a multidisciplinary team approach involving physicians, nurses, physiotherapy, dietetics, social work, occupational therapy, pharmacy, and psychological medicine. Transition and transfer to adult services is recognised as a critical phase in the life of a young adult with CF.

Table 1: Manifestations of cystic fibrosis.

- Respiratory disease
  - Bronchiectasis
  - Pneumothorax
  - Haemoptysis
  - Sinusitis
  - Nasal polyps
- Pancreatic insufficiency
- Cystic fibrosis related diabetes
- Liver disease
- Bone disease
- Infertility
- Anxiety
- Depression

3.1. *Pulmonary Complications*

The typical feature of CF-related lung disease is bronchiectasis, which is usually present from childhood and leads to recurrent infection and ultimately reduced lung function. Bronchiectasis is a pathological term that describes permanent dilatation and destruction of one or more bronchi. A chronic, productive cough is a common manifestation although people with milder phenotypes of CF may have minimal or no symptoms and signs. Exacerbations of CF-related lung disease present with increased sputum production and/or change in sputum colour. This can herald infection with a new organism, exacerbation due to the known chronic bacterial infection, a viral infection or allergic bronchopulmonary aspergillosis. Regimens with oral, nebulised and/or intravenous antibiotics are utilised to attempt to eradicate *Pseudomonas aeruginosa* when it is first isolated and to treat exacerbations. Physiotherapy and nebulised hypertonic saline and/or DNAase (pulmozyme) improve sputum clearance and expectoration. Guidance on the management of pneumothorax and haemoptysis has been published by Flume *et al.*

3.2. *Extrapulmonary Complications of CF*

3.2.1. *Pancreatic insufficiency and diabetes*

The majority of individuals with CF have pancreatic insufficiency. This manifests in early life as failure to thrive and gastrointestinal symptoms of meconium ileus or steatorrhoea. Pancreatic enzyme replacement ameliorates these symptoms and allows absorption of essential nutrients from the diet. Enzyme requirement can change over time and necessitate adjustment in adolescence. Dehydration or non-adherence to enzyme treatment can lead to distal intestinal obstruction syndrome.

The prevalence of CF-related diabetes increases with age. It is rare below the age of 10 and present in up to 30% of individuals by the age of 25 years. It occurs as a consequence of fatty infiltration and fibrosis of the pancreas along with a degree of insulin resistance. Impaired glucose tolerance and diabetes can be transient during infective episodes, corticosteroid therapy, or pregnancy. The decision to treat with insulin depends on a number of factors. These include the degree of impaired glucose tolerance as well as nutritional status and lung function, all of which are improved by treatment with insulin.

3.2.2. *Liver disease*

CF-related liver disease occurs as a result of thick, dehydrated mucus within the intra- and extra-hepatic bile ducts and gallbladder, causing obstruction and subsequent hepatocyte injury. Fatty liver, focal biliary cirrhosis, fibrosis, multilobular cirrhosis, and portal hypertension have all been described. Gallstones and cholecystitis are also recognised complications. The peak onset of liver disease is before or during puberty and severe disease has a median age of diagnosis of 12 years. The use of oral ursodeoxycholic acid is advocated in the treatment of CF-related liver disease and liver transplant has been successfully performed to treat liver failure.

3.2.3. *Bone disease*

Low bone mineral density in CF was first reported 30 years ago and is common in adults. Monitoring with regular bone densitometry, particularly if there is evidence of osteopaenia or rapid loss of BMD, is advocated. The pathogenesis of low BMD is complex and multifactorial. Corticosteroid use, pancreatic insufficiency, low vitamin D and K and calcium levels, hypogonadism, increased inflammation, and infection are all factors that influence bone health in CF. Various management strategies and treatment options have been suggested, which include vitamins D and K, and calcium supplementation, bisphosphonates, sex hormone replacement, and exercise.

3.2.4. *Fertility*

The majority of males with CF are infertile, usually secondary to congenital absence of the vas deferens. The testes are normal and spermatogenesis does occur. Sperm retrieval and *in vitro* fertilisation via assisted fertility techniques are available and have enabled a growing number of men with CF to father children. Women with CF are able to conceive naturally and, due to improved health status, young women with CF currently have higher fertility rates than ever before. Pregnancy should be planned and discussed with the relevant members of the CF team to ensure optimum health prior to conception. Counselling of young people with CF in early adolescence regarding fertility and sexual health issues is an extremely important part of the transition process.

3.3. *Lung Transplantation*

Lung transplantation for patients with end-stage CF lung disease has been available since 1985. The majority of centres now perform bilateral sequential lung transplants. The decision to refer for lung transplantation is based on severity of lung disease, a rapid rate of decline of lung function, frequent use of intravenous antibiotics, and deteriorating quality of life. Discussion regarding the need for transplantation should ideally be commenced a couple of years prior to it becoming essential. This allows time for assessment and the wait for donor lungs. It may, however, not be suitable for all individuals. Lung transplantation is high-risk major surgery and only appropriate when the affected young person is very unwell and not responding to conventional treatment. Life-long immunosuppression and monitoring are required and infection following transplant is a frequent complication. Acute and chronic rejection can occur. Despite these issues, patients with end-stage lung disease can benefit enormously from what is a life-saving procedure. Lung function and activity levels usually improve significantly and many patients are able return to work and enjoy a good quality of life. Published data for five-year survival rates following lung transplantation are between 50% (international) and 60% (in the UK).

Further information on CF can be found at www.cysticfibrosis.org.au, www.cff.org and www.cftrust.org.uk.

4. Non-CF Bronchiectasis

Bronchiectasis may also occur in young people who do not have CF. Other causes, of which the most common is 'idiopathic', are listed in Table 2. In recent years, immunisation programmes have led to a reduction in infection-related secondary causes. High resolution computerised tomography of the chest can be utilised to diagnose bronchiectasis. The aim of management is to reduce or prevent exacerbations and prevent further deterioration in lung function. Some conditions will require input from both a respiratory physician and an immunologist.

Table 2:   Aetiology of bronchiectasis.

- Idiopathic
- Recurrent aspiration
- Post infection: measles, pertussis, tuberculosis, adenovirus
- Traction with pulmonary fibrosis
- Allergic bronchopulmonary aspergillosis
- Atypical mycobacterial infection
- Primary ciliary dyskinesia
- Post-transplantation
- Bronchial obstruction-intrinsic or extrinsic
- Diffuse panbronchiolitis
- Tracheomegaly and polychondritis
- Immunodeficiency — both primary and secondary
- Others causes such as yellow nail syndrome and
    alpha-1-antitrypsin deficiency

4.1. *Recurrent Aspiration*

Recurrent aspiration may occur as a result of severe gastro–oesophageal reflux disease, structural abnormalities including trachea–oesophageal fistula and laryngeal cleft, or neurological disorders resulting in difficulty swallowing or inability to protect the airway. Typically, GORD is known to cause lower lobe bronchiectasis. Severe GORD can be treated with non-pharmacological methods which include weight loss, smoking cessation and raising the bed head, and pharmacological agents, including proton-pump inhibitors. In severe refractory cases fundoplication, a surgical procedure that tightens the lower oesophagus, may be necessary. Management of aspiration from any of the causes above may require different combinations of modified diet consistency, tube feeding, pharmacological agents such as glycopyrrolate, and surgery.

4.2. *Primary Ciliary Dyskinesia*

Primary ciliary dyskinesia is thought to contribute to up to 15% of all non-CF bronchiectasis. Cilia within the respiratory tract normally beat in a synchronised manner, moving mucus up the respiratory tract and removing bacteria and potentially harmful debris. Immotility or dyskinesia results in an absent or abnormal cilial beat pattern, which may lead to bronchiectasis. Ciliary dyskinesia, situs inversus, bronchiectasis and sinusitis is known as Kartagener syndrome. Measurement of nasal nitric oxide, where available, is a useful screening tool. A value >250 ppb effectively rules out a diagnosis of PCD. The diagnosis is confirmed by use of light and electron microscopic analysis of cilia from a nasal biopsy. Treatment involves aggressive management of respiratory infection and sinusitis.

4.3. *Primary Immunodeficiency*

This category includes hypogammaglobulinaemia (X-linked agammaglobulinaemia, severe combined and common variable immunodeficiency), functional antibody deficiency, complement pathway defects such as mannose binding lectin deficiency, and neutrophil function abnormalities. Patients with primary immunodeficiency will require joint input from immunology and respiratory teams. Treatment focuses on replacement therapy with immunoglobulin, if available, and aggressive management of respiratory infection.

5. Acute Lung Disease

Pneumonia is common in adolescents and young adults. Short, middle, and long term sequelae are seen in both the previously well and those with underlying disease (Table 3). Community acquired pneumonia encompasses both bacterial (extracellular and intracellular) and viral infections. *Pneumococcus* and *Mycoplasma* are the most common bacterial causes. Infections with *S. aureus* should be considered in those with severe disease. Mixed viral and bacterial infections are present in 10%–40%. Although the majority of cases are successfully treated, a small percentage will develop medium and long-term complications. Complicated pneumonia, with empyema, lung necrosis, and broncho–pleural fistulae in adolescents and young adults is most commonly caused by Pneumococcus and *S. aureus*. Influenza may also be implicated. Antibiotic treatment

Table 3: Complications of pneumonia.

- Respiratory failure requiring ventilation
- Pleural effusion and empyema
- Right middle lobe syndrome
- Bronchiectasis
- Obliterative bronchiolitis
- Fibrosis
- Necrotising pneumonia — necrosis of consolidated lung tissue
- Pneumatocoeles — air-filled intraparenchymal cysts that can result in pneumothorax and/or broncho-pleural fistulae

should be given according to local guidelines and in consultation with microbiology and infectious diseases services. Antibiotic resistance should always be considered, such as with penicillin-resistant *Pneumococcus* and methicillin-resistant *S. aureus*.

Complications are generally idiosyncratic but persistence of symptoms or radiological abnormalities following adequate treatment necessitates further investigation. Length of follow-up may extend into adulthood and is dependent on the type of complication.

6. Technology-Dependent Respiratory Disorders

An increasing number of children with neuromuscular disorders, such as congenital muscular dystrophy, Duchenne muscular dystrophy, and spinal muscular atrophy, are surviving into adolescence and young adulthood as a result of improvements in medical care and medical technology — in particular, the ability to provide non-invasive respiratory support at home. Often, respiratory disease is only one of a number of comorbidities with which these young people and their families have to deal, thus highlighting the importance of a multidisciplinary team approach, case-managed by a single coordinating member of the team.

Young people with neuromuscular disease usually require ventilation with biphasic positive airway pressure, rather than continuous positive airway pressure, which is used in conditions in which the primary aim is to maintain a patent airway such as obstructive sleep apnoea. Respiratory support can be delivered either via a mask or tracheostomy, with or without oxygen, as required. With the rise in the number of young people with severe obesity, CPAP is increasingly being used to manage adolescents with obstructive sleep apnoea secondary to obesity (Chapter 23).

7. Adult Consequences of Neonatal Lung Disease

As a consequence of the improvements in the quality of neonatal intensive care, an increasing number of infants born with extreme prematurity from as early as 23 weeks gestational age, now survive into adolescence and young adulthood. Chronic respiratory disease is one of a number of long-term consequences, with others being neurological, gastrointestinal, and cognitive, that may affect these young people in adolescence and adulthood. The combination of extreme prematurity, positive pressure ventilation, and infection results in abnormal lung development, primarily affecting alveolar development. In addition, impairment of airway growth is associated with low birth weight and maternal smoking in pregnancy. In infancy and early childhood, survivors of extreme prematurity are at increased risk of respiratory problems, particularly in association with viral respiratory tract infections. In adolescence, respiratory symptoms are less obvious, although on questioning and with objective testing, evidence of reduced exercise tolerance may be present. However, as a result of abnormal lung development, there is a *significant risk of the early onset of chronic obstructive airways disease in adulthood, which is further increased if the young person starts smoking.* Although the data demonstrating the long-term effects of extreme prematurity on adult lung disease are currently limited, it is likely that this will become an increasing health problem in the near future and one with which adult physicians will need to be familiar.

8. Smoking Cessation

The harmful effects of tobacco smoke are well recognised and damage to the respiratory system is related to both the amount smoked and individual genetic predisposition. A recent global report demonstrated a smoking prevalence of 9.5% in 13–15 year olds and almost 71% of adult smokers smoked daily before the age of 18 years. There is increasing evidence that suggests young adults with chronic disease are more likely than their healthy peers to participate in health risk behaviours, which include smoking, alcohol misuse, substance misuse, and risky sexual behaviour. As discussed above, smoking in those with chronic lung disease has a higher ascribed risk than in healthy individuals. The health risks associated with smoking include short-term increase in respiratory symptoms and long-term damage such as airflow obstruction and emphysema. The reasons why young adults with or without chronic respiratory disease smoke are complex. The risks associated with smoking may not be perceived in the short term and therefore do not prevent potential addiction.

Cannabis is the most commonly smoked substance after tobacco and the most commonly used illicit drug substance. The short-term effect is acute bronchodilation and longer-term use leads to airway inflammation and reduced macrophage activity along with increased cough, sputum, and wheeze. There are conflicting reports on the long-term effects on lung function, but an effect on airway function and subsequent obstruction, emphysema and pneumothorax has been described.

Preventative strategies such as a ban on tobacco advertising have been implemented in higher income countries. Healthcare activities such as the adoption of both the five As model (Table 4) and motivational interviewing into routine adolescent and young adult health care are important steps in reducing adolescent tobacco use.

Table 4:   The five As for smoking cessation.

- Anticipate tobacco use and risk factors for use
- Ask all patients about smoking status
- Advise about tobacco related health risks & encourage smokers to stop smoking and non smokers to abstain
- Assist smokers-self-help with smoking cessation materials plus quit date
- Arrange for routine follow up and support

References

Australian Institute of Health and Welfare. (2007) Young Australians: Their health and wellbeing 2007. Available online at: http://www.aihw.gov.au/publication-detail/?id=6442467991.

Beshay M, Kaiser H, Niedhart D, Reymond MA, Schmid RA. (2007) Emphysema and secondary pneumothorax in young adults smoking cannabis. *Eur J Cardio-Thorac Surg* **32**(6): 834–838.

British Thoracic Society Standards of Care. (2002) British Thoracic Society guidelines for the management of community acquired pneumonia in childhood. *Thorax,* **57**(1): i1–24.

Bush A, Alton EWFW, Davies JC, Griesenbach U, Jaffe A. eds. (2006) *Cystic fibrosis in the 21st century,* (Switzerland, S.Karger AG).

Flume PA, Mogayzel PJ Jr, Robinson KA, Rosenblatt RL, Quittell L, Marshall BC, Clinical Practice Guidelines for Pulmonary Therapies & Cystic Fibrosis Foundation Pulmonary Therapies. (2010) Cystic fibrosis pulmonary guidelines: Pulmonary complications: Hemoptysis and pneumothorax. *Am J Respir Crit Care Med* **182**(3): 298–306.

Lange P. (2007) Cannabis and the lung. *Thorax* **62**(12): 1036–1037.

Morton J, Glanville AR. (2009) Lung transplantation in patients with cystic fibrosis. *Semin Respir Crit Care Med* **30**(5): 559–568.

Pellegrino R, Viegi G, Brusasco V, Crapo RO, Burgos F, Casaburi R, Coates A, Van Der Grinten CPM, Gustafsson P, Hankinson J, Jensen R, Johnson DC, Macintyre N, Mckay R, Miller MR, Navajas D, Pedersen OF, Wanger J. (2005) Interpretative strategies for lung function tests. *European Respiratory J* **26**(5): 948–968.

Pohunek P, Tal A. (2004) Budesonide and formoterol in a single inhaler controls asthma in adolescents. *Int J Adolesc Med Health* **16**(2): 91–105.

Shah S, Peat JK, Mazurski EJ, Wang H, Sindhusake D, Bruce C, Henry RL, Gibson PG. (2001) Effect of peer led programme for asthma education in adolescents: Cluster randomised controlled trial. *Br Med J* **322**(7286): 583–585.

Simonds AK. (2006) Recent advances in respiratory care for neuromuscular disease. *Chest* **130**(6): 1879–1886.

Tsang KW, Bilton D. (2009) Clinical challenges in managing bronchiectasis. *Respirology* **14**(5): 637–650.

Tsang KW, Zheng L, Tipoe G. (2000) Ciliary assessment in bronchiectasis. *Respirology* **5**(2): 91–98.

Tyc VL, Throckmorton-Belzer L. (2006) Smoking rates and the state of smoking interventions for children and adolescents with chronic illness. *Pediatrics* **118**(2): e471–487.

Chapter 35

Common Adolescent Endocrine Disorders

Shubha Srinivasan

1. Introduction

This chapter will cover thyroid disorders, pituitary disease, cranio-pharyngiomas and adrenal disorders. Initial investigation and management is generally under the care of an endocrinologist but patients may present with non-specific symptoms to any clinician. Furthermore, once initial treatment has been established appropriate monitoring through the transition period from paediatric to adult care is important for long term well-being.

2. Thyroid disorders

2.1. *Hypothyroidism*

Hypothyroidism in adolescents is usually acquired and due to thyroid gland failure (primary).

2.1.1. *Clinical presentation*

Clinical presentation may be with goitre (thyroid enlargement), weakness, lethargy, constipation, cold intolerance, dry skin, decreased appetite, growth retardation, and weight gain. Patients may also present with delayed puberty, rarely precocious puberty, galactorrhoea in girls and macro-orchidism (large testicles) in boys. Disruptions to normal puberty occur due to chronic thyroid stimulating hormone releasing hormone stimulation of the pituitary gland resulting in hyperprolactinaemia and altered LH/FSH secretion. Adolescent girls who develop hypothyroidism after menarche may experience excessive and irregular menstrual bleeding. Presentation may mimic polycystic ovarian syndrome and hypothyroidism should be excluded in the workup of PCOS.

2.1.2. *Aetiology*

Beyond infancy the most common cause of hypothyroidism is chronic autoimmune thyroiditis (Hashimoto's thyroiditis). The disease occurs more frequently in girls than boys and in patients with other autoimmune mediated conditions such as type 1 diabetes mellitus as well as in Down, Turner, and Klinefelter syndromes.

Most adolescents with congenital hypothyroidism will have been detected through newborn screening programs, which detect elevated thyroid stimulating hormone levels. Very rarely inborn errors of thyroid hormone synthesis or mild structural thyroid abnormalities are detected much later in childhood.

Primary hypothyroidism may also be due to iodine deficiency, thyroidectomy and irradiation of the thyroid. Secondary (TSH deficiency) or tertiary (TRH deficiency) hypothyroidism usually occur in conjunction with other hypothalamic/pituitary hormone deficiencies.

2.1.3. *Investigations*

Serum TSH, free thyroxine, free triiodothyronine, thyroperoxidase antibodies and thyroglobulin antibodies are generally all that is required to diagnose autoimmune thyroiditis. TSH and antibodies will be elevated and thyroid hormone levels low. Some patients may require serial antibody measurements if negative on initial testing. Urine iodine levels are helpful if iodine deficiency is suspected. Ultrasound and a nuclear radioiodide scan may be helpful to identify a rare late presentation of inborn errors of thyroid metabolism. If the TSH is low/normal and FT4 is low, then hypothalamic–pituitary disease should be considered.

A TRH stimulation test and MRI of the hypothalamic-pituitary region may be required.

2.1.4. *Treatment*

Oral L-thyroxine at 100 mcg/m^2/day should be started once the diagnosis is established. Females on oestrogen replacement therapy or who are pregnant may require higher doses. Adolescents with secondary or tertiary hypothyroidism may require lower than anticipated doses. Thyroxine solution should not be given due to the instability of the preparation. Instead L-thyroxine tablets may be crushed and dissolved in milk or water for those unable to swallow tablets. Monitoring of treatment is with TSH and FT4 levels, aiming to keep both the TSH and FT4 levels in the normal range. Monitoring of TSH levels is unnecessary for patients with secondary or tertiary hypothyroidism, as these levels will always be low.

2.2. *Hyperthyroidism*

Over-activity of the thyroid in adolescents is most commonly due to Grave's disease, but may also occur transiently in Hashimoto's thyroiditis.

2.2.1. *Symptoms and signs*

These may include tachycardia, tremor, sweating, restlessness, poor sleeping, weight loss, diarrhoea, goitre, proximal muscle weakness, or cardiac arrhythmia. Exophthalmos and orbital muscle weakness are seen in Grave's disease. Severe thyrotoxicosis can cause a life-threatening thyrotoxic crisis or thyroid storm. Early specialist referral is required for evaluation and management of thyrotoxicosis.

2.2.2. *Investigations*

These should include TSH, FT4, FT3, and thyroid antibodies: thyroid stimulating immunoglobulin or human thyrotropin receptor antibody, TPO Ab, and TG Ab. Thyroid imaging is not routinely indicated in typical Graves cases, but is helpful in other situations especially when an autonomous thyroid nodule is suspected (asymmetric enlargement or palpable nodule), or sub-acute thyroiditis. The latter condition may be caused by a viral infection and excess thyroid hormone is released secondary to tissue damage. Unlike the increased uptake of radioisotope in Grave's disease or in a hyperfunctioning nodule, radioisotope uptake is absent.

2.2.3. *Therapy*

Anti-thyroid drug treatment with carbimazole at 0.2–1.0 mg/kg/day (converted to methimazole) is the common first line treatment. Dosage schedule may be either titration to achieve euthyroid state or in association with thyroxine in a 'block and replace' regimen. Serious side-effects are uncommon, but can include agranulocytosis, hepatotoxicity, or aplastic anemia. Propylthiouracil 5–10 mg/kg/day is less commonly used due to the higher risk of liver failure in adolescents and children (1 in 2,000), compared to adults (1 in 10,000). Beta-blockers may be used as an adjunct to treatment in the first few weeks for symptom control (used with caution if asthma is present). Thyroid storm may require additional therapy such as iodine or glucocorticoids and general supportive measures.

Radioactive iodine treatment is also a suitable first line option in mild disease after initial control by anti-thyroid drugs, or for definitive treatment if there is relapse after a course (usually 1–2 years) of anti-thyroid treatment.

Poor prognostic indicators for remission of Graves's disease include large thyroid gland, age less than 12 years, non Caucasian ethnicity, high hTRAb titres or high FT4 (>50 pmol/L).

I131 therapy (>150uCi I131 per g of thyroid tissue) with a goal to induce hypothyroidism has a remission rate of greater than 95%. The incidence of congenital anomalies in offspring of adolescents treated with I131 for Grave's disease is no greater than in the general population. Furthermore, the higher doses of radiation used to treat Grave's disease are not associated with future thyroid cancer.

Thyroidectomy is rarely used as first-line therapy but may be indicated as definitive therapy in adolescents with large goitres who have failed or do not consent to I131 therapy. Complications of surgery occur in 10%–20% and include hypocalcaemia, recurrent laryngeal nerve palsy, and haematoma. Surgery should only be performed by experienced head and neck surgeons.

2.3. *Thyroid Cancer*

Thyroid cancer is rare in adolescents unless they have been exposed to radiation either as therapy (Chapter 44) or accidentally as in the Chernobyl disaster. The presentation is a solid nodule which does not take up radioisotope on scanning ('cold'). A fine needle aspiration biopsy may indicate malignant change. The treatment is total thyroidectomy and ablative radioactive iodine therapy.

3. Growth Hormone Deficiency and Hypopituitarism

3.1. *Causes of Growth Hormone Deficiency*

This may occur with or without other pituitary hormone deficiencies — TSH, ACTH, LH, FSH, vasopressin — and may be due to congenital CNS malformations (empty sella, septo–optic dysplasia, pituitary hypoplasia, interrupted pituitary stalk), hereditary mutations of genes encoding pituitary transcription factors, or acquired causes including craniopharyngioma, other CNS tumours, histiocytosis, trauma, CNS infection, and CNS radiation for cancer treatment.

3.2. *Presentation in Adolescence*

There will be poor growth velocity in early adolescence if epiphyses are still open. There may be evidence of other pituitary hormone deficits. Failure of development of secondary sexual characteristics and an inadequate pubertal growth spurt may be other presenting features of hypopituitarism in adolescence.

3.3. *Therapy*

This is discussed in Section 4.4.2.

4. Craniopharyngiomas

These are rare, slow growing, and account for up to 9% of all childhood and adolescent brain tumours.

4.1. *Presenting Symptoms*

Symptoms are most commonly from raised intracranial pressure (headache and nausea), and visual defects. Slow growth and failure to enter puberty may be the presentation in adolescence, but symptoms of endocrine deficiencies may often go unnoticed. Deficiencies of GH, gonadotropins, ACTH, TSH, and ADH are present at diagnosis in 50%–85% of patients. Although survival rates are high, disturbances to the hypothalamic–pituitary axis may cause significant morbidity and impaired quality of life. Many patients suffer from obesity and features of the metabolic syndrome due to loss of appetite regulation. These features may be compounded by metabolic consequences of growth hormone deficiency and excess corticosteroid replacement.

4.2. *Neurological Morbidity*

This occurs in up to half of patients with symptoms including short-term memory loss, personality changes, specific brain function impairment, anosmia, and vertigo. Over half of patients report poor academic performance or time off work.

4.3. *Investigation*

Imaging with CT or MRI demonstrates a cystic tumour in the intrasellar and/or suprasellar region with most tumours containing areas of calcification. Hypothalamic–pituitary hormone axis evaluation is useful to establish the diagnosis of pre-operative hormone deficiencies.

4.4. *Treatment*

4.4.1. *Surgery and radiotherapy*

Because of the large size and extent of the tumour at diagnosis, transcranial surgery may be required, which in turn entails a higher risk of pituitary gland and stalk damage. Some centres favour complete removal of the tumour as the most effective method for preventing recurrence, accepting sacrifice of the pituitary stalk as a consequence. Others advocate transphenoidal resection in selected patients with good outcomes in terms of gross total resection, low recurrence risk, and visual improvement. Partial resection followed by radiotherapy may also be considered, although irradiation is also frequently associated with hypothalamic–pituitary function deficits.

4.4.2. *Pituitary hormone replacement*

Peri-operative dexamethasone therapy will provide adequate cortisol cover for adrenal insufficiency at the time of surgery. On discharge, patients are usually changed to maintenance hydrocortisone ($8–10$ mg/m^2/day). Patients and their families should be instructed on the use of stress doses of hydrocortisone at times of physical illness or other stress, and the use of parenteral doses of hydrocortisone (100 mg/m^2/day) if the adolescent is severely ill or vomiting. Most patients also require thyroxine replacement (100 mcg/m^2/day) and many require desmopressin if diabetes insipidus is present. Oral preparations of desmopressin are preferred due to more reliable dosing compared to intranasal or subcutaneous preparations. Growth hormone replacement, and pubertal induction/ pubertal hormone replacement are generally required (Chapter 20). Some patients with craniopharyngioma do not require growth hormone therapy despite a biochemical growth hormone deficiency. This is the 'growth without growth hormone' phenomenon whereby linear growth is thought to be driven by obesity and hyperinsulinaemia.

4.4.3. *Hypothalamic obesity and metabolic complications*

These are challenging long term management issues. The degree of hypothalamic damage often correlates with the degree of obesity.

Lifestyle measures to limit caloric intake and increase exercise are encouraged. A number of pharmacological therapies for obesity and insulin resistance (orlistat, dexamphetamine, octreotide and metformin) as well as bariatric surgery have all been trialled, but with no long-term proven positive effect.

5. Prolactinomas

These have an estimated prevalence in the adult population of 100 per million and are the most common hormone secreting pituitary tumour. Prolactinomas account for 50% of all pituitary adenomas in adolescents, with females having a higher incidence than males.

5.1. *Symptoms*

These are due to the effects of elevated prolactin resulting in delayed puberty, amenorrhoea, and galactorrhoea in females. Galactorrhoea is a presenting feature in 30%–50% of adolescents compared to 80% of adult females. Males present with delayed puberty, gynaecomastia, galactorrhoea, and due to the higher prevalence of macroadenomas (tumour >1 cm diameter), may also present with mass effects such as headaches and visual field defects.

5.2. *Investigations*

The diagnosis of prolactinoma requires documentation of sustained hyperprolactinaemia (at least two levels should be taken), as well as MRI evidence of a pituitary adenoma. Adolescents may have asymptomatic hyperprolactinaemia due to abnormal elevations of prolactin macromolecule isoforms (Big-PRL and Big Big-PRL). In addition any pituitary mass compressing the stalk may cause elevation of prolactin levels. Another confounding factor is that about 10% of the population have asymptomatic pituitary microadenomas, noted incidentally on imaging. Visual field testing is only required for a macroprolactinoma.

5.3. *Treatment*

5.3.1. *Dopamine agonists*

Dopamine agonists are the first line treatment for prolactinomas. Bromocriptine (5–7.5 mg/day split twice daily) is very effective in reducing prolactin levels and shrinking tumour mass, thereby restoring normal pubertal development. Side effects include nausea, vomiting, and postural hypotension. Carbergoline (0.3–3.5 mg/week) has a long half-life and hence is administered once or twice per week with good efficacy in adolescents. The main side effect is orthostatic hypotension. There are limited data in adolescents on the use of newer dopamine agonists such as pergolide and quinagolide. Pergolide is associated with exacerbation of pre-existing psychosis.

5.3.2. *Other therapies*

If dopamine agonist therapy is not tolerated or ineffective transphenoidal surgical excision of the prolactinoma may be required. Rarely, radiation therapy is required after failed surgery and/or drug therapy and may induce later hypopituitarism.

6. Adrenal Disorders

6.1. *Adrenal Insufficiency*

This may be:

- Primary as a result of congenital adrenal aplasia, hypoplasia or hyperplasia, adrenoleukodystrophy, adrenal haemorrhage, autoimmune destruction, and rare enzyme defects.
- Secondary to deficient corticotropin releasing hormone and/or adrenocoticotropic hormone secretion (hypopituitarism or after prolonged steroid therapy).
- Related to end-organ unresponsiveness (cortisol resistance, aldosterone resistance).

6.1.1. *Clinical features*

Clinical features of glucocorticoid (cortisol) deficiency include fasting hypoglycaemia, nausea, vomiting, and fatigue. Mineralocorticoid (aldosterone) deficiency results in muscle weakness, weight loss, fatigue, nausea, vomiting, salt craving, hypotension, hyponatraemia, and hyperkalaemia. Patients may also have decreased pubic hair, axillary hair, and libido due to adrenal androgen deficiency. Hyper-pigmentation due to increased beta-lipotropin levels (which is part of the ACTH peptide) occurs only in primary adrenal hypofunction.

6.1.2. *Investigations*

Investigations suggesting adrenal insufficiency include an inadequate cortisol response to hypoglycaemia or other stress. Patients should proceed on to a short ACTH stimulation test to rule out primary and overt secondary adrenal insufficiency. A normal result is a rise in cortisol from baseline by >190 nmol/L or a peak level >500 nmol/L. Patients with suspected partial secondary adrenal insufficiency may require a low-dose short ACTH simulation test or insulin tolerance testing in a specialised endocrine testing unit.

6.1.3 *Treatment*

Treatment for primary adrenal insufficiency requires both glucocorticoid replacement with oral hydrocortisone (10–20 mg/m^2/day) or prednisone (2–4 mg/m^2/day), and mineralocorticoid replacement with fludrocortisone (0.05–0.125 mg/day). For secondary adrenal insufficiency lower hydrocortisone doses (8–10 mg/m^2/day) are sufficient and mineralocorticoid replacement is usually not required. Mild androgenic preparations are sometimes used to improve libido and pubic hair growth in adolescent and adult women with adrenal androgen deficiency. Patients should be instructed in the use of stress doses of hydrocortisone (60–100 mg/m^2/day) and families/partners taught the use of intramuscular hydrocortisone for acute adrenal crises.

6.2. *Congenital Adrenal Hyperplasia*

The classical form of autosomal recessive CAH due to 21-hydroxylase deficiency is usually diagnosed in infancy with either female virilisation or potential life threatening salt wasting adrenal crisis. The worldwide incidence of classical CAH is 1 in 14,000 live births. In older children and adolescents, non-classical CAH may be diagnosed following investigation of premature adrenarche, advanced bone age, severe acne, androgenic alopecia, and menstrual irregularities. Boys may present with pubic hair and enlarged phallus despite relatively small testes. The frequency of non-classical CAH is about 1 in 1,000.

6.2.1. *Investigations*

Classical CAH is diagnosed by elevated plasma 17 hydroxy-progesterone levels. Some countries offer new born screening for CAH. If the results are borderline, elevation of the 17OHP to cortisol ratio following a short ACTH stimulation test can be diagnostic. Genetic testing detects approximately 95% of mutant alleles in the CYP21A2 gene. In non-classical CAH a random 17 OHP level may not be sufficiently elevated to allow diagnosis and an ACTH stimulation test may be required. Measurement of other adrenal steroids either on stimulation test or as a urine steroid profile may be helpful to confirm 21OHD and exclude other rarer forms of CAH.

6.2.2. *Treatment*

Glucocorticoid replacement therapy (hydrocortisone 10–20 mg/m^2/day) and if necessary mineralocorticoid therapy (fludrocortisone 0.05–0.125 mg/day) should commence as soon as the diagnosis is made. Adolescents with non-classical CAH may be treated with dexamethasone (0.25 mg/day), but care should be taken to avoid excess dosage.

Titration of the dose is aimed at suppression of 17OHP levels and maintaining androgen levels appropriate for age and gender. Inadequate treatment may lead to signs of hyperandrogenism such as acne, hirsutism, excess body odour, and rapid linear growth resulting in compromised final height. Adolescent females who are poorly treated may have irregular or absent menses. They may also develop PCOS due to excessive adrenal androgens disrupting cyclical gonadotropin release. Inadequately treated males may have reduced sperm counts, small testes, and intra-testicular adrenal rests, which present as nodular testes. Overtreatment of CAH can lead to growth suppression in the younger adolescent and iatrogenic Cushing syndrome.

7. Cushing Syndrome

This is a result of excess glucocorticoid and presents with moon facies, abdominal or central obesity, abdominal and axillary striae, hypertension, and osteoporosis, and growth failure in younger adolescents. Excess glucocorticoid may be endogenous (pituitary tumour, adrenal adenoma, or adrenal carcinoma) or exogenous. The latter is common in adolescents who are prescribed glucocorticoid for immunosuppression, including for autoimmune disease and post solid organ transplantation. The treatment of iatrogenic Cushing syndrome is to use the lowest dose of glucocorticoid which will maintain well-being, consider the use of alternative immunosuppressive agents/steroid sparers and supplement with calcium and Vitamin D.

Endogenous glucocorticoid excess is confirmed by an elevation of 24 hour urinary free cortisol. Cushing disease, which is Cushing syndrome of pituitary tumour origin, has elevated ACTH levels, whereas ACTH is suppressed in adrenal adenomas and carcinomas which secrete excess glucocorticoid. Investigation and treatment are the realm of the specialist endocrinologist and the treatment is surgical.

References

Colao A, Loche S. (2010) Prolactinomas in children and adolescents. *Endocrine Development* **17**: 146–159.

Dallas JS, Foley Jr TP. (2007) Hypothyroidsism. In: Lifshitz F. (ed.), *Pediatric Endocrinology.* Informa Healthcare, New York.

Lin-Su K, Nimkarn S, New MI. (2008) Congenital adrenal hyperplasia in adolescents: Diagnosis and management. *Annals N Y Acad Sci* **1135**: 95–98.

Mortini P, Losa M, Pozzobon G, Barzaghi R, Riva M, Acerno S, Angius D, Weber G, Chiumello G, Giovanelli M. (2011) Neurosurgical treatment of craniopharyngioma in adults and children: Early and long-term results in a large case series. *Journal of Neurosurgery* **114**(5): 1350–1359.

Muller HL. (2010) Childhood craniopharyngioma-current concepts in diagnosis, therapy and follow-up. *Nature Reviews Endocrinology,* **6**(11): 609–618.

Pereira AM, Schmid EM, Schutte PJ, Voormolen JHC, Biermasz NR, Van Thiel SW, Corssmit EPM, Smit JWA, Roelfsema F, Romijn JA. (2005) High prevalence of long-term cardiovascular, neurological and psychosocial morbidity after treatment for craniopharyngioma. *Clin Endocrinol* **62**(2): 197–204.

Ranke MB. ed. (2003) *Diagnostics of endocrine function in children and adolescents.* Karger Switzerland.

Rivkees SA (2010) Pediatric graves' disease: Controversies in management. *Hormone research in pdiatrics* **74**(5): 305–311.

Sharma ST, Nieman LK. (2011) Cushing's syndrome: All variants, detection, and treatment. *Endocrinology & Metabolism Clinics of North America* **40**(2): 379–391.

Srinivasan S, Ogle GD, Garnett SP, Briody JN, Lee JW, Cowell CT. (2004) Features of the metabolic syndrome after childhood craniopharyngioma. *Journal of Clinical Endocrinology & Metabolism* **89**(1): 81–86.

Chapter 36

Diabetes During Adolescence

Kristine Heels, Nuala Harkin and Kim C Donaghue

1. Introduction

For those with childhood-onset diabetes, adolescence is a time of increasing stress when medical and psychological problems can arise, each affecting the other. Hyperglycaemia, with its associated symptoms of nocturia, polyuria and polydipsia, abdominal pain, lethargy, and blurred vision can cause significant time off school and make learning more difficult. Subclinical microvascular disease can also manifest. Long-term complications of diabetes and other impacts on the lives of adolescents need to be discussed and addressed. This chapter focuses on the important management issues for adolescents and young adults.

2. Monitoring Diabetes

Modern treatments have facilitated glycaemic control closer to normoglycaemia, but this requires monitoring 4–6 times a day. During adolescence the monitoring may be suboptimal. Current targets for blood glucose are: pre-prandially 4–7 mmol/l, post-prandially 5–10 mmol/l and before bed 6–10 mmol/l. Monitoring diabetes control can be divided into the following categories:

- Monitoring of blood glucose levels throughout the day. It is advisable to check the BGLs at least four times a day, and include an overnight

467

check on a regular basis. Extra BGL checks are important during illness, and increased physical activity. The most common way of checking the BGL is by using an accurate blood glucose meter, and lancing device, which are inexpensive.

- Continuous glucose monitoring systems are available, but comparatively expensive. Their advantage is that a glucose reading every five minutes for up to six days is provided, via a sub-cutaneous sensor, and attached to a transmitter which stores the glucose levels. The disadvantage is that it has to be worn continuously, and some adolescents do not want to have an obvious device attached to them, as it is a constant reminder of their diabetes, and may also be visible to others. The optimal goal would be to have a non-invasive blood glucose monitoring system, and although research continues in this field, there are no devices available for use at this time.

- Monitoring of blood or urine ketones when the BGL is elevated, or the adolescent is unwell. If the BGL is >15 mmol/l, it is important to check for ketones. If ketones are present more insulin is required. Appropriate sick day management will reduce the risk of, or prevent the progression to a diabetic ketoacidotic state or coma.

- Monitoring long-term control with the Haemoglobin A1c test. HbA1c monitors glycaemic control over the previous 12 weeks and should be performed three monthly. The target is <7.5%. For those on an insulin pump HbA1c targets can be lower and the target blood glucose for the pump can be set at 5–6 mmol/l.

- Monitoring for complications of diabetes. This should be carried out at 1–2 yearly intervals.

The challenges that adolescents and health care professionals face in the management of a chronic illness is well documented in the literature. The daily diabetes routines are no exception, and this is often a time when monitoring BGLs is not a high priority for adolescents. The health professional needs a high level of negotiation skills, should be non-judgmental, and will do well if the adolescent agrees to check their BGLs one to two times a day.

The development of a trusting relationship between the adolescent and the health care team is paramount.

3. Growth and Puberty

Persistently poorly controlled diabetes can result in delay in growth and maturation. Mauriac syndrome was described as short stature, with hepatomegaly and poor diabetes control. Non-alcoholic hepatic steatosis (fatty liver) is now a well described complication of poorly controlled diabetes. Fatty liver is also seen in obesity and Type 2 diabetes. It can cause right upper quadrant abdominal pain and is often diagnosed by elevated hepatic transaminases during routine testing.

More recently, with the increase in obesity and insulin resistance now recognised with Type 1 diabetes, polycystic ovarian syndrome is more commonly diagnosed (Chapter 50). This is likely due to non-physiological delivery of insulin, sometimes at supra-physiological levels. Overweight adolescents with Type 1 diabetes may omit insulin for weight loss, by inducing ketonuria. Common symptoms are abdominal or calf pain, nausea, and diarrhoea. Also common are eating disorders (Chapter 24).

4. Insulin Pump Therapy

The insulin pump, or continuous subcutaneous insulin infusion is a small computerised device that delivers continuous subcutaneous insulin. CSII is currently the closest to physiological insulin delivery (islet cell transplant excluded). The pump is programmed to deliver approximately 40%–50% of the total daily dose of insulin continually over 24 hours (basal insulin). When carbohydrate food is eaten, the pump is manually activated to deliver extra insulin (meal bolus). The pump can also be manually activated to give extra insulin if the BGL is elevated (correction bolus). The insulin pump set and site should be changed every three days. During bathing, swimming, and combative sports, the pump can easily be disconnected. A temporary basal rate reduction can be used during and after other exercise to avoid hypoglycaemia. Access to insulin pumps is often limited by financial costs; however the pumps have potential benefits over multiple daily insulin injections. Insulin pumps may be a treatment option for the management of Type 1 diabetes in the adolescent. Adolescence is a time of rapid physical growth and pubertal hormonal activity, which causes insulin resistance. Insulin requirements during this time are increased, and can range from 1–2 units/kg/day. The flexibility offered to cover food at any time of the day is a great advantage, and similarly the adolescent can reduce food intake by only eating when hungry rather than eating to cover excess insulin. Hence CSII can be of benefit in controlling excessive weight gain. The total insulin dose is usually 10% less on the pump compared to MDIs. During the transition from childhood to adolescence, and adolescence to young adulthood the insulin pump has the potential to offer more convenience and flexibility, more patient satisfaction, greater precision, and potentially better diabetic control than MDIs. Insulin pump therapy has also been found effective in recurrent ketoacidosis, presumably because of the ease of giving correction boluses for high glucose readings caused by insulin omission or miscalculations of food intake — both common occurrences in adolescence. Adolescent issues, such as non-adherence and risk taking behaviours, need special attention if considering the introduction of an insulin pump.

5. Diabetic Ketoacidosis

DKA results from insulin deficiency, and is caused by increasing levels of circulating ketones in the absence of insulin. Increased ketones lead to a drop in the pH of the blood and triggers the buffering system associated with metabolic acidosis. Adolescents are at an increased risk of developing DKA, as they become more independent, and parents are less involved in the usual diabetes routines of monitoring BGLs, supervising insulin injections, or management of the insulin pump. Chronic sub-optimal diabetes control may also lead to rapid deterioration in times of increased stress, especially illness. Adolescents who use an insulin pump can rapidly develop DKA when insulin delivery fails for any reason, including inadvertent disconnection or kinking of tubing. DKA may occur at diagnosis, or if insulin is omitted, or as a result of an intercurrent illness. *Recurrent* DKA in adolescents is almost always caused by insulin omission. There is usually an important psychosocial reason for insulin omission, and a comprehensive review is necessary to exclude an eating disorder, clinical depression, or a difficult social circumstance that requires intervention. Intravenous rehydration is usually required for initial management of ketoacidosis.

The severity of DKA is categorised by the severity of acidosis. Mild: venous pH <7.3 or bicarbonate <15 mmol/l; moderate: venous pH <7.2, bicarbonate <10 mmol/l; severe: venous pH <7.1, bicarbonate <5 mmol/l.

Clinical symptoms and signs may include dehydration, hypotension and shock, frequent vomiting, hyperventilation (Kussmaul respiration), acetone detected on the breath, or ketones present in the blood, polyuria despite dehydration, polydipsia, and altered level of consciousness. Patients with moderate to severe DKA should be managed in centres with specialised nursing, medical, and laboratory facilities. In non-expert hands, potential complications of the treatment can occur. The management of DKA is described in the International Society for Pediatric and Adolescent Diabetes Clinical Practice Consensus Guidelines 2009.

In order to prevent DKA, advice on what to do during periods of hyperglycaemia, and sick day management should be an integral part of any diabetes education program. However as many adolescents may have been diagnosed at an early age, education may have been directed at the parents. It is advisable to re-educate the adolescent prior to transition to the adult diabetes services. The importance of checking for blood ketones when the blood glucose level is persistently >15 mmol, and administering extra insulin via injection pen when the blood ketones are >0.6 mmol, are paramount in reducing the risk of progression to DKA. Insulin pump users who fail to administer insulin via pen when ketones are high can rapidly progress to DKA, as ketones signal a likely problem with the delivery of insulin. Appropriate follow-up care with a diabetes team is recommended. In times of uncertainty, access to a 24-hour telephone helpline may also avoid the progression to DKA. SMS and email are often more clinically useful communication tools in adolescents.

6. School

School for a young person living with diabetes can represent a place of wonderful support or a place of ongoing anxiety. Diabetes education and planning can help to enhance the positives whilst containing the negative aspects of the school experience. Planned, routine interactions between all parties involved can often help to alleviate or resolve issues before potential health threatening problems arise. Better glycaemic control and quality of life occur when school personnel and friends receive some training in diabetes and its management.

7. Diabetes Camps

The bringing together of a common group, living with the same condition, provides many positive experiences for the participants. Camps are thought to work on many levels, providing respite for carers, whilst providing opportunities for the adolescent to develop social contact with other young people living with the same issues and to realise that they are not alone. The 'real life setting' can provide insights they may not have previously considered and camp is also often the first time that many young people will attempt to take control of the daily demands of their diabetes.

8. Diabetes and Surgery

The gold standard treatment for surgery has been the intravenous insulin infusion commenced a few hours before surgery and monitored with hourly BGLs. The long-acting analogue insulin which would be active during this time is omitted or significantly reduced if overlapping with insulin infusion. The infusion rate can be started at 0.02 units/kg/hour and adjusted for a target BGL of 5–10 mmol/l. For those on an insulin pump the basal rates do not generally need to be altered and the pump is equivalent to an intravenous insulin infusion. For those not on an insulin pump or if an insulin infusion is difficult to supervise or maintain, the background long-acting insulin can usually be given without any short or rapid acting insulin. Extra short-acting insulin can be given if BGLs are too high whilst fasting. When the adolescent resumes eating short-acting insulin boluses can be recommenced.

9. Long Term Complications

The diagnosis of diabetes brings with it long term risks for macrovascular disease and microvascular disease — retinopathy, nephropathy, and neuropathy. Diabetes also confers an increased mortality due to both acute and chronic complications. Microvascular complications of diabetes are

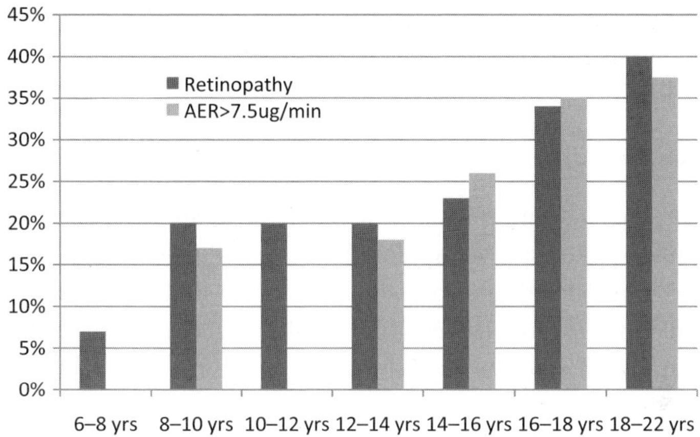

Fig. 1: Retinopathy and early elevation of albumin excretion in a population cohort after six years diabetes duration in NSW (from Donaghue *et al.* Diabet Med 2005).

usually subclinical during adolescence, with early retinopathy changes and urinary microalbuminuria. Nevertheless, visual loss in early adult years and macroalbuminuria in late adolescence are possible (see Fig. 1). For those who do not access health care frequently, chronic complications are more likely to develop. Troubling painful neuropathy can considerably reduce quality of life, as can disabling gastroparesis with nausea and vomiting due to autonomic neuropathy.

The Diabetes Control and Complications Trial was a landmark study — a randomised controlled trial of intensive insulin therapy versus conventional insulin therapy which demonstrated a clear difference in outcome measures for the IIT versus CIT group at a mean follow-up of 6.5 years. The major differences were a 66% reduction in retinopathy, a 53% reduction in microalbuminuria and a 60% reduction in neuropathy for the IIT group. Concerns that greater hypoglycaemia in IIT may manifest in cognitive or quality of life differences were not realised. It is noteworthy that higher HbA1c was associated with a decline in psychomotor and mental efficiency, with the CIT group doing less well with cognitive performance than the IIT after 6.5 years.

Both high and low BGLs can affect cognitive function. As modern technology has allowed the achievement of glycaemic targets closer to the normal range, it has become apparent that hyperglycaemia can affect mood, behaviour, and cognitive performance.

10. Other Autoimmune Disease

Coeliac disease is commonly diagnosed prior to adolescence in the child with diabetes. The rate in adolescence is still above that of the non diabetic population. Adherence to the gluten free diet can be more difficult to achieve during adolescence than to the diabetic diet itself. Thyroid disease usually presents as Hashimoto's hypothyroidism. Grave's disease (thyrotoxicosis) may also occur and will interfere with tight diabetic control.

11. Risky Behaviours

The presence of diabetes often enhances the damaging effects of risk behaviours. Tobacco use is a clear risk factor for progression of microvascular complications and future macrovascular disease. Alcohol is an inhibitor of hepatic gluconeogenesis, the endogenous protection against hypoglycaemia in Type 1 diabetes. Adolescents with Type 1 diabetes should be given both standard advice about safe drinking and in addition the following instructions:

- Always eat carbohydrate if drinking alcohol.
- Check BGL at the end of the evening, adjust the next dose of insulin if low and eat extra carbohydrate.
- Ask family or friends to wake the next morning — being left to 'sleep it off' may result in severe hypoglycaemia.

The effect of alcohol on BGL is also modified by the type of drink consumed, as the highly sweetened alcoholic drinks marketed specifically to youth may cause hyperglycaemia. Caution should be used with corrective insulin doses in the presence of alcohol. Marijhuana may increase appetite, with consequent high BGLs. Any substance use which impairs cognition will interfere with the adolescent's ability to manage self-care. Adolescent females with diabetes should be counselled about the risk of malformations if they become pregnant with poorly controlled diabetes and advice about contraception provided. There is no contraceptive method contra-indicated in Type 1 diabetes. The oral contraceptive is unlikely to cause significant insulin resistance or variability in insulin dose during the menstrual cycle (as may be seen in normal ovulatory cycles).

12. Other Forms of Diabetes

The peak time of new onset of Type 1 (autoimmune) diabetes is puberty. It is also the time when Type 2 diabetes starts to manifest, and is more common in non-Caucasian adolescents. The rarer monogenic diabetes can also be diagnosed in this time period. The treatments are different (Table 1). The majority of adolescents presenting with diabetes will have Type 1 diabetes.

Classification of diabetes has become more difficult with the increase in childhood obesity. The overweight adolescent of non-Caucasian background who is found to have asymptomatic hyperglycaemia is most likely to have Type 2 diabetes. However he or she could also have Type 1 diabetes, especially if there has been weight loss. Obesity itself may induce

Table 1: Classification of diabetes during adolescence modified from ISPAD Clinical Practice Consensus Guidelines 2009.

	Type 1	**Type 2**	**Monogenic**
Ketosis.	Common.	Uncommon, occurs during severe physiological stress.	Rare.
Pancreatic antibodies.	Present.	Rare.	Absent.
C peptide.	Low.	High.	Often in normal range.
Body mass index.	Within normal range.	Mostly overweight.	Within normal range.
+ve parental history.	2–4%	High.	90%
Treatment.	Insulin	Lifestyle modification, metformin.	Sulfonylureas.

autoimmunity, so that positive diabetes-associated autoantibodies (IA2, GAD and insulin antibodies) may be found in both forms of diabetes. Indeed Type 2 diabetes can also present with ketoacidosis, especially with an intercurrent infection.

Recent Australian data confirm that Indigenous adolescents have a six times greater rate of type 2 diabetes than non-Indigenous adolescents, but have a similar incidence of Type 1 diabetes as non-Indigenous adolescents (15.5 versus 21.4 per 100,000). The adolescent group with Type 2 diabetes has a high rate of comorbidities, especially psychiatric disease and developmental delay. Type 2 diabetes is also seen as a result of newer psychotropic drugs which can cause rapid weight gain. Adolescents with Type 2 diabetes have higher rates of microalbuminuria and hypertension than those with Type 1 diabetes, despite shorter diabetes duration and generally lower HbA1c levels.

Monogenic diabetes can also present during adolescence and may be exquisitely sensitive to sulphonylureas. There is usually a strong family history and inheritance is autosomal dominant.

In a metabolically unstable adolescent, treatment of hyperglycaemia must start with insulin therapy, especially when significant ketonuria or ketonaemia is present, as these may signal impending ketoacidosis. Delay in treatment of hyperglycaemia with ketonaemia may result in life threatening DKA.

13. Transition from Paediatric to Adult Care

It is common for this event to occur around the ages of 16–18 years, at a time of great change for the young person in many other aspects of their life. Evidence exists that many young people with diabetes will 'drop out' of care if the process is not well initiated by the paediatric team and supported by the adult team. The end result is often recurrent admissions with DKA, and representing to adult facilities with new microvascular complications. Young adult/adolescent diabetes centres in adult services that provide a sick day call service, flexible appointment times, and follow up of nonattenders have prevented DKA admissions and improved diabetic control.

References

Amin R, Widmer B, Prevost AT, Schwarze P, Cooper J, Edge J, Marcovecchio L, Neil A, Dalton RN, Dunger DB. (2008) Risk of microalbuminuria and progression to macroalbuminuria in a cohort with childhood onset type 1 diabetes: Prospective observational study. *BMJ,* **336**(7646): 697–701.

Betts P, Brink S, Silink M, Swift PGF, Wolfsdorf J, Hanas R. (2009) Management of children and adolescents with diabetes requiring surgery. *Pediatr Diabetes* **10**(12): 169–174.

Codner E, Cassorla F. (2009) Puberty and ovarian function in girls with type 1 diabetes mellitus. *Horm Res* **71**(1): 12–21.

Craig ME, Femia G, Broyda V, Lloyd M, Howard NJ. (2007) Type 2 diabetes in indigenous and non-indigenous children and adolescents in New South Wales. *Med J Aust* **186**(10): 497–499.

Donaghue KC, Craig ME, Chan AKF, Fairchild JM, Cusumano JM, Verge CF, Crock P A, Hing SJ, Howard NJ, Silink M. (2005) Prevalence of diabetes complications 6 years after diagnosis in an incident cohort of childhood diabetes. *Diabet Med* **22**(6): 711–718.

Eppens MC, Craig ME, Cusumano J, Hing S, Chan AKF, Howard NJ, Silink M, Donaghue KC. (2006) Prevalence of diabetes complications in adolescents with type 2 compared with type 1 diabetes. *Diabet Care* **29**(6): 1300–1306.

The Diabetes Control and Complications Trial Research Group (1993) The effect of intensive treatment of diabetes on the development and progression of long-term complications in insulin-dependent diabetes mellitus. The diabetes control and complications trial research group. *N Engl J Med* **329**(14): 977–986.

Holmes-Walker DJ, Llewellyn AC, Farrell K. (2007) A transition care programme which improves diabetes control and reduces hospital admission rates in young adults with type 1 diabetes aged 15-25 years. *Diabet Med* **24**(7): 764–769.

Jacobson AM, Musen G, Ryan CM, Silvers N, Cleary P, Waberski B, Burwood A, Weinger K, Bayless M, Dahms W, Harth J, Diabetes C, Complications Trial/Epidemiology of Diabetes, I. & Complications Study Research, G. (2007) Long-term effect of diabetes and its treatment on cognitive function. *New Engl J Med* **356**(18): 1842–1852.

Misso ML, Egberts KJ, Page M, O'Connor D, Shaw J. (2010) Continuous subcutaneous insulin infusion (CSII) versus multiple insulin injections for type 1 diabetes mellitus. *Cochrane Database Syst Rev* 1 CD005103.

Rewers M, Pihoker C, Donaghue K, Hanas R, Swift P, Klingensmith GJ. (2009) Assessment and monitoring of glycemic control in children and adolescents with diabetes. *Pediatr Diabetes* **10**(12): 71–81.

Skinner TC, John M, Hampson SE. (2000) Social support and personal models of diabetes as predictors of self-care and well-being: A longitudinal study of adolescents with diabetes. *J Pediatr Psychol* **25**(4): 257–267.

Wolfsdorf J, Craig ME, Daneman D, Dunger D, Edge J, Lee W, Rosenbloom A, Sperling M, Hanas R. (2009) Diabetic ketoacidosis in children and adolescents with diabetes. *Pediatr Diabetes* **10**(12): 118–133.

Chapter 37

Adolescent Bone Health

Craig Munns

1. Introduction

This chapter provides a background into the mechanisms controlling bone health and some of the disorders that can adversely affect it for clinicians who look after adolescents and young adults. The chapter also outlines a strategy for the investigation and management of these disorders.

During growth, bones not only get longer but also wider and thicker, through a process known as modelling. During adolescence, young people undergo a significant growth spurt prior to the attainment of final height. In the two years either side of the peak height growth velocity (approximately 12 years for females and 13 years for males), young people accrue almost 40% of their maximum attained bone mass. This percentage is equivalent to the amount of bone lost with normal ageing. As such, ensuring maximal accrual of bone mass and strength through adolescence may to a great degree prevent osteoporosis in later adult life.

The strength of the bone is governed by its size, shape, mineral density, and material properties. Genetics are responsible for determining approximately 80% of bone mass (a proxy for strength). Of the remaining 20%, 15% is determined by muscle mass. The residual 5% is determined by factors such as pubertal hormones, calcium intake, and

479

serum vitamin D levels. Health professionals can help maximise bone health in all adolescents by:

- Encouraging physical activity.
- Providing to ensure adequate dietary calcium intake.
- Maintaining serum vitamin D concentrations within the normal range.
- Ensuring that there are no barriers to adequate and timely pubertal progression.

2. Osteoporosis

2.1. *Definition*

Osteoporosis in adolescents is defined as a bone mineral content or areal bone mineral density age adjusted z-score of <-2.0 plus a clinically significant fracture. A clinically significant fracture is defined as a lower extremity long fracture, vertebral compression fracture, or two or more upper extremity long bone fractures.

2.2. *Diagnosis*

2.2.1. *Bone mass/density*

To diagnose osteoporosis by this definition it is necessary to have access to dual X-ray absorptiometry. It is equally important to understand the utility and pitfalls of this investigation. DXA does not provide a true volumetric BMD but rather it is the mass of bone mineral per projection area (gm/cm^2), termed aBMD.

Areal BMD is a size dependent measure, with shorter adolescents having a reduced aBMD compared to taller aged-matched controls. This is not because there is anything inherently abnormal with their bones, but simply because they are small. Adolescents with chronic illness frequently have short stature resulting from their primary disease or its treatment, and may therefore have a resultant reduction in aBMD. Despite these issues with DXA, it is the preferred method of assessment of reduced bone mass and density as it is estimated that an adolescent will have to have a 30% reduction in bone mass before it can be appreciated on plain radiographs.

However, if BMD is not available, second metacarpal cortical thickness is a recognised method of assessing for reduction of cortical long bone thickness, and can be easily attained from a bone age X-ray. A lateral thoraco–lumbar spine X-ray is also useful for the assessment of bone mass, as well as the detection of vertebral crush fractures.

2.2.2. *Biochemical markers*

In adolescents with a suspected abnormality of bone health, as well as for an assessment of bone mass/density, evaluation of mineral homeostasis and secondary causes of osteoporosis should be undertaken where possible.

Mineral homeostasis: serum calcium, magnesium, phosphorus, alkaline phosphatase, 25-hydroxy vitamin D, parathyroid hormone and urinary calcium: creatinine ratio.

Secondary causes of osteoporosis: full blood count, coeliac screen, renal function, thyroid function, gonadotropins and sex hormones — testosterone or oestradiol (if pubertal delay). Unlike in adults, bone turnover markers in adolescents are more a reflection of growth and are of limited clinical use outside the research setting.

3. Primary Osteoporosis

3.1. *Osteogenesis Imperfecta*

OI is the most common primary bone disorder with an incidence of approximately 1:20,000. OI most commonly results from a mutation in the Type I collagen gene. Recent reports from families of African descent have described severe forms of OI that arise from mutations in non-COL1 genes. The treatment of OI does not rely on the presence or otherwise of a COL1 mutation, but rather on the phenotype of the child. Response to bisphosphonate treatment has been shown to be similarly effective for all groups other than Type VII who respond poorly. There are various forms of OI, from the neonatally lethal OI Type II to the milder variants of OI Types I and IV. It is not unusual for the diagnosis of mild OI to be made in an adolescent who may present with recurrent fracture following low level trauma. The chapter does not have the scope to discuss the management of OI in great detail, but it should be remembered that adolescents with all forms of OI experience the psychosocial problems common to many adolescents with a chronic illness.

Intravenous bisphosphonates remain the mainstay of medical therapy for moderate to severe OI. In children and adolescents, bisphosphonates have been shown to increase bone density, improve growth, reduce fracture rate, and allow for improved motor function. The use of oral bisphosphonates, and the administration of bisphosphonates to children and adolescents with mild OI remains an area of active research and at this time cannot be recommended as standard practice. Approximately 80% of adolescents will experience an acute 'flu-like reaction' (fever, myalgia, nausea and vomiting) following the first dose of intravenous bisphosphonate. A similar percentage will become temporarily hypocalcaemic and it is essential that all adolescents receiving bisphosphonates are vitamin D replete (25-hydroxy vitamin D >50 nmol/L) throughout treatment. Due to these side effects and the lack of long term safety data for these medications, centres experienced with their use should supervise administration. Bisphosphonates cross the placenta and have been shown to result in abnormal bone development in animal models. As such, their use during pregnancy is contraindicated. There are no data that their administration prior to conception is detrimental to the mother or foetus. During growth, bisphosphonates are administered at regular intervals. Once final height is attained, the treatment interval can often be extended and in some situations suspended for a period of time.

Transition of the adolescent with OI to adult care requires careful planning. All will require monitoring of their bone health with regular BMD scans and bloods for mineral homeostasis including vitamin D. Many will require ongoing bisphosphonate therapy. These services can often be performed through adult endocrinology services. These youth may also need an action plan in case of fracture and often regular orthopaedic follow-up outside these times. It can be difficult to identify adult orthopaedic surgeons with experience in managing OI. A physician with an understanding of the medical issues specific to OI, for example basilar invagination and joint hypermobility, is also required and regular

Table 1: Causes of secondary osteoporosis in adolescents.

Endocrine.	Glucocorticoid excess, hypogonadism, hyperthyroidism, hyperparathyroidism.
Deficiencies.	Calcium, vitamin D, malnutrition.
Inflammation.	Juvenile idiopathic arthritis, inflammatory bowel disease.
Immobilisation.	Paraplegia, cerebral palsy, Duchenne muscular dystrophy.
Neoplasia.	Leukaemia.
Medication.	Glucocorticoids, methotrexate, anti-convulsants.
Inborn errors of metabolism.	Glycogen storage disease, Gaucher disease.
Haematological disorders.	Thalassaemia, sickle cell disease.
Renal.	Chronic renal failure, chronic metabolic acidosis.

monitoring is advised. Pre-conception genetic counselling should be offered through a clinical genetics service for all couples where one partner has OI.

4. Secondary Osteoporosis

Following the attainment of final height the ability to positively influence bone mass and strength is greatly diminished when compared to that possible during the adolescent growth spurt. As such, the management of secondary causes of osteoporosis is of paramount importance during adolescence. A chronically ill adolescent will usually have multiple factors influencing bone health and strength, with the number increasing with the severity of the illness.

4.1. *Reduced Mobility*

Bones develop to withstand the mechanical forces applied to them in every-day life. The magnitude of these forces and the skeleton's ability to sense and respond to them is the major influence on the mineral content and architectural design of bone, and therefore its strength. In the normally ambulatory adolescent, the major bone strains result from muscle pull and growth. Efforts to increase bone mass and strength in adolescents should therefore concentrate on increasing physical activity.

In the chronically ill adolescent with reduced mobility, bone development is often abnormal and bone strength reduced. Pathological fracture becomes more common with age in adolescents with reduced mobility from disorders such as cerebral palsy, Duchenne muscular dystrophy, and acquired spinal injury. Trans-iliac bone biopsies from adolescents with various neurological disorders and immobility have shown that the reduced mass results from small bone size, thin cortices, and a reduced trabecular bone volume.

The most common site of fracture in adolescents with immobility is the distal femur. This is because their long bones tend to be slender with thin cortices and reduced trabecular density, and the lower extremities are subject to trauma from accidents or manual handling. Vertebral crush fractures are less frequent, but can be complicated by the development of scoliosis.

To prevent immobilisation bone loss in adolescents with chronic illness, weight-bearing activity should be maximised, which in both healthy adolescents and in those with cerebral palsy, has been shown to increase bone mineral accrual and bone size. For adolescents with extreme bone fragility, swimming and hydrotherapy may be beneficial. In ambulant and non-ambulant adolescents with spastic cerebral palsy, weight bearing activity has been shown to significantly improve femoral neck bone mineral content and volumetric BMD when compared to controls.

4.2. *Pubertal Delay*

During puberty, not only is there impressive longitudinal growth of bone but there are also changes to the structure of bone. Trabecular bone comprises the majority of flat and cuboid bones, and also the epiphysis and metaphysis of long bone. Through puberty, there is increased trabecular thickness and density. Cortical bone makes up the majority of bone mass. It is the outer shell of all bone and makes up the mid section (diaphysis) of long bones. With puberty there is an increase in cortical density, most pronounced in females. During puberty, males achieve a greater periosteal radius and females a relatively smaller endosteal radius. Due to oestrogen, females are able to accrue a greater amount of calcium into their skeleton in relation to their amount of muscle and develop bones that have a greater cross sectional area per muscle mass than males.

Delayed or arrested pubertal development may occur as a result of an underlying chronic illness and/or its treatment, and unless assessed prospectively may be easily overlooked in the care of the chronically ill adolescent. As noted above, pubertal hormones, oestradiol in females and testosterone in males, influence longitudinal bone growth and bone mineral accrual, with their appropriate timing being important for normal skeletal development and the attainment of normal BMD.

There are no data on the minimal level of pubertal hormones required for normal bone development during adolescence. It is unclear if the induction of puberty in otherwise normal children with constitutional delay of puberty positively influences bone mass at final height. There are however data that delayed puberty in both males and females is associated with reduced bone mass later in life and increased fracture rate. The situation is even less clear for adolescents with a chronic illness, where osteoporosis is associated with low bone turnover and small bone size.

Short term (six month) androgen therapy, has been demonstrated to progress puberty without adversely affecting final height in males with CDGP. Androgen therapy however has not been shown to positively affect bone mass.

No data on sex steroid 'priming' are available in females. Here, if there is no pubertal development by age 13.5 years, it is recommended to introduce low dose oestrogen with a gradual increase in dose over 2–3 years. Once pubertal development has been achieved, it may be possible to withdraw therapy to see if puberty can be maintained spontaneously.

In the disabled adolescent with osteoporosis, pubertal induction may exacerbate behavioural difficulties and raise concerns about menstrual hygiene. These are important issues and need to be addressed appropriately, but given the potential beneficial effects of puberty hormones on bone health, there are very few clinical situations where the withholding of these hormones would be justified.

5. Nutrition and Low Body Weight

Adequate nutrition is essential for normal growth and development. It is not surprising therefore that osteoporosis is associated with nutritional and low body weight disorders such as anorexia nervosa, inflammatory bowel disease, malignancy, and cystic fibrosis. The aetiology of the osteoporosis in such disorders is multifactorial with interplay between low body weight, reduced lean tissue mass, low calcium, vitamin D and protein intakes, and gonadal deficiency, functional growth hormone resistance, and malabsorption.

5.1. *Anorexia Nervosa*

Anorexia nervosa and other eating disorders affect approximately 10% of young Australian women. It is most common amongst adolescent women, a time of maximal bone mass accrual. One of the most serious long term consequences of AN, which persists even after successful management of the eating disorder, is the severe loss of bone mass, resulting in osteoporosis in up to 40% and low bone density (osteopaenia) in over 90%. The abnormal bone development has a negative effect on bone strength, with a cumulative incidence of fracture 40 years after the diagnosis of AN greater than 50%. The optimal management of bone health in AN is the restoration of weight. Oestrogen supplementation in the face of primary or secondary amenorrhoea is of little benefit. Ensuring adequate calcium and vitamin D intake is important, but this in itself is likely to be of little benefit in the absence of adequate dietary management.

5.2. *Calcium and Vitamin D*

An adequate intake of calcium and vitamin D is essential for skeletal mineralisation. In adolescents, a dietary calcium intake of approximately 1100 mg/day is associated with peak calcium accretion rates of 350 mg/day in boys and 300 mg/day in girls. In healthy adolescents, short-term gains in BMD have been achieved through calcium supplementation. It is unclear however, whether such gains are sustainable, improve peak bone mass or most importantly, increase bone strength. Given this, the recommended daily intake of calcium for healthy adolescents is 1,300 mg. Further studies are required to assess if the calcium needs are similar for adolescents with a chronic illness.

Vitamin D is essential for normal skeletal development especially during adolescence when growth is rapid. Adolescence and infancy are the two time points when the complications of vitamin D deficiency — rickets, poor growth, bone fragility, and hypocalcaemic seizures — are most common. Vitamin D deficiency and associated rickets are again emerging as major public health issues worldwide. The majority of vitamin D is synthesised in the skin from the ultraviolet B radiation in sunlight, with dietary sources contributing only a small percentage of total daily requirements. There is also increasing evidence for non-skeletal roles of vitamin D, including in autoimmune disease, cardiovascular disease, and cancer, making the maintenance of adequate vitamin D levels even more important. Risk factors for vitamin D deficiency during adolescence include increased skin pigmentation, clothing that limits exposure of skin to sunlight, chronic disability, and obesity. The definitions of vitamin D deficiency are:

- Mild — 25-hydroxyvitamin D level 25.1–50 nmol/L.
- Moderate —12.5–25 nmol/L.
- Severe — less than 12.5 nmol/L.
- Those at risk of vitamin D deficiency should be on preventative vitamin D supplementation of 400–600 IU daily. When vitamin D levels are low, treatment doses of vitamin D should be given, 2000–5000 IU daily for three months or oral high dose stoss therapy (400,000–600,000 IU) given in 2–4 divided doses.

6. Glucocorticoids

Glucocorticoids are commonly prescribed to adolescents with chronic inflammatory and autoimmune disorders. Even at low doses, glucocorticoids may result in osteopaenia by decreasing bone formation and increasing bone resorption. In the majority of situations there will be multiple factors responsible for the deterioration in bone health of adolescents receiving glucocorticoid therapy including the medication itself, inflammatory cytokines, decreased mobility, poor nutrition and impaired calcium absorption, suppression of gonadotropins and hepatic IGF-1 and reduced local growth factor production.

Vertebral crush fractures are the most prevalent fractures associated with glucocorticoid use in adolescents. A prednisolone dose of 0.62 mg/kg/day in young people with juvenile idiopathic arthritis is associated with a mean time to vertebral collapse of 2.6 years. Intermittent steroid use may also predispose to fracture, with a recent study reporting an increased fracture incidence in children and adolescents who received over four courses of glucocorticoids. It is however difficult to differentiate between glucocorticoid induced bone loss and that associated with the primary disorder and its associated increase in inflammatory cytokines, malnutrition, and decrease in weight bearing.

The role of calcium and vitamin D supplementation in the prevention of glucocorticoid induced osteoporosis remains controversial. Until further data are available, adolescents on glucocorticoid therapy should receive the recommended daily intake of calcium (1,300 mg) and vitamin D supplementation, 400–800 IU/day.

7. Inflammatory Cytokines and Growth Factors

Systemic inflammatory disorders are frequently associated with osteopaenia and osteoporosis. The aetiology of the bone loss is multifactorial, but increased circulating and focal concentrations of inflammatory cytokines (IL-1, IL-6, IL-7, TNF-alpha and –beta, and RANKL- receptor activator of nuclear factor kappa-B ligand) and growth factors (including platelet derived growth factor) are likely to play an important role. Cytokines have been shown to stimulate osteoclastogenesis, suppress osteoblast recruitment, and induce resistance to 1,25-dihydroxyvitamin D_3, thus increasing bone resorption and decreasing bone formation.

8. Treatment of Osteopaenia/Osteoporosis

Treatment aims to optimise weight bearing activity, and vitamin D and calcium status, together with inducing and maintaining puberty if required, in a window of opportunity when health is relatively good and corticosteroid needs are low.

These measures are frequently inadequate in preventing the development of osteoporosis with chronic bone pain or fragility fractures. In these situations, specific anti-osteoporosis therapy should be considered, where available. Bisphosphonates are the most widely used medications for the treatment of adolescent osteoporosis in regimens similar to those used to treat OI (Section 3.1). Similar clinical and densitometric outcomes have been demonstrated in small numbers of adolescents with osteoporosis associated with various chronic illnesses including glucocorticoid induced osteoporosis, cystic fibrosis, cerebral palsy, Duchenne muscular dystrophy, spina bifida, and Gaucher disease. As with OI, oral bisphosphonates remain an area of active research and cannot be recommended for routine use. Here again it is essential that adolescents on bisphosphonate therapy have a vitamin D level >50 nmol/L.

References

Adams JS, Hewison M. (2010) Update in vitamin D. *J Clin Endocrinol Metab* **95**(2): 471–478.

Bailey DA, Martin AD, Mckay HA, Whiting S, Mirwald R. (2000) Calcium accretion in girls and boys during puberty: A longitudinal analysis. *J Bone Miner Res* **15**(11): 2245–2250.

Batch JA, Couper JJ, Rodda C, Cowell CT, Zacharin M. (2003) Use of bisphosphonate therapy for osteoporosis in childhood and adolescence. *J Paediatr Child Health* **39**(2): 88–92.

Garn SM, Poznanski AK, Nagy JM. (1971) Bone measurement in the differential diagnosis of osteopenia and osteoporosis. *Radiology* **100**(3): 509–518.

Greenway A, Zacharin M. (2003) Vitamin D status of chronically ill or disabled children in Victoria. *J Paediatr Child Health* **39**(7): 543–547.

Leonard MB, Feldman HI, Shults J, Zemel BS, Foster BJ, Stallings VA. (2004) Long-term, high-dose glucocorticoids and bone mineral content in childhood glucocorticoid-sensitive nephrotic syndrome. *N Engl J Med* **351**(9): 868–675.

Munns C, Zacharin MR, Rodda CP, Batch JA, Morley R, Cranswick NE, Craig ME, Cutfield WS, Hofman PL, Taylor BJ, Grover SR, Pasco JA, Burgner D, Cowell CT, Paediatric Endocrine G, Group Paediatric Bone Australasia. (2006) Prevention and treatment of infant and childhood vitamin D deficiency in Australia and New Zealand: A consensus statement. *Med J Aust* **185**(5): 268–272.

Munns CF, Cowell CT. (2005) Prevention and treatment of osteoporosis in chronically ill children. *J Musculoskelet Neuronal Interact* **5**(3): 262–272.

Munns CFJ, Sillence DO. (2007) Disorders predisposing to bone fragility and decreased bone density. In: Rimoin DL, Connor JM, Pyeritz RE, Korf BR (eds), *Principles and practice of medical genetics.* Elsevier, Churchill Livingstone, Philadelphia.

Rauch F, Plotkin H, Dimeglio L, Engelbert RH, Henderson RC, Munns C, Wenkert D, Zeitler P. (2008) Fracture prediction and the definition of osteoporosis in children and adolescents: The ISCD 2007 pediatric official positions. *J Clin Densitom* **11**(1): 22–28.

Zacharin M. (2004) Current advances in bone health of disabled children. *Curr Opin Pediatr* **16**(5): 545–551.

Chapter 38

Common Neurological Disorders

Richard Webster

1. Introduction

Neurological disease in adolescence presents a range of challenges different from those seen in younger children and adults. The management of adolescents with neurological disease is complicated by less reliable compliance with medication and poorer adherence to management plans. The establishment of independence can be particularly difficult for adolescents with neurological disorders that produce severe disability such as neuromuscular disorders. Throughout adolescence, education about the nature of their disorders and any potential genetic implications becomes increasingly important, as do decisions about transition to the care of adult neurology services.

2. Headache

2.1. *Evaluation of Headache*

It is important to differentiate adolescents with a primary headache disorder (for example migraine) from those whose headache is secondary to another disorder (for example raised intracranial pressure).

2.1.1. *Migraines*

Migraines are characterised by recurrent episodes of, usually, throbbing headache with complete recovery. In older adolescents the headache is commonly unilateral; however in younger adolescents it may be bilateral. Migraine usually comes on gradually and may be preceded by an aura (such as visual disturbance, hemiplegia). Photophobia, phonophobia, and anorexia are common. Resolution of symptoms with sleep is an important diagnostic clue. There is usually a family history.

2.1.2. *Tension type headaches*

These are commonly seen in adolescence. Tension headaches are dull and poorly localised and are not associated with the development of neurological symptoms or signs. While not usually as disabling as migraine, these may occur frequently or become constant and may co-occur in adolescents with typical migraine.

2.1.3. *Headache with raised intracranial pressure*

This is often associated with a constant **progressively worsening** headache sometimes exacerbated by coughing, straining, or sneezing. The headache is often dull and poorly localised. Headache occurring early in the morning (particularly when associated with vomiting) or which wakes an adolescent from sleep is a concerning sign and raises the possibility of raised intracranial pressure. Focal headache may occur with unilateral lesions.

2.1.4. *Examination*

It is important to check blood pressure. The neurological examination should aim to identify focal signs. The presence of papilloedema or strabismus suggests benign intracranial hypertension or a space-occupying lesion.

2.1.5. *Imaging*

Imaging is not mandatory in uncomplicated migraine, however imaging is indicated if the history or examination is atypical, if the headaches are of recent onset, or exclusively occipital. Sometimes, in order to address the anxiety caused by an ongoing headache disorder, imaging may be required to allow management to progress.

2.2. *Treatment of Primary Headache Disorders*

2.2.1. *Migraine*

The treatment of migraine depends upon the pattern and severity of headaches and its effect on the adolescent's quality of life. For adolescents with infrequent headaches, acute treatments are indicated; whereas for frequent headaches that limit activity and participation, preventive treatments are important. The identification and avoidance of triggering factors (such as dehydration, sleep deprivation) and treatment of comorbid psychological problems may decrease the frequency of headaches.

Ibuprofen (7.5–10 mg/kg/dose — maximum dose 400 mg) and paracetamol/acetaminophen (15 mg/kg/dose — maximum dose 1 g) are the first line treatments for migraine. These should be taken at the first sign that an adolescent is going to have a migraine (often during the aura). Triptans are the next line of treatment for migraine, although there are limited data about their effectiveness in adolescents. Sumatriptan nasal spray and almotriptan have been shown to be significantly better than placebo in producing headache relief. Triptans should be taken with headache onset and should be avoided in conditions where vasoconstriction might be dangerous such as hemiplegic or basilar migraine.

2.2.2. *Preventive treatment*

The choice of preventive treatments is limited by the absence of good clinical studies in adolescence. Usually prophylactic medications are started at a low dose and titrated upwards according to side effects and migraine control. Propanolol is one of the most commonly used medications for migraine prevention in adults. There is mixed evidence about its effectiveness in adolescents who should be started at a low dose (10–20 mg bd) and then titrated upwards based on response. Precautions need to be taken in adolescents with asthma. There is evidence that flunarizine, a calcium channel blocker, is effective in treating adolescent migraine. There is some evidence that low dose anti-epileptics, in particular topiramate (50 mg bd) and sodium valproate are effective in treating adolescent migraine. Side effects such as cognitive difficulties (topiramate) and weight gain (sodium valproate) may limit the use of these medications. Limited evidence also supports the use of cyproheptadine and amitriptyline as treatments of migraine in this age group.

2.2.3. *Chronic daily headaches*

Chronic daily headaches represent a major management problem during adolescence. These are often associated with psychosocial stressors. Treatment often requires multidisciplinary input to address mental health problems, to re-establish physical exercise and to re-integrate adolescents back into school and their peer groups. Headaches in this group are sometimes exacerbated by the overuse of simple analgesics. Medicines that prevent migraine are usually ineffective, however sometimes the use of a tricylic anti-depressant (such as amitriptyline) can be very helpful and allow the adolescent to resume normal activities.

3. Paroxysmal Disorders

3.1. *Evaluation of Paroxysmal Disorders*

Adolescents commonly present with paroxysmal episodes of real or apparent neurological disturbance. Because these episodes are often infrequent and the individual usually appears to be well in between the events, the diagnosis usually relies on obtaining a detailed history of the event from the adolescent as well as an observer. The key diagnostic features when evaluating a paroxysmal event (both from observers and the patient) are summarised in Table 1.

3.2. *Syncope*

Syncope is defined as a transient loss of consciousness usually resulting in a loss of muscle tone followed by collapse. Syncope results from a

Table 1: Important pieces of information about paroxysmal events.

1. The circumstances preceding the event for example hot day, blood collection, physical health, exercise, sleep, cough, urination.
2. Posture (standing, recumbent) prior to the event.
3. The symptoms/signs immediately preceding an event for example feelings of nausea, light headedness, visual disturbance, pallor, sweatiness.
4. The level of consciousness during the event; for example recall of event.
5. The nature of any movements/behaviours during the event.
6. The nature, duration and speed of recovery.
7. Evidence of neurological dysfunction after the event.
8. Family history — syncope, sudden death, arrhythmia.

global decrease in blood supply to the brain in which the cerebral perfusion pressure decreases to a point where consciousness is lost.

3.2.1. *Neurocardiogenic syncope*

In adolescence, the most common cause of syncope is fainting or neurocardiogenic syncope.

Typically the event occurs after a prolonged period of standing although sometimes there is a clear trigger. A prodrome associated with visual disturbance and a sensation of dizziness and/or nausea is common. Observers note increasing pallor or a greenish/grey colour preceding the collapse. Loss of consciousness then occurs. Observers may note that the eyes roll up and sometimes there is brief period of tonic posturing. The event is usually of relatively short duration, unless the adolescent is prevented from becoming recumbent. After this, there is a rapid return of consciousness. Often adolescents can recall having the pre-syncopal feeling at other times and sometimes the symptom can be reproduced. Symptoms that suggest an event may not have a benign cause are:

- Exercise/excitement precipitation — long QT syndrome.
- Palpitations preceding the event — cardiac arrhythmia.
- Events from sleep — epilepsy/cardiogenic syncope.
- Clonic jerking — epilepsy.
- Prolonged period of sleep post event — epilepsy.

3.2.2. *Evaluation*

The initial clinical evaluation should include a general physical examination concentrating on a detailed cardiac and neurological examination, supine and upright blood pressure, and an ECG. In the absence of cardiac disease, prolonged tilt table testing may provide information that helps establish a diagnosis by showing an abrupt fall in heart rate and/or blood pressure or an abnormal increase in heart rate.

3.2.3. *Treatment*

Neurocardiogenic syncope is usually a benign problem that improves with age. Adolescents should be taught to try to avoid situations that provoke syncope and to lie down as soon as they develop pre-syncopal symptoms. Strategies such as increasing fluid and salt intake may help. Medical treatments such as the use of beta-blockers, alpha agonists, selective serotonin re-uptake inhibitors and the use of mineralocorticoid drugs have been used, although there is a limited evidence base.

3.3. *Epilepsy*

3.3.1. *Evaluation of epilepsy*

A detailed history of the nature of the event (Table 1) and in particular a history from an observer is critical. This helps with the identification of seizure type, appropriate choice of medication, and guides further investigation. The neurological examination aims to identify signs (usually focal, such as hemiparesis) indicating an underlying neurological cause for the seizure.

Baseline investigations (electrolytes, calcium, magnesium, phosphate, glucose) aim to exclude secondary metabolic causes for seizures. An EEG (most often performed after sleep deprivation) may provide very useful diagnostic information. Imaging the brain, preferably with an MRI, should be considered in adolescents with evidence of focal epilepsy, with a history or neurological signs suggesting an underlying structural lesion or when the classification of epilepsy is in doubt.

3.3.2. *Juvenile myoclonic epilepsy*

JME most often presents during adolescence. This syndrome is characterised by generalised tonic-clonic seizures in 90% (sometimes preceded by myoclonic jerks) and often exacerbated by sleep deprivation. Photosensitivity is common and may lead to seizures induced by video games. Absence seizures are seen in a substantial number of adolescents. Myoclonus often occurs in the morning and is noted when an adolescent is brushing his/her teeth or eating breakfast — a history of myoclonus is frequently not volunteered and so it is important to ask specifically about this. Characteristically the EEG shows 4–6 Hz poly-spike and wave complexes, although 3–4 Hz spike and wave complexes may be seen. JME usually responds well to sodium valproate; however in adolescent girls, other medications such as lamotrigine and levetiracetam may be reasonable alternatives because of teratogenicity and weight gain.

3.3.3. *Choice of anti-epileptic medications in adolescence*

This involves balancing the probable efficacy of a medication with the likelihood and severity of its side effects. Particular medications (for example carbamazepine in JME) may exacerbate epilepsy. Compliance is a major issue. Adolescents are less likely to take medications that they feel are producing side effects. Checking blood levels of medications (for those drugs where assays are available) helps monitor compliance.

Potential teratogenic risks of anti-epileptic medication are an important consideration in adolescent girls. The use of sodium valproate and phenobarbitone is associated with a significantly increased risk of congenital malformations. Carbamazepine, lamotrigine, and phenytoin are also associated with a slightly increased risk of congenital malformations. Currently there are little data on the potential teratogenic effects of the newer anti-epileptic medications.

3.3.4. *Lifestyle in adolescents with epilepsy*

Adolescents with epilepsy need help to make informed decisions about the balance between the risks of epilepsy and their lifestyle choices. This is particularly important for activities (for example swimming) where a seizure might result in death. Most adolescents with epilepsy should only swim if they are in a place where there are persons able to supervise and/or assist. Similar considerations apply to other activities where a seizure might have fatal consequences. Given the stigma associated with a diagnosis of epilepsy, the decision to inform peers about this is often very difficult and we usually leave the adolescent to make this decision based on whom they feel they can trust with this information. We would encourage an adolescent with epilepsy to inform whoever is supervising them in activities where a seizure may have serious consequences about their diagnosis. On occasion this might require telling a friend about their diagnosis. The use of alcohol and other drugs poses extra risks for adolescents with epilepsy. Alcohol and other drugs may provoke seizures in some seizure disorders, such as the exacerbation of JME with alcohol ingestion. Alcohol and other drugs may interfere with the metabolism of other anti-epileptic medication (for example phenytoin) and may enhance the sedative effects of some medications (for example benzodiazepines, phenobarbitone).

3.3.5. *Contraception*

Interactions between certain anti-epileptic medications, particularly enzyme inducing medications such as carbamazepine and hormonal contraception (both oral and injectable) may diminish the effectiveness of these methods. Other methods such as barrier contraception may be required.

3.3.6. *Driving*

The independence that driving brings is very important for most adolescents. Broadly speaking adolescents with poorly controlled epilepsy are not permitted to drive. Different jurisdictions have differing rules as to how long a person has to be free of seizures before being deemed safe to drive and physicians need to be familiar with local restrictions.

3.3.7. *Employment*

There are a number of occupations that exclude people with epilepsy. Adolescents with epilepsy (even well-controlled epilepsy or sometimes only a history of epilepsy) may be not allowed to undertake jobs such as being a pilot, commercial driving, diving or military service. Physicians may need to play a strong advocacy role if they believe that the adolescent or young adult is being unfairly discriminated against because of their diagnosis.

4. Neuromuscular Disorders

4.1. *Acute Neuromuscular Disorders*

4.1.1. *Assessment*

Assessment of an adolescent with acute weakness requires the localisation of the disorder to either the lower motor unit or less commonly the upper motor neuron. The absence of reflexes in a weak adolescent usually suggests that there is a problem with the lower motor unit although occasionally an acute spinal cord injury can produce similar signs. In situations where there is doubt, an MRI of the spine may be needed to rule out treatable spinal causes.

4.1.2. *Guillain–Barré syndrome*

Guillain–Barré syndrome (acute inflammatory demyelinating polyneuropathy) is the most common cause of acute weakness in adolescence in developed countries. While Guillain–Barré syndrome is most frequently associated with weakness and areflexia, often a sensory neuropathy predominates at presentation and pain can be a major symptom. Sometimes, if autonomic nerves are involved, autonomic problems such as hypertension or arrhythmias may complicate the disorder. Guillain–Barré can usually be diagnosed on nerve conduction studies (best performed more than a week after onset) and responds well to treatment with intravenous immunoglobulin.

4.1.3. *Autoimmune myasthenia gravis*

Autoimmune myasthenia gravis in adolescence may present with either acute or chronic weakness. The hallmark of this disorder is fluctuating and fatigable weakness. Ptosis and ophthalmoplegia (common presenting symptoms) may sometimes suggest an intracranial pathology. However on examination adolescents usually show fatigable weakness upon sustained use of involved muscles, such as up gaze. Diurnal variation in muscle strength, particularly if the adolescent is seen when strong, may suggest a conversion disorder until the patient is seen at another time. Diagnosis can usually be confirmed using specialised neurophysiological techniques such as repetitive nerve stimulation or by close observation after the administration of short-acting cholinesterase inhibitors, such as neostigmine.

4.2. *Chronic Neuromuscular Disease*

The transition from childhood to adolescence to young adulthood comes with significant challenges for young people with chronic neuromuscular disease. These problems are magnified for those diseases such as Duchenne muscular dystrophy that show relentless progression and for those disorders such as fascioscapulohumeral muscular dystrophy that manifest during adolescence. Important neuromuscular management issues in adolescence are listed below in Table 2.

The transition from adult to paediatric services is a major problem for adolescents with progressive neuromuscular disorders. Ideally adult services for adolescents with neuromuscular disease should be based upon a multidisciplinary model with input from allied health, neurologists, rehabilitation, respiratory physicians, orthopaedic surgeons, and cardiologists. The rigid application of age based transition is particularly difficult for boys with Duchenne muscular dystrophy. After having built close relationships with multidisciplinary management teams during their childhood and adolescence, the inexorable decline in muscle strength often results in major medical crises (such as respiratory failure) occurring at the time when they are in transition. Without detailed planning and good liaison with adult medical services, adolescents with Duchenne muscular dystrophy often present to adult medical services in respiratory failure without adequate plans to manage this emergency. Where possible, transition should be avoided in adolescents who have a short life expectancy.

Table 2: Important neuromuscular management issues in adolescence.

1. Independence
   - Provision of adequate aids e.g. power wheel-chair.
   - School/home assessment to evaluate access.
   - Aids to assist with activities of daily living e.g. hoists.
   - Provision of appropriate mattresses (e.g. air mattress) to address sleep related discomfort and frequent awakening.
2. Respiratory muscle weakness
   - Early treatment of respiratory infection.
   - Monitor for clinical signs of nocturnal hypoventilation.
   - Sleep studies to identify nocturnal hypoventilation.
   - Nocturnal non-invasive ventilation for adolescents and young adults with nocturnal respiratory failure.
3. Kyphoscoliosis
   - Monitor for the development of scoliosis.
   - Early referral for consideration of surgery in adolescents with progressive scoliosis.
4. Cardiomyopathy
   - Regular cardiology review to detect the development of cardiomyopathy in diseases associated with cardiomyopathy (Becker and Duchenne muscular dystrophy).
5. Physiotherapy/orthopaedic interventions
   - Prevention of contractures by limb stretching and splints.
   - Orthopaedic surgery to address functional impairments due to contractures.
6. Preparation for adult life
   - Discussion about suitable careers.
   - Assessing understanding of the disorder and its management.
   - Discussion about causes and genetics of disorder.
   - Discussion about relationships and sexuality.

5. Neurodegenerative Disorders

The diagnosis of neurodegenerative disorders in adolescence can present major difficulties. Often the onset is insidious and may involve one neurological system before the typical range of symptoms and signs develop. Psychiatric symptoms may predominate at the onset and this may lead to the mistaken diagnosis of a psychiatric disorder prior to the manifestations of other neurological features. Conversely, psychiatric disorders, such as depression, may present with apparent cognitive regression leading to concerns about a neurodegenerative disorder. Neurodegenerative disorders may also present with epilepsy that early on is indistinguishable from other more common forms of adolescent epilepsy.

5.1. *Evaluating the Adolescent with a Possible Neurodegenerative Disorder*

It is important to differentiate those adolescents with neurological disease from those with pseudo-regression due to other causes (psychological illness, substance abuse, sleep disorders). In the case of adolescents presenting with neurological signs such as ataxia or spasticity this is not usually difficult. However, the assessment of adolescents presenting with apparently isolated cognitive regression can be more challenging. It is important to obtain as much objective information as possible about previous cognitive function from school reports and previous psychological testing, especially when adolescents have a pre-existing cognitive/intellectual disability. Specific questions should be asked about psychological health, the use of alcohol and other drugs, and sleep disturbance. A formal neuropsychological assessment can provide information about the likelihood of a degenerative disorder and provide a useful baseline assessment.

Evidence of sensory impairments (in particular vision), spasticity, neuropathy, cerebellar involvement, dystonia, and other movement disorders are important clues to the underlying aetiology of the disorder. While an exhaustive review of neurodegenerative disorders of adolescence is beyond the scope of this chapter, some of the findings in important neurodegenerative diseases in adolescence are summarised in Table 3. It is important to realise that at the onset of these diseases the full range of symptoms is often not present.

5.1.1. *Investigation*

Investigation of an adolescent with a regressive disorder is predicated on the clinical findings. Thus clinical evidence of a peripheral neuropathy such as absent or diminished reflexes or sensory impairments should be investigated with nerve conduction studies. A brain MRI and/or spinal cord MRI is a very useful test. MRI may identify lesions suggestive of a leucodystrophy in an adolescent with spasticity, changes in the basal

Table 3: Important neurodegenerative disorders of adolescence.

Disease	Clinical	Investigations
Friedreich ataxia.	Ataxia, neuropathy (sensory), spasticity, dysarthria, scoliosis, cardiomyopathy, diabetes.	Nerve conduction study, *frataxin* gene.
Metachromatic leukodystrophy.	Academic impairment, behavioural/ gait disturbance, peripheral neuropathy, dysarthria, seizures.	MRI brain — leukodystrophy, nerve conduction studies, neuropathy, Leucocyte enzymes — decreased arylsulfatase A.
Adreno-leucodystrophy/ Adreno-myeloneuropathy	ALD — males, cognitive disturbance, loss of vision and hearing, dysphasia, hemiparesis. AMN — males, slowly progressive paraparesis, impaired position and vibration sense, urinary/ sexual dysfunction.	MRI — parieto-occipital demyelination, primary adrenal failure, NCS-neuropathy.
Wilson disease.	Movement disorder — tremor, chorea, micrographia, dystonia — esp. face, pharynx, and tongue. Psychiatric disturbance.	Slit lamp examination — Kayser Fleischer rings, low serum ceruloplasmin, elevated timed urine copper.
Juvenile Huntington disease.	Clumsiness, rigidity, bradykinesia, oropharyngeal dysfunction, cognitive decline, psychiatric disturbance, chorea, motor restlessness, seizures, family history.	MRI — caudate atrophy, *HTT* gene — trinucleotide CAG expansion.

ganglia in an adolescent with dystonia, and may also help identify structural changes such as a Chiari 1 malformation or a slowly progressive tumour. For a number of neurodegenerative disorders, assessment by a skilled ophthalmologist may identify diagnostic optic or retinal changes, for example optic atrophy in Freidreich ataxia.

6. Stroke

The sudden onset of a new focal neurological deficit (in particular hemiplegia) in an adolescent should raise the possibility of stroke. The risk of a stroke is increased by the presence of underlying disorders such as haemo-globinopathies (sickle cell disease), heart disease (particularly cyanotic), coagulation disorders, vasculitis, diseases associated with vasculopathy (homocystinuria, Down syndrome), cerebrovascular malformations, and the use of cocaine. Stroke in adolescence is a medical emergency. The clinical examination should aim to clinically localise the site of the stroke as well as identify predisposing factors (such as signs of sub-acute bacterial endocarditis). The assessment should also aim to identify evidence of raised intracranial pressure (decreased level of consciousness, hypertension, bradycardia, pupillary dilatation, papilloedema).

6.1. *Investigation*

The investigation of an adolescent with a suspected stroke requires urgent neuroimaging. An MRI (preferably with MR angiography) is the most sensitive imaging modality for identifying a stroke; however if there are delays in obtaining this or an MR scanner is not readily available, a CT scan should be obtained particularly if there is concern about intracerebral haemorrhage. Depending upon the likely cause of the stroke (embolic versus vasculitic/vasculopathic) and the appearance of the stroke on imaging (thrombotic versus haemorrhagic) further investigation, such as echocardiography and screening for vasculitic and prothrombotic disorders, is indicated.

6.2. *Treatment*

The optimal treatment of an adolescent with stroke is controversial. In adults the use of thrombolytic therapies for acute thrombotic stroke is well established; however the safety and effectiveness of this in adolescents has not yet been demonstrated, largely because of limited studies in this age group. The same reservations apply to intravascular techniques such as clot retrieval. Acutely, adolescents with stroke should be managed in high dependency areas where they can be closely monitored. Adolescents with large haemorrhages may need neurosurgical intervention. For adolescents with thrombotic stroke, anticoagulation is usually recommended. Rehabilitation is critical to optimise recovery. Detailed guidelines for stroke investigation and management have been published by the American Heart Association.

7. Infectious and Inflammatory Disorders

While the incidence of infectious disorders of the CNS in adolescence is lower than in early childhood, meningitis and infectious encephalitis remain important causes of neurological morbidity.

7.1. *Meningitis*

Meningitis typically presents with headache, drowsiness, neck-stiffness, photophobia, and fever. However this presentation can be modified in an adolescent who has been taking antibiotics or where the infection is caused by a more indolent pathogen (such as *Mycobacterium tuberculosis, Cryptococcus neoformans*). A lumbar puncture is essential for the diagnosis of meningitis, however in situations where there is concern that this may be risky (signs suggestive of a focal neurological lesion, severely raised intracranial pressure, coagulopathy), empiric treatment with antimicrobial therapy should be instituted prior to performing a lumbar puncture.

7.2. *Encephalitis*

Encephalitis usually presents with a disturbance in the level of consciousness, often associated with seizures and focal neurological signs. Sometimes the onset is insidious and fever may be minimal or absent. Usually a lumbar puncture will show a CSF pleocytosis although the evidence of inflammation may be difficult to identify unless specific inflammatory markers are sought (for example, CSF pterins). MRI imaging may provide confirmatory evidence of the diagnosis. Herpes simplex is an important and treatable cause of viral encephalitis and patients with encephalitis are frequently treated for this until the diagnosis is excluded. It is sometimes difficult to differentiate viral encephalitis from post-infectious inflammatory disorders such as acute disseminated encephalomyelitis.

7.3. *Immunologically Mediated Inflammatory Disorders of the CNS*

These are an increasingly recognised cause of neurological disease in adolescence. These disorders may present acutely with the new development of focal neurological signs (acute disseminated encephalomyelitis or multiple sclerosis) or insidiously with psychiatric disease, movement disorders, or epilepsy (such as anti NMDA receptor encephalitis). While the manifestations of these disorders are protean, it is important to consider such diagnoses as these disorders are amenable to treatment with immunosuppressive therapies.

8. Evaluation of Suspected Conversion Disorders

The accurate diagnosis of a conversion disorder is sometimes difficult and often investigations are needed to exclude alternative diagnoses. Moreover neurological disorders such as movement disorders, epilepsy and neuro-metabolic disease can have paroxysmal presentations that may appear on history to be non-organic. Not infrequently, conversion disorders are comorbid with organic problems such as headache and syncope. With the increasing availability of devices capable of recording video, there are more opportunities to document the nature of paroxysmal events. Sometimes if events are occurring frequently, video-telemetry is very helpful in confirming that events are not epileptic.

While the management of conversion disorders is beyond the scope of this chapter, the way a diagnosis is conveyed is important in order to allow the adolescent and their family to engage in therapy. It is important to be honest about the diagnosis and admit uncertainty, should this exist. It is helpful if the family understands the diagnosis, as sometimes the response to the diagnosis of a conversion disorder is the development of new symptoms or a worsening of the pre-existing problems.

References

Chen-Scarabelli C, Scarabelli TM. (2004) Neurocardiogenic syncope. *BMJ* **329** (7461): 336–341.

Divasta AD, Alexander ME. (2004) Fainting freshmen and sinking sophomores: Cardiovascular issues of the adolescent. *Curr Opin Pediatr* **16**(4): 350–356.

Hershey AD, Kabbouche MA, Powers SW. (2010) Treatment of pediatric and adolescent migraine. *Pediatr Ann* **39**(7): 416–423.

Jentink J, Dolk H, Loane MA, Morris JK, Wellesley D, Garne E, De Jong-Van Den Berg L, EUROCAT Antiepileptic Study Working Group. (2010) Intrauterine exposure to carbamazepine and specific congenital malformations: Systematic review and case-control study. *BMJ* **341**: c6581.

Jentink J, Loane MA, Dolk H, Barisic I, Garne E, Morris JK, De Jong-Van Den Berg LTW, EUROCAT Antiepileptic Study Working Group. (2010) Valproic acid monotherapy in pregnancy and major congenital malformations. *N Engl J Med* **362**(23): 2185–2193.

Lewis D, Ashwal S, Hershey A, Hirtz D, Yonker M, Silberstein S. (2004) Practice parameter: Pharmacological treatment of migraine headache in children and adolescents: Report of the American Academy of Neurology Quality Standards Subcommittee and the Practice Committee of the Child Neurology Society. *Neurology* **63**(12): 2215–2224.

Lewis DW, Ashwal S, Dahl G, Dorbad D, Hirtz D, Prensky A, Jarjour I. (2002) Practice parameter: Evaluation of children and adolescents with recurrent headaches: Report of the Quality Standards Subcommittee of the American Academy of Neurology and the Practice Committee of the Child Neurology Society. *Neurology* **59**(4): 490–498.

Macleod S, Appleton RE. (2007) Neurological disorders presenting mainly in adolescence. *Arch Dis Childhood* **92**(2): 170–175.

Prasad A, Kuzniecky RI, Knowlton RC, Welty TE, Martin RC, Mendez M, Faught RE. (2003) Evolving antiepileptic drug treatment in juvenile myoclonic epilepsy. *Arch Neurol* **60**(8): 1100–1105.

Roach ES, Golomb MR, Adams R, Biller J, Daniels S, Deveber G, Ferriero D, Jones BV, Kirkham FJ, Scott RM, Smith ER, American Heart Association Stroke and the Council of Cardiovascular Disease in the Young (2008) Management of stroke in infants and children. *Stroke* **39**(9): 2644–2691.

Wheless JW, Kim HL. (2002) Adolescent seizures and epilepsy syndromes. *Epilepsia* **43**(3): 33–52.

Chapter 39

Common Gastrointestinal Disorders of Adolescence

Annabel Magoffin

1. Introduction

Gastrointestinal symptoms are a common reason for the adolescent to seek medical attention. The skill is to distinguish the more common functional gastrointestinal disorders from relatively infrequent organic disease. Organic diseases seen in adolescence include oesophagitis, peptic ulcer disease and gastritis, coeliac disease, inflammatory bowel disease, pancreatitis, and acute or chronic liver disease. Most require referral for specific investigation and management by a specialist gastroenterologist. In the adolescent with organic disease, it is crucial to maintain normal growth and pubertal development, and also to allow normal psychosocial development and maintain quality of life.

2. Functional Gastrointestinal Disorders

2.1. *Diagnosis of FGIDs*

Gastrointestinal symptoms in the adolescent are frequently due to functional gastrointestinal disorders. These disorders, as defined using the Rome III criteria, are described in the following sections.

2.1.1. *Adolescent rumination syndrome*

Repeated painless regurgitation and re-chewing of food.

2.1.2. *Functional dyspepsia*

Persistent or recurrent discomfort or pain in the upper abdomen, which is not relieved by defaecation, or associated with change in bowel habit.

2.1.3. *Irritable bowel syndrome*

Abdominal discomfort or pain associated with at least two of the following: improvement with defaecation, onset associated with change in stool frequency, or onset associated with change in stool appearance.

2.1.4. *Abdominal migraine and cyclical vomiting syndrome*

Paroxysmal episodes of intense acute peri-umbilical pain and/or nausea/vomiting lasting one hour or more with intervening periods of usual health lasting weeks to months. The pain and vomiting interfere with normal activities and are associated with at least two of the following: anorexia, nausea, headache, photophobia, or pallor.

2.1.5. *Adolescent functional abdominal pain*

Episodic or continuous abdominal pain, without criteria for other FGIDs.

2.1.6. *Functional constipation and incontinence*

Retentive constipation with infrequent stooling and non-retentive faecal incontinence with inappropriate defaecation.

In the diagnosis of a functional gastrointestinal disorder, no evidence for an inflammatory, anatomic, metabolic, or neoplastic process should be present. Symptoms and signs which should alert the clinician to organic disease include:

- Nocturnal pain and/or diarrhoea, dysphagia, persistent vomiting, gastrointestinal bleeding, fever.

- Pubertal delay, arthritis, peri-anal disease, weight loss.
- A family history of inflammatory bowel disease, Crohn's disease, peptic ulcer.

Psychosocial stressors are important precipitating factors in the adolescent with FGIDs. The onset of a FGID may follow an infection, inflammatory disorder or trauma and is frequently associated with anxiety and depression.

2.2. *Investigations for FGIDs*

Clinical evaluation and explanation has an important therapeutic role. Simple investigations that may be considered include a full blood count, erythrocyte sedimentation rate or C-reactive protein, liver and renal function tests, amylase and lipase, iron studies, and coeliac serology. An ultrasound of the abdomen/pelvis may be performed when indicated to assess for structural abnormalities. Endoscopy is usually performed when there are localising or concerning symptoms.

2.3. *Treatment of FGIDs*

Psychological therapy including cognitive behavioural therapy is the most effective therapy for the adolescent with a FGID. Specialised diets, use of probiotics, and pharmacological therapy, such as acid suppressive agents for dyspepsia, may be used but have not been validated in controlled clinical trials. Care must be taken to avoid restrictive diets where there is no confirmed evidence of intolerance or allergy in order to avoid the risk of inadequate nutrition during pubertal growth. Many of these young patients can have severe symptoms with a significant impact on quality of life, including reduced school attendance. For the adolescent with ongoing symptoms, referral to a specialised adolescent unit or psychological service for review, consideration of psychotropic medication, and rehabilitation may be required.

3. Oesophagitis

The adolescent with oesophagitis presents in a similar manner to adults with complaints of epigastric pain, heartburn, acid regurgitation, and vomiting. It is most commonly due to gastro-oesophageal reflux disease or eosinophilic oesophagitis. Infections including cytomegalovirus and fungus are rare causes of oesophagitis which should be considered in the immuno-suppressed patient. Caustic ingestion is uncommon in this age group.

3.1. *Gastro–Oesophageal Reflux Disease*

GORD is the most common cause of oesophagitis. Retrograde movement of gastric contents into the oesophagus results in symptoms and inflammation. Most adolescents with GORD are responsive to pharmacotherapy.

3.1.1. *Diagnosis*

The young person requiring ongoing therapy for more persistent symptoms or complications, such as haematemesis or for dysphagia, requires referral for specialist review and consideration of endoscopy to confirm the diagnosis by oesophageal biopsy.

3.1.2. *Treatment*

The use of a proton pump inhibitor is recommended as initial therapy, although H2 antagonists may also be used. PPIs are often used empirically for four weeks in the adolescent with typical symptoms. In patients with confirmed erosive oesophagitis longer term therapy may be necessary. Surgery (fundoplication) is rarely necessary except in more severe cases requiring long term therapy. This situation often occurs with an associated anatomical abnormality such as hiatus hernia or with an associated disorder such as cerebral palsy. Complications of GORD such as fibrotic stricture or Barrett's oesophagus are rare in adolescence but have been reported. Adolescents with persistent disease will need to be transitioned to an adult gastroenterologist for ongoing care, including follow up endoscopy.

3.2. *Eosinophilic oesophagitis*

Eosinophilic oesophagitis is an increasingly recognised cause of oesophagitis. Adolescents complain of epigastric pain and odynophagia with a characteristic history of dysphagia for solid foods and/or intermittent severe food impaction. Response to PPIs is poor.

3.2.1. *Diagnosis*

Upper gastrointestinal endoscopy and oesophageal biopsy is required. Endoscopy may reveal the classic appearance of patchy white exudate, mucosal thickening, and prominent linear furrows in the oesophagus, but it may also appear normal or similar to GORD. Histology demonstrates a typical eosinophilic infiltrate.

3.2.2. *Treatment*

Management requires a multidisciplinary approach with input from both gastroenterologists and immunologists. Treatment may include topical steroids (fluticasone proprionate or budesonide, swallowed rather than inhaled) and dietary restriction. The young person with this condition requires continuing specialist care into adulthood to avoid potential complications of long term inflammation of the oesophageal mucosa, including fibrotic stricture.

4. Peptic Ulcer Disease and Gastritis

Concern about the possibility of peptic ulcer disease and *Helicobacter pylori* infection in the adolescent with abdominal pain is a frequent reason for referral. Although the infection is generally acquired in the first years of life, *H. pylori*-induced gastritis and peptic ulcer disease are relatively uncommon in adolescence.

4.1. *H. pylori Infection*

In adolescents the clinical presentation and natural history of peptic ulcer disease are comparable to those observed in adults. Teenagers complain of epigastric and nocturnal pain and frequently have a positive family history of peptic ulceration. There may be unexplained anaemia. They may present acutely to hospital with upper gastrointestinal haemorrhage. Duodenal ulceration is most common in association with *H. pylori* infection and is typically accompanied by a chronic active gastritis.

There is controversy regarding the potential for *H. pylori* gastritis to cause significant symptoms in the absence of peptic ulcer disease. In these adolescents, symptoms may be due to functional gastrointestinal disorders including functional dyspepsia and chronic abdominal pain. This must be considered in the patient with chronic symptoms despite effective eradication therapy.

4.1.1. *Diagnosis*

The diagnosis is made by upper gastrointestinal endoscopy and gastric biopsy. *H. pylori* infection can also be diagnosed non-invasively with breath testing using the stable isotope ^{13}C or radiolabelled ^{14}C (the stable isotope ^{13}C being preferred for use in adolescents). The gastritis and ulcers resolve with successful eradication of *H. pylori* infection.

4.1.2. *Treatment*

Treatment is usually a combination of a PPI (such as omeprazole), plus two antibiotics (amoxicillin and either clarithromycin or metronidazole), in a twice daily dosage regimen over seven days. Successful eradication occurs in 80% of patients. Repeat endoscopy is not usually required, except in complicated disease. Eradication of the infection is confirmed with breath testing. Resistant disease needs specialist referral. Alternative treatment regimens may be necessary after endoscopy and culture to determine *H. pylori* antibiotic resistance.

4.2. *Gastritis and Gastric or Duodenal Ulcer Without H. pylori Disease*

Gastritis and gastric or duodenal ulcer may be due to the administration of medication including non-steroidal anti-inflammatory drugs, which are commonly used in adolescents for pain management. Crohn's disease may cause a focal acute gastritis. Gastritis may also be seen in association with acute viral illness, such as cytomegalovirus infection. Gastritis and gastric ulcers occur in the acutely ill young person, for example with burns or on chemotherapy and during treatment with pharmacological doses of glucocorticoids. Treatment strategies include addressing the causative agent and the use of an acid suppressive medication such as a PPI.

5. Coeliac Disease

Coeliac disease is an immunologically mediated chronic inflammatory disorder of the small intestine. It develops with exposure to gluten in the genetically susceptible individual, with susceptibility determined by expression of HLA DQ2 and DQ8. It has a prevalence of 1% in most populations, noting that many affected persons are undiagnosed.

5.1. *Presentation*

The presentation of the adolescent with coeliac disease is varied. Higher risk groups may be diagnosed after screening, including young persons with autoimmune disease such as Type 1 diabetes mellitus and autoimmune thyroiditis, chromosomal disorders such as Down and Turner syndromes, or an affected first-degree relative. These persons are frequently asymptomatic. Common symptoms include abdominal pain, anorexia, bloating, constipation and diarrhoea. Constitutional symptoms associated with coeliac disease may include weight loss, pubertal delay, arthritis and arthralgia, neurological symptoms, and anxiety or depression.

5.2. *Diagnosis*

Serological tests are a sensitive and specific way to screen for coeliac disease. If serology is positive (IgA tissue transglutaminase antibody or IgA anti-endomysial antibody) the diagnosis must be confirmed by upper gastrointestinal endoscopy and small intestinal mucosal biopsy while on a gluten containing diet. Diagnosis requires the characteristic findings on biopsy of intraepithelial lymphocytosis, crypt hyperplasia and villous atrophy.

5.3. *Treatment*

A lifelong gluten free diet is required which results in complete healing of the intestinal mucosa. The risk of complications is reduced when the patient is compliant. This is not easy and yearly follow up with coeliac disease is advisable. The adolescent patient and their parents require education by an experienced dietitian. Coeliac disease associations also provide excellent support for affected persons.

5.4. *Complications*

Osteoporosis occurs in all age groups and can be reversed by a gluten free diet. Peak bone mineralisation may be reduced in those diagnosed or nonadherent during late adolescence and these patients may have an increased risk of osteoporosis and fracture in adult life. Autoimmune disorders occur more frequently in persons with coeliac disease including Type 1 diabetes, thyroiditis, and autoimmune hepatitis. An increased risk of sepsis has also been reported. Although the overall risk is low, coeliac disease is associated with an increased risk of cancer, including T and B cell lymphoma and adenocarcinoma of the small intestine. This risk is estimated at twice the usual population risk, and compliance with a gluten free diet is considered protective. Refractory coeliac disease, which is not responsive to a gluten free diet, is a rare complication reported in young adults.

6. Inflammatory Bowel Disease

Around 20%–30% of cases present before the age of 20 years. The majority of these present in adolescence, with an incidence of 3–10/100,000 and a prevalence of 20–30/100,000.

6.1. *Types*

Ulcerative colitis is characterised by diffuse mucosal inflammation limited to the colon. Disease involves the rectum and may affect part of or the entire colon (pancolitis) in a continuous manner. Crohn's disease is associated with transmural or full thickness inflammation, which most commonly involves the ileum and colon, but can potentially affect any region of the gastrointestinal tract, from the mouth to the anus. Disease may be patchy with skip lesions. Indeterminate colitis is reserved for colitis where findings are not sufficient for either a diagnosis of UC or CD.

6.2. *Diagnosis*

This is the province of a specialist gastroenterologist and typically colonoscopy and/or endoscopy with biopsy will be required. Symptoms include abdominal pain, diarrhoea, rectal bleeding, weight loss, lethargy, and anorexia. Pubertal delay is frequent, particularly in CD. Examination may identify oral ulceration, pallor and finger clubbing. Extra-intestinal manifestations include erythema nodosum, iritis, and arthritis. It is essential to examine for perianal disease (abscess, fissure or perianal tags) as this may be an important clue to the diagnosis.

Laboratory investigations include full blood count looking for anaemia or thrombocytosis, inflammatory markers (ESR and C-reactive protein) which may be raised, liver function tests, and serum albumin which may be low. Stool cultures should be performed to exclude infectious diarrhoea. A technetium white cell scan is a useful screening test for IBD and for localisation of the site of intestinal disease. MRI scanning is frequently used to assess both disease extent and location and for complications, including stricture and perianal fistula. A Mantoux test and chest X-ray should be performed to exclude tuberculosis. The assessment of immunisation status with history and serology is important, given the likely requirement for immunosuppressive therapy.

6.3. *Treatment*

This aims to achieve remission and prevent relapse, and for the younger adolescent, the achievement of normal growth and pubertal development. First line therapy for UC and CD is usually glucocorticoids (prednisolone) given at high dose for 4–6 weeks and then gradually weaned. Exclusive enteral nutrition with a polymeric liquid feed (oral or naso-gastric tube) for 6–8 weeks is also effective for achieving remission in CD, and is particularly useful in the patient with malnutrition and pubertal delay. EEN avoids the complications of steroid therapy, but patients need significant support to achieve compliance.

Continuing therapy to prevent relapse requires supervision by a specialist gastroenterologist. Aminosalicylates, including sulphasalazine and mesalazine may be effective in mild disease, and are most useful in UC. Immunomodulators including azathioprine or 6-mercaptopurine, methotrexate or biological agents (including the anti tumour necrosis factor agents infliximab and adulimumab) may be required. Close monitoring is required as all these therapies present significant acute and long-term side effects, including hepatitis, pancreatitis, bone marrow failure, infection, and lymphoma.

Surgery may be required in refractory or complicated disease. Where the adolescent is unwell and affected by complications of the disease and medication, well timed surgery may be critical to allow the adolescent to achieve their full growth potential and normal progression through puberty. Colectomy is curative in UC. A two stage operation is usually required with subtotal colectomy and temporary ileostomy, followed by formation of a J-pouch and stoma closure. Surgery may be required urgently with fulminant colitis or toxic megacolon. Surgery in adolescents with CD cannot be regarded as curative. It is undertaken when severe disease has proven refractory to medical therapies, or with a life threatening complication. Complications may require drainage of collections or abscesses, and surgery to manage fibrotic strictures. If colectomy is required, a permanent ileostomy is likely in Crohn's disease — a difficult decision for the adolescent and their family. A permanent stoma has a significant impact on quality of life for the adolescent and into young adulthood.

Case History: James was referred at 14 years of age. He was easily fatigued, and had a poor appetite and recent onset of intermittent diarrhoea and lower abdominal pain. He was concerned that he was not growing. On examination, James was pale, thin (weight third percentile) and small (height 10th percentile). He was completely pre-pubertal. He was anaemic, with raised inflammatory markers and a low serum albumin. Colonoscopy identified CD of the ileocaecal region. James was initially treated with a course of prednisolone, but relapsed early during weaning, and had significant steroid side effects. He tolerated a six week course of

EEN and during this period began to gain weight. He developed pain on recommencement of a normal diet, despite the commencement of long term immunomodulator therapy with azathioprine. Abdominal ultrasound identified an inflammatory phlegmon at the caecum and MRI identified a stricture. After a period of total parental nutrition, James required surgery at 15 years of age to remove a short segment stricture in the ileocaecal region associated with a fistula. After surgery he remained well on maintenance azathioprine, and experienced a dramatic increase in growth velocity and began to progress through puberty.

7. Hereditary Polyposis Syndromes

Inherited polyposis syndromes are rare in adolescence, but when they occur, carry significant lifetime risks of malignancy. Those presenting in adolescence include familial adenomatous polyposis, Peutz–Jegher syndrome and juvenile polyposis syndrome. These are generally identified because of an affected first degree relative, but may occasionally be identified following colonoscopy for abnormal bowel habit or rectal bleeding. The hamartomatous lesions of PJS are typically located in the small intestine and the patient may present with abdominal pain, bowel obstruction, gastrointestinal bleeding, or intermittent intussusception. Patients with PJS may have characteristic facial hyperpigmentation, most commonly on the lips and buccal mucosa.

Hereditary polyposis syndromes are rare, and screening protocols vary according to the condition involved. Screening colonoscopy every 1–2 years may be required from as early as 10 years of age in FAP and prophylactic colectomy required in early adolescence due to the high risk of colon cancer with multiple polyps. The adolescent with PJS or JPS requires upper endoscopy and colonoscopy every 2–3 years. PJS is associated with a significant lifetime risk of malignancy (over 80%) and screening guidelines have been developed to monitor for cancers of other organs including the breast, testes, uterus, ovaries, and pancreas.

8. Pancreatitis

This may be acute or chronic in adolescence. Symptoms include acute epigastric pain, anorexia, nausea, and vomiting. In adolescence the most common causes of *acute pancreatitis* are biliary tract disease (usually cholelithiasis), trauma, infection such as enterovirus and mycoplasma, and drugs. The latter includes azathioprine, tetracyclines, sodium valproate, and asparaginase. Structural disorders such as pancreas divisum and annular pancreas are additional aetiologies. Causes of *chronic/recurrent pancreatitis* include hereditary pancreatitis, including mutations of cystic fibrosis transmembrane conductance regulator, serine protease inhibitor (SPINK1), and serine protease 1 (PSSR1) genes, autoimmune pancreatitis (associated with autoimmune disease including IBD), or metabolic disease such as hypercalcaemia, mitochondrial disease, hyperlipidaemia, and urea cycle defects. An increasing incidence of binge drinking and heavy use of alcohol in adolescents and young adults places them at risk of acute and chronic alcohol induced pancreatitis.

Treatment depends on the underlying cause and whether pancreatitis is complicated, for example by a pseudocyst (a collection of pancreatic fluid), severe necrosis or infection. The adolescent may require a period of gut rest along with pain relief. If symptoms are persistent or prolonged the patient will need investigation in a tertiary centre, with facilities for advanced investigation such as MRI and endoscopic retrograde cholangiopancreatography. Management includes nutritional support with jejunal feeding or parenteral nutrition.

9. Acute Liver Disease

In the adolescent this may be due to:

- An acute infective hepatitis, including hepatitis A, B, C and E, non A–G and EBV.
- Drugs, including paracetamol, sodium valproate, isoniazid.
- Toxins, including amanita phalloides (death cap) mushroom.
- Metabolic disease, including Wilson disease; an early diagnosis of Wilson disease, which is an abnormal accumulation of copper in the body resulting in liver and neuro-psychiatric disease, may allow a cure.
- Autoimmune hepatitis.
- Fatty liver of pregnancy.

In the initial assessment of the patient, fulminant liver failure needs to be considered as this requires urgent transfer to a centre with access to a liver transplantation program. Symptoms include lethargy and poor appetite, nausea, vomiting and diarrhoea, abdominal pain, and weight loss. On examination the patient may be jaundiced and have an enlarged and tender liver. Clinical signs such as finger clubbing, spider naevi, and splenomegaly, suggest chronic liver disease. Oedema, ascites, prominent bruising and encephalopathy suggest liver synthetic dysfunction and a need for urgent specialist management.

Worldwide, HAV is the commonest cause of viral hepatitis and is endemic in the developing world, where it is a significant cause of fulminant liver failure. Infection is sporadic in the developed world, where it is usually a self-limiting illness. HEV is an increasingly common cause of acute infective hepatitis in the developing world. HBV and HCV are most commonly associated with chronic and silent disease, acquired through vertical (mother to child) or horizontal (sexual, parenteral, or household) transmission, but may have an acute presentation. EBV is frequently associated with hepatitis in the adolescent patient, with a more severe course in an immunocompromised patient.

In the adolescent with fulminant liver failure, paracetamol toxicity (both acute overdose and chronic dosing) is a common cause and important to diagnose, as it is usually treatable with prompt use of N-acetyl cysteine infusion.

10. Chronic Liver Disease

Chronic liver disease is uncommon in the adolescent patient and has a spectrum of disease similar to that seen in an adult population. Although rare, it is important not to miss the diagnosis of chronic liver disease, as correct diagnosis and treatment are important to reduce long term morbidity. Presentation of chronic liver disease may include asymptomatic persons, identified by an incidental finding of abnormal liver function tests, or screening due to risk of viral hepatitis such as a family history of HBV. Some young people have an insidious onset of symptoms, which may include symptoms of fatigue, weight loss, abdominal discomfort, increasing jaundice, pruritis, bruising or oedema. Others present acutely unwell with fulminant hepatic failure, with a sudden onset of symptoms including jaundice, coagulopathy and encephalopathy.

10.1. *Causes of Chronic Liver Disease in the Adolescent*

- Congenital liver disease such as biliary atresia, progressive familial intrahepatic cholestasis and Allagille syndrome (which also has cardiac and renal abnormalities).
- Viral hepatitis is the most frequent cause worldwide, most commonly due to HBV and HCV.
- Autoimmune liver disease such as autoimmune hepatitis and sclerosing cholangitis.
- Wilson disease and other metabolic liver disease.
- Non alchoholic steatohepatitis: more frequent with the increasing prevalence of overweight and obese adolescents.
- Haemochromatosis may occur in adolescents receiving frequent blood transfusions for disorders such as thalassaemia, especially if adherence to chelation is poor. Hereditary haemochromatosis is an iron storage disorder resulting in liver disease in adult patients, and rarely associated with liver disease in adolescents. Adolescents, however, may be identified at risk of the disease by genetic screening after identification of affected parents and need to be monitored with iron studies to avoid iron overload, which when identified early is treatable with regular phlebotomy.

10.2. *Liver Transplantation*

Most patients do well with close to 80% long term survival. Compliance with long term immunosuppressive therapy is required to avoid graft rejection and may be problematical in adolescence. Most patients post liver transplantation in adolescence are in good health, but need ongoing regular monitoring. Increasing numbers of women transplanted in childhood have now achieved successful pregnancies.

11. Transitional Issues

Specialist to specialist transition is essential for the adolescent with a chronic gastrointestinal disorder, in particular IBD and chronic liver disease. Loss to follow up may have disastrous health consequences including relapse of disease with severe malnutrition in patients with IBD, liver failure in chronic liver disease or graft rejection post liver transplantation. There are specific issues for the adult physician caring for the adolescent with chronic gastroenterological disease. IBD has a significant impact on sexuality, pregnancy, and fertility. Chronic malnutrition, pubertal delay, the presence of severe perianal disease or a stoma will all have a major impact on body image and the adolescent's developing sexual identity and sexual function. The clinician should be proactive in seeking psychological assistance and in seeking ways through illness support groups to help young people work through such confronting issues.

Care also needs to be taken to avoid unwanted pregnancy. Contraception is mandatory when taking potentially teratogenic drugs such as mycophenylate mofetil for post transplant immunosupression and autoimmune hepatitis, and methotrexate for IBD. When disease is well controlled fertility in patients with IBD should be normal. Previous surgery and active disease can however impact on sexual function. In females, disease should be inactive prior to conception and potentially teratogenic therapy discontinued. Males will need medical care reviewed to avoid drugs such as methotrexate, and sulphasalazine because of effects on sperm motility (reversible).

Surveillance colonoscopy for bowel cancer may be required in the adolescent with longstanding IBD, particularly for UC when disease has been present for more than 10 years. This is best performed by an adult gastroenterologist experienced in screening colonoscopy and adenoma detection.

Education and management of risk taking behaviours in the context of chronic gastrointestinal disease is essential. Smoking has a significant negative impact on Crohn's disease. Alcohol intake, especially binge drinking, may worsen chronic liver disease and exacerbate recurrent pancreatitis.

Patients who are chronic carriers of HBV or HCV need to be educated about risks of transmission to others through sexual activity, and the sharing of toothbrushes and razors.

References

Blumberg R, Cho J, Lewis J, Wu G. (2011) Inflammatory bowel disease: An update on the fundamental biology and clinical management. *Gastroenterology* **140**(6): 1701–1703.

Di Sabatino A, Corazza GR. (2009) Coeliac disease. *Lancet* **373**(9673): 1480–1493.

Forsmark CE, Baillie J, AGA Institute Clinical Practice and Economics Committee. AGA Institute Governing Board (2007) AGA Institute technical review on acute pancreatitis. *Gastroenterology* **132**(5): 2022–2044.

Garza JM, Kaul A. (2010) Gastroesophageal reflux, eosinophilic esophagitis, and foreign body. *Pediatr Clin North Am* **57**(6): 1331–13245.

Huertas-Ceballos AA, Logan S, Bennett C, Macarthur C. (2008) Pharmacological interventions for recurrent abdominal pain (RAP) and irritable bowel syndrome (IBS) in childhood. *Cochrane Database Syst Rev* 2008, Issue 1. Art. No.: CD003017.

Hyams JS. (2004) Irritable bowel syndrome, functional dyspepsia, and functional abdominal pain syndrome. *Adolesc Med Clin* **15**(1): 1–15.

Jasperson KW, Tuohy TM, Neklason DW, Burt RW. (2010) Hereditary and familial colon cancer. *Gastroenterology* **138**(6): 2044–2058.

Koletzko S, Jones NL, Goodman KJ, Gold B, Rowland M, Cadranel S, Chong S, Colletti RB, Casswall T, Elitsur Y, Guarner J, Kalach N, Madrazo A, Megraud F, GO. (2011) Evidence-based guidelines from ESPGHAN and NASPGHAN for helicobacter pylori infection in children. *J Pediatr Gastroenterol Nutr* **53**(2): 230–243.

McColl KEL. (2010) Clinical practice. Helicobacter pylori infection. *N Engl J Med* **362**(17): 1597–604.

Nydegger A, Couper RTL, Oliver MR. (2006) Childhood pancreatitis. *J Gastroenterol Hepatol* **21**(3): 499–509.

Chapter 40

Common Dermatological Problems in Adolescents

Anuja Elizabeth George

1. Introduction

Adolescence is the time when skin and hair become more greasy, a body odour develops and disorders such as acne make their appearance for the first time, with effects on self-image and self-esteem. Although a variety of dermatological disorders can occur during adolescence, certain conditions like acne and dandruff are more common and affect almost all adolescents at some time, because these are due to normal development.

2. Dermatological Conditions Which Mainly Occur in Adolescence

2.1. *Acne*

Acne is the most common skin disorder of adolescents, affecting about 85% of teenagers. It is more physiological than a disease process, and generally self limiting. Picking and squeezing of acne leads to scarring called 'acne excorie' which may persist for life.

525

2.1.1. *Pathogenesis*

Androgens play a major role in the development of acne. More than 75% of circulating androgens are bound to sex hormone binding globulin, 15%–20% to albumin and the rest is free. It is the free androgen that acts on the end organs. Oestrogens increase the plasma SHBG, thus reducing free androgens. Androgens stimulate sebaceous glands to secrete sebum which is responsible for the increased oiliness in areas with the most sebaceous glands like the scalp, face, and upper trunk. The exact mechanism of formation of the primary lesion in acne, the comedo, is unknown. Altered keratinisation and retention hyperkeratosis in sebaceous follicles, either *de novo* or due to effects of circulating sex hormones; the amount and quality of sebum secreted; follicular microbial flora; immunological factors; and environmental factors all affect development of acne. There is increased colonisation of *Propionibacterium acnes* in sebaceous glands. These metabolise the sebum to form free fatty acids, which cause inflammation resulting in the clinical picture of acne. *P. granulosum* and *Staphylococcus epidermidis* also play a role. Premenstrual flare is due to changes in hydration of pilosebaceous epithelium. Stress also has a significant role in increasing acne.

2.1.2. *Clinical features of acne*

Acne is characterised by closed comedos or white heads, open comedos or black heads (due to presence of oxidised melanin in the keratinous material blocking the sebaceous canal), papules, pustules, nodules, and cysts. Other lesions are icepick scars and atrophic macules, due to decreased collagen synthesis and keloidal scars. Post-inflammatory hyperpigmentation also occurs. Acne may be arbitrarily graded into:

Grade. 1 (Mild) where there are comedos and occasional papules.
Grade. 2 (Moderate) with papules, comedos, and a few pustules.
Grade. 3 (Severe) with predominant pustules, nodules, and abscesses.
Grade. 4 (Cystic) with mainly cysts, abscesses, and widespread scarring.

- Acne vulgaris is the most common variant in adolescents.
- Acne conglobata is a chronic inflammatory type of acne seen more in men.
- Acne fulminans is an acute ulcerative type with systemic features such as fever, musculoskeletal pain, and even osteolytic changes. Differential diagnoses of acne include acneform eruptions, usually induced by drugs, and acne rosacea.

2.1.3. *Problems associated with acne*

Acne may lead to loss of self-image and self-esteem, and is associated with an increased incidence of depression, suicidal ideation and suicidal attempts. Treatment failures may be due to the lack of education of the patient regarding acne management, resistant *P. acnes*, and the apparent flare due to Gram negative folliculitis.

2.1.4. *Management*

Mild acne needs topical therapy alone. Mild to moderate acne may require the addition of oral agents. Moderate to severe acne requires both topical and oral medication, while severe acne and nodulocystic acne are managed with oral isotretinoin, with or without antibiotics and topical agents.

2.1.4.1. Topical therapy in acne

Topical agents may be grouped based on their predominant action.

Anti-comedogenic agents: these include adapalene (the only retinoid with anti-inflammatory effects within the first few days); all-trans-retinoic acid; azelaic acid; isotretinoin and tazarotene. Isotretinoin and tazarotene are to be avoided in pregnancy.

Antimicrobial agents: azelaic acid; benzoyl peroxide; erythromycin and clindamycin. Zinc may be an added ingredient with beneficial effects.

Anti-inflammatory agents: adapalene; antibiotics and salicylic acid.

In mixed infections, anti-comedogenic agents may be given at night and the anti-inflammatory agent with antibacterial agents in the morning. All topical agents can produce irritant dermatitis, which may require steriods and moisturisers for management. Topical agents may have to be continued for some years.

2.1.4.2. Oral therapy in acne

Antibiotics: these are indicated in moderate to severe acne. Treatment can be given for six months, but if no improvement is seen within three months, treatment should be changed. The commonly used antibiotics belong to the tetracycline group: tetracycline 1 gm/day initially and maintained at 250–500 mg/day, doxycycline (100–200 mg/day) and minocycline (50–100 mg/day). The latter two have better compliance as a once a day dosage. Side effects include phototoxicity, fixed drug eruption, onycholysis, and benign intracranial hypertension. Minocycline can also induce bluish pigmentation especially on sun exposed areas. Since tetracyclines are contraindicated in pregnancy, erthyromycin (same dose as tetracycline) can be used in pregrancy.

Hormones: this therapy is used in females with severe acne not responding to usual treatment measures. These include the oral contraceptive pill (taking care to use a progestogen which is not androgenic) and spironolactone, at a dose of 100–200 mg/day for six months. Cyclical ethinylestradiol (30 µg/day) with medroxyprogesterone acetate (5 mg/day) for seven days of the cycle is also used. Side effects include weight gain and melasma (skin pigmentation) with the contraceptive, and menstrual irregularities with spironolactone.

Retinoids: isotretinoin at a dose of 0.5–1 mg/kg/day for 20 weeks will give long term remission in 70% of patients. It is the only treatment effective against all aetiological factors, as it reduces sebum secretion, *P. acnes* colonisation, comedo formation, and inflammation. It is indicated where conventional treatment fails, in severe acne, scarring, Gram negative folliculitis and dysmorphogenesis. The most serious side effect is teratogenicity. Counselling and adequate contraception are essential, and written informed consent obtained. However, retinoids are better avoided in women of reproductive age. Other unwanted effects are acne flare; muco-cutaneous changes which include crusting, flaking, cheilitis, and conjunctivitis; arthralgia; hyperlipidaemia and hepatotoxicity (regular liver function tests to be done).

Miscellaneous: zinc has beneficial effects. Ibuprofen, clofazimine, oral vitamin A and anxiolytics have been tried with variable results.

2.1.4.3. Physical modalities for acne treatment

These include mechanical extraction of the comedo, superficial freezing, cryosurgery for nodules older than a week, and intralesional triamcinolone for nodules less than a week old. Cosmetic procedures like camouflage and chemical peels; dermatosurgical procedures for treatment of scars by excision, subcision, dermabrasion, collagen injection, gelatin matrix implants, and keloid surgery are now widely accepted modalities for treatment of acne.

2.2. *Dandruff and Seborrhoeic Dermatitis*

Seborrhoeic dermatitis is a common superficial eczematous dermatitis affecting the areas of the body with maximum seborrhoeic activity, and with the onset around puberty. Dandruff is the mildest form of seborrhoeic dermatitis and is considered to be its precursor. It affects 3%–5% of young adults. It is characterised by visible desquamation of the scalp skin without signs of inflammation.

2.2.1. *Pathogenesis*

The major aetiological factor responsible for seborrhoeic dermatitis is androgen and so it is more common in males. Patients with seborrhoeic dermatitis, have reduced cell mediated immunity to *Malassezia furfur*, the aetiological agent of pityriosporum versicolor.

2.2.2. *Clinical features*

A distinct pattern of distribution is seen with involvement of areas with maximum sebaceous gland activity. Pruritus is common. The commonest and earliest change is pityriasis sicca or dandruff without inflammation, which may progress through perifollicular redness, irritation, and increased scaling. Loss of hair is significant, but is reversible in the early stages. On the face, the nasolabial area, eyebrows, eyelid margins, below the lips and beard area, forehead and chin are involved. On the trunk, the presternal and interscapular areas as well as the hairy flexures are involved. The differential diagnosis of seborrhoeic dermatitis includes psoriasis, infective dermatitis due to Pediculosis capitis and rosacea.

2.2.3. *Treatment*

Although there is no permanent cure, most patients respond well to conventional treatments. These include twice a week use of shampoos containing selenium sulfide, zinc pyrithione, ketoconazole 2%, terbinafine 1%, tar, steroids, fluconazole, or cyclopirox olamine. For seborrhoeic dermatitis of face and body, topical hydrocortisone 5% with ketoconazole 2%; benzoyl peroxide creams and UVB therapy are used. Oral ketoconazole (200 mg daily for two weeks); itraconazole (100 mg daily for three weeks) and in severe cases, systemic steroids and isotretinoin have been found to be beneficial for generalised or exfoliative dermatitis. Seborrhoeic dermatitis is usually self limiting with age.

2.3. *Disorders of Hair Growth*

Testosterone and its metabolism to 5-alpha-dihydrotestosterone by 5-alpha-reductase play a role in the development of hair in a male pattern distribution, including temporal recession which commences during male puberty. There are strong genetic influences on hair growth and distribution.

2.3.1. *Hirsutism*

Excessive unwanted terminal hair growth in unacceptable sites in women is termed hirsutism. The hair follicles in different regions of the body respond variably due to the differences in the number of androgen receptors or their sensitivity to androgens or due to differences in androgen metabolism. The amount of hair that causes anxiety and depression in one adolescent, may be seen as within the normal range for female family members by another.

2.3.1.1. Causes of hirsutism

For the majority of women, no clear cause is found and it is labelled idiopathic. Polycystic ovarian syndrome is a common pathological cause in adolescents and young adults. The occurrence of hirsutism along with features of virilisation or menstrual irregularities, should make one suspect endocrine pathology and referral for further endocrine investigation and management is essential.

2.3.1.2. Management of hirsutism

The primary aim is to treat any underlying cause and prevent further hair growth. Cosmetic modalities include bleaching the hair, shaving, plucking, and waxing or using depilatory creams, electrolysis and laser therapy. Electrolysis gives a permanent result but it is both painful and costly if large areas require treatment. Laser therapy also gives a permanent result and is also costly. The best laser results are seen with the combination of dark hair on light coloured skin. It is advisable to trial a patch of skin first.

Oral contraceptives act directly by reducing androgens and indirectly by increasing SHBG, which in turn reduces the bioavailability of androgens, and are suppressive rather than curative. Systemic anti-androgens take 6–12 months for sufficient miniaturisation of terminal hairs, and signs of improvement, such as slower and finer hair growth, take about three months. The agents commonly used are cyproterone acetate (in combination with ethinyl estradiol) and spironolactone. Pure anti-androgens such as flutamide and nilutamide are useful in idiopathic hirsutism, but their availability varies from country to country. Finasteride is a 5-alpha-reductase inhibitor and results in reduction of facial hair diameter within three months. Eflornithine applied topically reduces hair growth by blocking the formation of putrescine from ornithine that is necessary for the growth of hair follicles.

2.3.2. *Hypertrichosis*

Hypertrichosis is excess hair in normal locations, which is not as thick or pigmented as that seen in hirsutism. Cyclosporin, minoxidil, diazoxide, glucocorticoids, phenytoin, streptomycin, and interferons are recognised causes. POEMS (polyneuropathy, organomegaly, endocrinopathy, monoclonal gammopathy, skin changes) syndrome, juvenile dermatomyositis, hypothyroidism, malabsorption syndrome, and malignancies are also associated with hypertrichosis. Adolescents and young adults who have had solid organ transplants often have generalised hypertrichosis due to cyclosporin and glucocorticoid therapy. Adolescents with anorexia nervosa develop a covering of fine downy hair on the body called lanugo hair which disappears when healthy eating habits are resumed. The treatment of hypertrichosis is along the same lines as that for hirsutism.

2.3.3. *Alopecia*

Alopecia refers to loss of hair and may be localised (alopecia areata) or diffuse. Seborrhoeic dermatitis, fungal infections, anaemia, protein and vitamin deficiencies, thyroid dysfunction, PCOS, post-infection and febrile illness, haematological and other metabolic disorders and psychological stress have all been implicated in its aetiology. Treatment is aimed at the underlying cause.

2.4. *Disorders of Sweat Glands*

2.4.1. *Bromhidrosis (osmidrosis)*

This is excessive offensive odour of the skin. It may be *apocrine* bromhidrosis due to the degradation of the axillary apocrine sweat by gram positive bacteria or *eccrine* bromhidrosis due to alteration of the eccrine sweat. Apocrine bromhidrosis has its onset only in adolescence due to the dormant nature of these glands prior to puberty. Apocrine sweat which is sterile and odourless when it first appears on the skin develops the classic acrid odour within one hour by the bacterial degradation of sweat. Eccrine bromhidrosis occurs at all ages. Bromhidrosis may be controlled with regular cleansing of the axilla with germicidal soaps, shaving of axillary hair, and use of axillary deodorants and antiperspirants. Q-switched Nd:YAG laser and botulinum toxin A are recently introduced successful treatments.

2.4.2. *Chromhidrosis*

This is the secretion of coloured sweat due to increased secretion of lipo-fuschins in sweat. Apocrine chromhidrosis occurs only at puberty or early adult life, and is noticed as either yellow or less commonly green, blue, or blue black staining of undershirts and even the axillary skin. There is no effective management, but it may be controlled with repeated washing of the area with soaps or organic solvents.

2.4.3. *Fox–Fordyce disease or apocrine miliaria*

This is a chronic itchy, smooth, round papular eruption affecting the apocrine gland bearing areas like the axilla and pubis, and also the mammary areola, and which has its onset after puberty. It is due to obstruction of the intra-epidermal part of the apocrine sweat gland which then ruptures resulting in inflammation. There is no permanent cure, though antibiotic and steroid lotions, intra-lesional triamcinolone, and retinoids are of some use.

2.4.4. *Hidradenitis suppurativa*

This is a chronic suppurative, scarring disease of axillae, inframammary area, buttocks, and ano–genital areas. It starts as simple acne like boils which then develop into abcesses which rupture, yielding a seropurulent discharge. This heals with scarring but recurs and forms sinus tracks with thick bands of fibrosis. Axillary, inguinal, and mammary hidradenitis are more common in females, while perianal involvement is more common in males. Treatment in the early stages is mainly medical, while in the later stages scarred and fibrotic lesions with sinus tract formation often require surgical management.

2.4.5. *Hyperhidrosis*

Excessive sweating of palms, soles, and axillae is common in adolescents and young adults, and is mostly due to emotional or neural stimulation. Primary hyperhidrosis is inherited as an autosomal dominant disorder and usually has an onset during adolescence. Secondary hyperhidrosis may start at any age and may be due to endocrine disorders such as hyperthyroidism or growth hormone excess or drugs such as zinc supplements, desipramine, nortryptyline, and paracetamol, ciprofloxacin, and omeprazole. The current therapy with local injections of botulinum toxin is very effective.

2.5. *Disturbances of Melanin Pigmentation*

2.5.1. *Naevi*

Certain naevi are peculiar by their development in puberty. Becker's naevus is usually seen in males as a uniform segmental hyper-pigmentation of the pectoral area. Hypertrichosis of the overlying skin with smooth muscle hamartomas, skeletal defects, and acneform papules may be seen. Laser removal of the naevus is effective. Naevus spilus has small deeply pigmented macules on a background of light tan pigmentation.

2.5.2. *Other pigmentation disorders*

Reticular acropigmentation of Kitamura, reticulate pigmented anomaly of the flexures (Dowling–Degos disease) and hereditary acanthosis nigricans are disorders with autosomal dominant traits which tend to develop during adolescence. Naevus of Ito involving the areas innervated by the trigeminal nerve and naevus of Ota in the distribution of the supraclavicular and lateral brachiocutaneous nerves develop and darken during adolescence. Erythema dyschromicum perstans (ashy dermatosis) is a progressive, symmetric blue grey pigmentation of the face, arms, and trunk with an onset in the first or second decade of life.

3. Other Dermatological Conditions which Occur in Adolescence

3.1. *Infections*

3.1.1. *Fungal infections*

Common superficial mycosis seen in the adolescent are dermatophytosis, tinea versicolor, piedra, candidiasis, and tinea nigra. Among the dermatophytoses, the involvement of the groins (tinea cruris) and pressure sites on the trunk (tinea corporis) are common. Heat, humidity, excessive perspiration, use of tight synthetic occlusive undergarments, and lack of hygiene all encourage fungal growth. A diagnosis can easily be confirmed by microscopic examination of the scrapings from the skin lesions. Treatment with topical azoles (clotrimazole, miconazole, econazole, ketoconazole), terbinafine, Whitfield's ointment, or ciclopirox olamine usually controls the infection. Systemic fluconazole 150 mg once weekly for 4–6 weeks, or itraconazole 200 mg/day for six weeks, may be needed in severe forms to attain complete cure.

Pityriasis versicolor presents as macules and patches of different colours with fine bran-like scales on the upper trunk and upper arms. Diagnosis is confirmed by skin scrapings. Topical selenium sulfide 2.5% applied daily for 10 minutes for 7–10 days, clotrimazole, ketoconazole, miconazole, and ciclopirox olamine creams or lotions are all beneficial.

Piedra is a superficial fungal infection of the hair shaft or scalp. *Piedraia hortae* causes black piedra with distinct brownish black, hard, gritty pin head sized nodules firmly attached to hair with eventual breakage of hair. Less common is white piedra caused by *Trichosporon asahii*. There is no complete cure. Clipping or shaving of hair, and drying and steaming of hair along with topical antifungals give relief.

3.1.2. *Viral infections*

Verruca vulgaris or warts is a common viral infection caused by the human papilloma virus. Lesions are most often seen on the hands, feet and forearms. On the face, the smooth flatter hyper-pigmented papules termed verruca plana or plane warts are more common. Electrosurgical or cryosurgical removal of warts is the usual treatment. Molluscum contagiosum is a viral infection caused by the pox virus and presents as shiny, pearly white or erythematous dome shaped papules with a central umbilication. Trichloroacetic acid or phenol cautery along with curettage of the lesions is curative.

3.2. *Infestations*

3.2.1. *Scabies*

Scabies is a parasitic infestation of skin caused by the itch mite *Sarcoptes scabei* var. hominis. Close contact with an infected person for as little as

15–20 minutes, and overcrowding, lead to rapid spread of the disease. There is intense itching, which is worse at night. The characteristic sites of involvement are the inter-digital spaces, flexors of wrist, elbow, anterior axillary folds, inner thighs, umbilicus, external genitalia in males, and the nipple and areola in females. The presence of burrows in the web space, wrists, or penis, and the demonstration of mites as well as an exposure history form the criteria for diagnosis. Post streptococcal glomerulonephritis arising from secondary pyoderma of the lesions, eczematisation, lichenification, and urticaria are known complications. Treatment is using permethrin 5% or gamma benzene hexachloride 1% applied all over the body a single time and washed off after 12 hours. Benzyl benzoate 25%, with three consecutive applications 12 hours apart, is a cheaper option. Single oral use of ivermectin, 2 µg/kg body weight, is also effective.

3.2.2. *Pediculosis capitis*

Pediculosis capitis or louse infestation of the scalp presents with intense pruritus of the scalp. Lice are seen more often on the post auricular area and lower hair margin but mostly it is only the nits (eggs) which can be seen, as shiny oval bodies firmly attached to the hair shaft. Secondary pyoderma and cervical lymphadenopathy are common complications. Permethrin 1% or gamma benzene hexachloride 1% lotion application to hair and scalp help to cure the condition.

3.2.3. *Pediculosis pubis*

Pediculosis pubis (phthiriasis) is a common infestation of the pubic area, eyelashes, and axilla by crab louse or *Phthirus pubis*, which may be seen as greyish specks, firmly attached to skin, or its nits may be seen attached to the hair. Treatment is using lindane cream 1% or shampoo, and clothes should be laundered and ironed. Pediculosis pubis is a sexually transmitted disease, and treatment of any sexual contacts is required.

3.2.4. *Larva migrans*

Larva migrans is a creeping eruption due to the cat and dog hookworm larvae. It starts as local itching, papules followed by thin tortuous lines which migrate at the rate of 2 cm per day. Thiabendazole for two days, and extraction of larva with a needle give good results.

3.3. *Eczema*

3.3.1. *Atopic dermatitis*

Atopic dermatitis is an endogenous eczema of no definite aetiology. Diagnostic criteria include four major and 23 minor criteria, from among which, if any three of either group are positive, atopic dermatitis may be diagnosed. *Major criteria* include pruritus; typical morphology, and distribution with flexural lichenification; chronic or chronically-relapsing dermatitis and a personal or family history of atopy (asthma, allergic rhinitis, atopic dermatitis). *Minor criteria* include xerosis, ichthyosis, immediate (type 1) skin-test reactivity; raised serum IgE; eczema of the nipples; keratoconus, anterior subcapsular cataracts; itch when sweating, and intolerance to wool and lipid solvents; food intolerance, and white dermographism or delayed blanch. There are three phases in atopic dermatitis, of which the adolescent phase is a transition period to the adult phase, and is characterised by pruritic lichenification with flexural predilection. Treatment is by keeping the skin well hydrated with emollients, the judicious use of topical steroids, and avoidance of known triggers.

3.3.2. *Contact dermatitis*

Both irritant and allergic types may occur in adolescence. Allergic contact dermatitis to nickel containing ear and neck jewellery, nail polishes, cosmetics, footwear, and deodorants are a few examples.

3.3.3. *Photodermatitis*

Photodermatitis is an abnormal skin reaction to UV rays, either as an eczematous allergic response to a sensitising agent such as perfume or as a toxic sun burn response to drugs including tetracyclines, sulfonylureas, tricyclic antidepressants and retinoids. Reducing sun exposure is the most important part of prevention and of treatment.

3.3.4. *Sun damage, including solariums*

While most young people are aware of the risk of sun damage, a large percentage fail to follow the public health messages about sunscreen, covering up, sunglasses and hats, and shade. Thus they place themselves at risk of long term sun damage which includes early skin ageing, cataracts, skin cancers, and melanoma. Melanoma is the most lethal skin cancer and is related to early onset sun exposure and severe sun burn. A history of sun exposure should be part of a risk taking history and premature skin ageing may be an incentive to reduce sun exposure. There should be specific discussion about the absolute danger of sun beds and solariums, whatever the proprietors claim about safety. The use of self-tanning sprays and creams is a safe alternative.

3.4. *Papulosquamous Disorders*

3.4.1. *Pityrasis rosea*

This is a self limiting skin rash of possible human herpes virus aetiology (HHV-6,7). A single large round erythematous herald patch is followed about 10 days later by multiple smaller oval lesions. There is usually a history of a preceding upper respiratory infection. There may be itching and spontaneous resolution which usually occurs within which six weeks. Antihistamines and emollients are useful.

3.4.2. *Psoriasis*

Psoriasis is a chronic disorder with genetic predisposition and which has an unpredictable course with remissions and exacerbations affecting mainly the skin and joints. It is a T-cell mediated inflammatory disorder of skin with a multilocus model of inheritance with specific HLA-cw6 association. Streptococcal infection, lithium, beta blockers, and antimalarial drugs are known precipitating factors. It has a varied clinical presentation with well-defined erythematous plaques and papules covered with silvery white micaceous scales with an extensor predilection. Nail lesions include pitting, subungual hyperkeratosis, onycholysis, and yellowish discoloration.

Psoriatic arthritis classically affects distal interphalangeal joints. Treatment is with topical keratolytics and anitimitotics, tetracyclines, omega-3 fatty acids, dapsone, clofazimine, methotrexate, cyclosporin, retinoids, phototherapy, retinoids in combination with PUVA therapy, and hydroxyurea. Biological drugs such as etanercept, infliximab, alefacept, and efalizumab which specifically affect immunological targets responsible for psoriasis have proved useful.

3.4.3. *Lichen planus*

Lichen planus is a disease of unknown aetiology, characterised by the presence of intensely pruritic, flat papules with a violaceous hue, mainly affecting the flexural aspects of the forearm, lower limbs, abdominal walls, and oral mucosa. Treatment is symptomatic with antihistamines and topical emollients. Steroids, including systemic steroids, and anxiolytics are used in the more generalised eruptive form.

3.5. *Urticaria*

Urticarias are vascular reactions characterised by oedematous, evanescent, erythematous or whitish lesions on the skin and mucosa called wheals. Angioedema refers to the giant wheals on skin or mucosal surfaces which involve the subcutaneous tissue. The causes of urticaria are varied and may follow infections (viral, streptococcal), helminthic infestations, use of drugs or certain foods. Urticaria may also be associated with connective tissue disorders, or may be physically triggered by heat, sweating, cold, sunlight and the use of vibratory equipment. Hereditary angioedema and papular urticaria are specific types of urticaria. Treatment is difficult as long as the definite cause remains obscure. Antihistamines and steroids and sometimes other immunosuppressives are used to control the wheals.

3.6. *Tattooing and Piercing*

While not strictly a skin disorder, tattooing and body piercing are important conditions which involve adolescent and young adult skin. Both these forms of skin decoration have been practised for centuries and have often been used to define cultural sub-groups. Clinicians should ask young people about their views and intentions as these relate to body decoration. This allows them to counsel the young person and help them to think through their attitudes and plans before they are placed in a situation of risk.

Tattooing is permanent, and many adolescents and young adults have their first tattoo while under the influence of alcohol or other drugs, or while on vacation when they are less likely to be able to ensure aseptic techniques. Fresh equipment, disposable needles, surgical gloves, and proper sterilising equipment all reduce the risk of blood borne viral transmission, including hepatitis and HIV/AIDS. Laser therapy can be used to remove tattoos with variable results.

At least a third of adolescents have their first piercing before the age of 18 years. There are a number of complications which may result. The common ones are hypersensitivity reactions and local infection, which need prompt treatment to avoid serious sepsis particularly in the immuno-compromised adolescent. Abscess formation and blood borne disease due to lack of aseptic technique, chondritis, and keloid formation can also occur.

4. Conclusion

Almost all the skin diseases affecting the adult population can present during adolescence and young adulthood. Adolescence, with the specific hormone changes of puberty, heralds the onset of skin conditions different to those of childhood. As skin is the most visible of body organs, conditions which affect it may have a major impact on psychosocial well-being. As many dermatological conditions are not curable, the adolescent will need considerable clinician and family support to continue with treatments over months or years.

References

Ayer J, Burrows N. (2006) Acne: More than skin deep. *Postgrad Med J* **82**(970): 500–506.

Bhidayasiri R, Truong DD. (2008) Evidence for effectiveness of botulinum toxin for hyperhidrosis. *J Neural Transm* **115**(4): 641–645.

Gollnick H, Cunliffe W, Berson D, Dreno B, Finlay A, Leyden JJ, Shalita AR, Thiboutot D. Global Alliance to Improve Outcomes in Acne. (2003) Management of acne: A report from a global alliance to improve outcomes in acne. *J Am Acad Dermatol* **49**(1): S1–37.

Hay RJ, Graham-Brown RA. (1997) Dandruff and seborrhoeic dermatitis: Causes and management. *Clin Exp Dermatol* **22**(1): 3–6.

Heckmann M, Teichmann B, Pause BM, Plewig G. (2003) Amelioration of body odor after intracutaneous axillary injection of botulinum toxin a. *Arch Dermatol* **139**(1): 57–59.

Holt DC, Mccarthy JS, Carapetis JR. (2010) Parasitic diseases of remote indigenous communities in Australia. *Int J Parasitol* **40**(10): 1119–1126.

James W, Berger D, Timothy G, Elston D. (2006) *Andrews' Diseases of the Skin: Clinical Dermatology*. Elsevier, Saunders.

James WD. (2005) Clinical practice. Acne. *N Engl J Med* **352**(14): 1463–1472.

Johnson BA, Nunley JR. (2000) Treatment of seborrheic dermatitis. *Am Fam Physician* **61**(9): 2703–2710, 2713–2714.

Purvis D, Robinson E, Merry S, Watson P. (2006) Acne, anxiety, depression and suicide in teenagers: A cross-sectional survey of New Zealand secondary school students. *J Paediatr Child Health* **42**(12): 793–796.

Sellheyer K, Krahl D. (2005) "Hidradenitis suppurativa" is acne inversa! An appeal to (finally) abandon a misnomer. *Int J Dermatol* **44**(7): 535–540.

Chapter 41

Common Haematological Conditions
in Adolescence

Julie Curtin

1. Haematological Changes in Adolescence

Under the influence of pubertal hormones, the total red cell mass increases, as well as the haemoglobin and mean cell volume. The higher testosterone in adult males is the reason that there is the observed adult differential in haemoglobin between males and females. Whilst most laboratories report reference ranges in relation to chronological age, it is important to also consider pubertal development in the assessment of full blood count results from an adolescent. As an example, a male with significant pubertal delay may have a haemoglobin level below the lower limit of an age defined range. Furthermore, the physiological changes that occur in puberty can result in haematological symptoms or abnormalities. For example, the rapid expansion of red cell mass in males may unmask a borderline deficient iron status, including iron deficiency anaemia. The dysfunctional uterine bleeding seen in some teenage girls at menarche may also lead to anaemia. Very occasionally the presumed menorrhagia of dysfunctional uterine bleeding may be the first presentation of a mild bleeding disorder, such as von Willebrand disease, which has previously gone undiagnosed.

543

2. Anaemia in Adolescents

Whilst there are many possible causes, both inherited and acquired, that may cause anaemia, iron deficiency remains the most common cause of anaemia in this population. Symptoms of anaemia will depend on the rapidity of onset and degree of anaemia. Other causes of anaemia include blood loss, thalassaemia and other haemoglobinopathies, autoimmune disease with haemolysis, marrow failure and marrow infiltration, inherited membrane and enzyme defects, and the anaemia of chronic disease.

2.1. *Iron Deficiency*

2.1.1. *Aetiology*

Adolescents are at particular risk for iron deficiency, mainly because their increased needs for iron during physical growth may not be met by their dietary intake. For males, the iron requirements are highest during peak height growth spurt in late puberty as a result of the expansion of the total blood volume, and the increase in lean body mass and muscle myoglobin. For females, as well as having increased requirements during peak height growth spurt in early puberty, the onset of menses means that their iron requirements remain high after menarche. Furthermore irregular and heavy periods may not be reported to care providers, placing females at increased risk of developing iron deficiency anaemia. Adolescents who undertake intensive physical training or endurance sports are at increased risk of iron deficiency, as a result of both skin and gut iron loss. Adolescents who are overweight or obese are also at increased risk of iron deficiency. The suggested mechanism is an increase in hepcidin levels derived from adipose tissue which inhibit the absorption of dietary iron and the release of iron from storage sites. Other underlying diseases such as inflammatory bowel disease and coeliac disease are rare but important causes of iron deficiency in adolescents.

Certain groups of adolescents are particularly at risk for iron deficiency because their increased needs may not be met by their diet. These groups include those who restrict their intake of red meat for moral (such as choosing vegetarianism) or cultural reasons, those who undertake frequent dieting and restrictive eating, skipping of meals and macrobiotic or other fad diets. Iron deficiency in a pre-menarchal adolescent may indicate a restrictive eating disorder, particularly if the anaemia is associated with loss of body weight or failure to gain weight.

2.1.2. *Prevalence*

Population studies suggest that only one quarter of adolescent females and women of childbearing age meet the recommended dietary allowance for iron through diet. Iron deficiency is the most prevalent nutrient deficiency in the world. There is some variation in reported incidences due to inconsistency in definitions and criteria used. The recent HELENA study, using the approach recommended by the WHO for defining iron status, looked at 940 adolescents without evidence of inflammation across 10 European cities. This study found that 17.6% of adolescents were iron depleted with females affected more than males (21.0% versus 13.8%). Iron deficiency was seen in 5.4% of females and 3.9% of males, and iron deficiency anaemia was seen in 0.5% of males and 2.0% of females.

2.1.3. *Symptoms of iron deficiency*

Iron deficiency is usually minimally symptomatic until iron deficiency anaemia occurs. Then symptoms include tiredness, fatigue, reduced aerobic sports performance, lack of concentration, and impaired memory and cognitive performance.

2.1.4. *Diagnosis of iron deficiency*

Examination of the FBC and blood film will usually suggest the diagnosis. The classical picture is that of a hypochromic/microcytic anaemia, although in the early stages of iron deficiency careful examination of the blood film may show a small population of hypochromic/microcytic cells in a patient with normal red cell indices. It should be emphasised that not all hypochromic/microcytic anaemias are due to iron deficiency, as haemoglobinopathies such as thalassaemia minor may produce a similar picture.

Serum ferritin is the most useful test in the diagnosis of iron deficiency. In healthy people, it accurately reflects iron stores; a level below normal is diagnostic of iron deficiency. However, ferritin is an acute phase reactant and may be raised into the normal level despite the presence of iron deficiency. In adolescents with indeterminate ferritin levels a therapeutic trial of oral iron may be instituted. Iron deficiency is confirmed by the presence of a reticulocytosis at one week and a rise in haemoglobin, usually in the order of 0.5–1.0 g/week.

2.1.5. *Treatment of iron deficiency*

Treatment of iron deficiency in adolescents involves iron replacement as well as addressing dietary causes of iron deficiency. Iron replacement should be given in divided doses of 150–200 mg of elemental iron per day. Combination of iron with vitamin C improves the absorption of iron.

2.2. *Haemoglobinopathies*

Haemoglobinopathies are disorders in the production of the alpha- or beta-globin chains of haemoglobin. These disorders may result in the production of an abnormal Hb molecule (for example Hb S) or reduced production of a normal globin chain (thalassaemic disorders). Major haemoglobinopathies such as sickle cell disease and thalassaemia major are usually diagnosed in childhood. However, milder disorders such as thalassaemia minor, or trait, may remain undiagnosed into adolescence. Classically thalassaemia trait causes microcytic, hypochromic red cells. Anaemia if present is usually mild. Thalassaemia trait is an important differential in the diagnosis of iron deficiency. The diagnosis of β thalassaemia trait (due to reduced production of beta-globin chains) is usually straightforward with a raised Hb A_2 seen on Hb EPG. Alpha thalassaemia trait (due to reduced production of alpha-globin chains) may be more difficult to diagnose, and is often a diagnosis of exclusion. DNA analysis gives a definitive diagnosis but is not routinely performed. Thalassaemia trait is usually of no consequence to the patient, but as these conditions are due to mutations in the alpha- or beta-globin genes, these may be passed onto the patient's offspring. If their partner also has a haemoglobinopathy the couple need to be counselled regarding the risks of a serious haemo-globinopathy in their offspring.

2.2.1. *Thalassaemia major*

This is a severe transfusion dependent anaemia that typically presents in late infancy in patients who are homozygous or compound heterozygous for two β thalassaemic mutations. These patients are typically transfused every four weeks and this treatment must continue for life. Whilst regular transfusions correct the anaemia, these unfortunately lead to iron loading of the patient with potentially serious consequences. The iron deposits, in particular in the liver, endocrine glands and heart, lead to problems with growth and pubertal progression, and the development of cirrhosis, diabetes mellitus, and ultimately arrhythmias and heart failure. Without chelation, iron overload will eventually lead to the demise of the patient. Therefore all patients with thalassaemia major on regular transfusions also require iron chelation to remove the excess iron. In some adolescents with thalassaemia major, compliance with iron chelation can become an issue. It is important that adolescents are monitored closely, measuring their iron burden and looking for complications of iron overload, as well as monitoring for side effects of iron chelation.

2.2.2. *Sickle cell disease*

This is a group of disorders that are caused by inheritance of an abnormal beta-globin subunit of haemoglobin, Hb S. In its commonest form, sickle cell anaemia patients are homozygous for Hb S. However, sickle cell disease may also result from compound heterozygosity of Hb S with other beta-globin mutations such as thalassaemia, Hb C and Hb D. Typically patients with sickle cell disease are diagnosed in infancy or early child-hood; occasionally some of the milder variants (for example Hb SC) may not be diagnosed until later, even into adolescence and adulthood. Sickle cell disease is a lifelong disease which, when the abnormal Hb S becomes deoxygenated and polymerises, results in the red blood cells distorting into a sickle shape. This sickling of red blood cells causes chronic haemol-ysis as well as episodic blockage of blood vessels. These acute episodes result in tissue and organ damage with painful crises, acute chest syndrome (infiltrate, fever, hypoxia), and stroke. By adolescence, most patients with sickle cell disease will be functionally asplenic, and therefore have an increased risk of infection. They are also at an increasing risk of developing pulmonary hypertension which is secondary to chronic haemolysis, asplenia, recurrent chest crises, and iron overload. Pulmonary hypertension seriously increases mortality. Management requires regular review, which may be difficult to achieve during adolescence.

For painful crises, adequate analgesia is the mainstay of therapy and opiates may be required. For chest crises, exchange transfusion is often indicated. For patients with recurrent painful crises or chest crises, oral hydroxyurea has been shown to reduce the frequency of crises. Adolescents on hydroxyurea need to be aware of the importance of contraception to prevent its potentially teratogenic effects. Oral contraceptives, injectable contraceptives, and barrier methods are all suitable for females with sickle cell disease. While few studies have evaluated oral contraceptives in this population there is no evidence of adverse effects. For some patients, including those with a previous stroke or pulmonary hypertension, a chronic transfusion program to maintain the Hb S level between 30% and 50% is indicated.

2.3. *Other Anaemias*

Adolescents may develop autoimmune haemolytic anaemia as a primary event or secondary to other underlying autoimmune disorders such as systemic lupus erythematosus. Females of Asian descent are particularly at risk.

Bone marrow failure may occur at any age and may be due to an inherited bone marrow failure syndrome (Fanconi anaemia, dyskeratosis congenita) or as an acquired predominantly autoimmune disorder. Marrow failure typically presents with a macrocytic anaemia, accompanied by thrombocytopaenia and leucopaenia. Marrow failure requires supportive therapy with platelets and red cell transfusion and judicious use of antibiotics. Definitive treatment depends on the underlying causes. Inherited marrow failure syndromes may respond to androgen treatment, such as oxymetholone, but often stem cell transplant is indicated. For patients with acquired aplastic anaemia and a fully matched sibling donor, stem cell transplant is the first line of treatment. For those without a sibling match, immunosuppression with anti-thymocyte immunoglobulin, steroids, and cyclosporine is usually used, keeping alternative donor stem cell transplant in reserve for those who fail immunosuppressive treatment.

Adolescents with underlying conditions such as renal failure, inflammatory bowel disease, juvenile arthritis, and immunodeficiency, may have anaemia of chronic disease. This is typically normocytic with reduced reticulocytes and the treatment is directed at the underlying condition.

3. Disorders of Haemostasis

3.1. *Bleeding Disorders in Adolescence*

Both congenital and acquired bleeding disorders may be present in the adolescent period. Excessive menstrual bleeding may be the first symptom of milder disorders such as VWD where the prevalence of menorrhagia is reported as between 5%–36%, and also with platelet function defects, thrombocytopaenia, and clotting factor deficiency. Mild haemophilia may present with prolonged bleeding following a tooth extraction. The commonest acquired bleeding disorder presenting in adolescence is immune thrombocytopaenic purpura.

3.2. *Congenital Bleeding Disorders*

3.2.1. *Haemophilia*

Haemophilia is an inherited bleeding disorder resulting from a deficiency of Factor VIII (Haemophilia A) or Factor IX (Haemophilia B). Haemophilia is classified as:

- Severe <1% baseline factor.
- Moderate 1–5% baseline factor.
- Mild 5–40% baseline factor.

Severe haemophilia is usually diagnosed in early childhood. Moderate haemophilia tends to present slightly later and mild haemophilia may remain undiagnosed into adolescence and adulthood. Most patients with severe haemophilia are managed with prophylactic factor replacement 2–3 times per week from a young age. The aim of this prophylaxis is to prevent bleeding and allow the patients to grow up with normal joints. Because of the effectiveness of this treatment regimen, many of these patients have few bleeds and are able to participate fully in age related activities. During adolescence, compliance with regular factor therapy often diminishes and adolescents may question the ongoing need for therapy. Many patients elect to only treat themselves at times of risk, such as when on holidays or when playing sports. Up to 50% of adolescent and young adult patients with severe haemophilia may be able to reduce or stop their prophylaxis without serious impact on their quality of life. Adolescents who have had repeated joint bleeds in the past or who are non-compliant may begin to show symptoms and signs of haemophilic arthropathy with joint pain and wasting. These patients require a multidisciplinary approach with involvement from haematology, rheumatology, physiotherapy, and orthopaedics.

3.2.2. *Von Willebrand disease*

VWD is the most common inherited bleeding disorder and is generally less severe than other bleeding disorders. Patients with VWD have reduced levels or functional activity of von Willebrand factor. VWF is a multimeric protein that mediates the attachment of platelets to exposed tissues and is therefore an essential component of haemostasis, particularly under conditions of high shear. There are three main types of VWD:

- Type 1 VWD is the most common form and is characterised by reduced levels of VWF and its activity.
- Type 2 VWD is due to a defect in the function of the VWF molecule.
- Type 3 VWD is very rare and is the most severe form, due to an almost complete absence of VWF and its activity.

Young people without a family history of VWD often present in adolescence and young adulthood. The index case of VWD, described by Erik Von Willebrand in 1926, bled to death from her fourth menstrual period. There is a variety of bleeding history scores currently being developed to assess the likelihood of VWD.

A haemostatic agent which may be used is desmopressin. While initially developed to treat central diabetes insipidus, it causes the release of endogenous VWF from endothelial cells. It is useful in the treatment of type 1 VWD, some cases of type 2 VWD and some cases of platelet dysfunction. It can be administered intravenously, subcutaneously, or intra-nasally (where the concentrated preparation is available). Desmopressin has side effects of headache, flushing, and water retention and therefore should be used under the guidance of a haematologist. Occasionally females with severe VWD or other factor deficiencies may require clotting factor concentrates, such as plasma derived Factor VIII, recombinant Factor VIII or recombinant Factor IX, to control bleeding.

3.2.3. *Inherited bone marrow failure syndromes*

Inherited bone marrow failure syndromes are rare genetic disorders, including Fanconi anaemia, dyskeratosis congenita, Shwachman Diamond syndrome, thrombocytopaenia absent radii, and severe congenital neutropenia. These disorders are associated with an overlapping spectrum of birth defects and a wide spectrum of haematological abnormalities from single cytopaenias to full blown marrow failure (aplastic anaemia). Some of these conditions may present later in adolescence and adulthood with the onset of thrombocytopaenia, and with bruising and bleeding being the first sign of bone marrow failure. Many of these disorders are associated with an increased risk of leukaemia and cancer and these may be the presenting feature. Initial management of patients presenting with bone marrow failure is supportive with blood product transfusion and antibiotics. Typically the patient with inherited bone marrow failure will not respond to immunosuppressive therapy and will often require a stem cell transplant.

3.3. *Acquired Bleeding Disorders in Adolescence*

3.3.1. *Immune thrombocytopaenic purpura*

ITP is an autoimmune disease seen at all ages. ITP in adolescence is more common in females than males and is more likely to follow the adult pattern of disease with an increased likelihood of chronicity. ITP in adolescents may be primary or secondary to other autoimmune disorders such as SLE and all adolescents with ITP need to be investigated for possible secondary causes. The bleeding seen in adolescents is quite variable but many patients will have minimal bleeding despite platelet counts less than 20×10^9/L. Most adolescents with ITP do not require treatment unless there is severe bleeding and most adolescents with ITP will improve whether they are given treatment or not. Most treatments aim to temporarily increase the platelet count and do not cure the underlying condition itself. The commonest problematic bleeding for adolescents with ITP is menorrhagia (Section 3.5). The mainstays of treatment for patients with acute ITP with serious bleeding are steroids and intravenous gammaglobulin. For patients with chronic problematic ITP rituximab and splenectomy may be used. Newer agents such as thrombopoietin mimetics may be useful.

3.3.2. *Other acquired bleeding disorders presenting in adolescence*

These include Vitamin C deficiency, which is relatively common when dietary intake is poorly balanced, and thrombocytopaenia secondary to acquired marrow failure or infiltration.

3.4. *Investigation of Bleeding Disorders in Adolescents*

This includes a FBC, film and coagulation screen (APTT, PT, fibrinogen). In many of the milder bleeding disorders these first line coagulation screening tests may be normal. Therefore, additional studies are often indicated, such as VWD disease screen — which includes Factor VIII coagulant activity, VWF antigen level, VWF: ristocetin cofactor activity and VWF-collagen binding assay, platelet function and vitamin C. Secondary causes need to be considered.

3.5. *Management of Bleeding Disorders*

Management of bleeding in the adolescent involves identification of the underlying defect and use of therapies directed to correct the defect wherever possible. The use of an anti-fibrinolytic agent, such as tranexamic acid may be useful in many of these conditions for mild bleeding symptoms. For menorrhagia oral contraceptives may be added to stabilise the endometrium and reduce the menstrual loss.

4. Thromboembolic Disorders

By adolescence, the rate of diagnosis increases. Typically thromboembolism is provoked by the presence of multiple risk factors which include the use of central venous lines, inherited prothrombotic mutations, immobilisation, dehydration, infection, the use of the oral contraceptive pill and pregnancy. Many adolescents with thrombosis have more than one inherited prothrombotic condition in addition to an acquired risk factor.

4.1. *Inherited Prothrombotic Disorders*

The inherited prothrombotic disorders are a heterogeneous group of disorders associated with an increased risk of venous thromboembolism. Excess activity of normal coagulation factors or deficiency in natural anticoagulants or their activity, predispose to thrombosis. The commonest hereditary prothrombotic disorder is the Factor V Leiden mutation, present in about 5% of the Australian population. There is an abnormal Factor V coagulation factor, which is resistant to the action of activated protein C, so that the clotting process continues for longer and increases the chance of an abnormal clot forming. Factor V Leiden mutation is a relatively mild risk factor, increasing the risk of thrombosis by approximately seven fold over baseline. The prothrombin gene G20210A mutation is also a mild risk factor for thrombosis. Deficiency of any of the natural anticoagulants (protein C and S, antithrombin) are more likely to result in a thrombosis. The diagnosis of inherited prothrombotic conditions is made by measuring protein C and S and antithrombin levels and by genetic testing for the prothrombin gene mutation and Factor V Leiden mutation. Dysfibrinogenaemias are diagnosed using thrombin times. Persons with hereditary prothrombotic states are also at increased risk of venous thromboembolism and recurrent miscarriage. These patients may require anticoagulation throughout pregnancy. Warfarin is teratogenic and typically low molecular weight heparin is used.

In adolescents with a known prothrombotic risk the relative risk of thrombosis on the combined oral contraceptive is three to five-fold, whereas the absolute risk for a healthy adolescent on this therapy is only 0.05% per year. Being heterozygous for Factor V Leiden mutation increases this risk 35 fold. The risk of VTE associated with the use of oral contraceptives needs to be balanced against the risk of VTE associated with an unintended pregnancy resulting from the use of less effective contraceptive methods.

4.2. *Management of an Acute Thrombotic Event*

This is similar whether an inherited prothrombotic state is present or not. Patients with acute thrombosis will need anticoagulation with unfractionated or low molecular weight heparin initially, followed by oral anticoagulation with warfarin. Treatment for an unprovoked deep vein thrombosis should continue for six months. A shorter time period of three months may be sufficient if there was no identified prothrombotic state.

5. Transition to Adult Care in Established Haematological Disease

The aim of care for adolescents with chronic haematological conditions such as thalassaemia, haemophilia, and sickle cell disease is to make them independent and responsible for their own treatment. For those with severe haemophilia this involves learning to perform their own venipuncture and administer their own Factor VIII, learning to recognise the need for additional treatment and to gain the confidence to speak with their haemophilia treatment centre on their own. Patients on regular transfusions will have regular contact with their adult carers and to a degree this makes the transition a little easier. They do, however, need to be responsible for their own iron chelation and if compliance is an issue in adolescence, the patient will be at risk of increased complications soon after transition to adult care. All adolescents and young adults with sickle cell disease, especially those not on regular transfusions, need to establish a process of seeking help for crises. For many young adults this is difficult and results in delays in presentation for treatment which may have devastating consequences.

References

Beard JL. (2000) Iron requirements in adolescent females. *J Nutr* **130**: 440S–442S.

Chalmers E, Ganesen V, Liesner R, Maroo S, Nokes T, Saunders D, Williams M. (2011) Guideline on the investigation, management and prevention of venous thrombosis in children. *Br J Haematol* **154**(2): 196–207.

Daniel WA Jr. (1973) Hematocrit: Maturity relationship in adolescence. *Pediatrics* **52**(3): 388–394.

Ferrari M, Mistura L, Patterson E, Sjostrom M, Diaz LE, Stehle P, Gonzalez-Gross M, Kersting M, Widhalm K, Molnar D, Gottrand F, De Henauw S, Manios Y, Kafatos A, Moreno LA, Leclercq C, Group HS. (2011) Evaluation of iron status in European adolescents through biochemical iron indicators: The HELENA study. *Eur J Clin Nutr* **65**(3): 340–349.

James AH. (2009) Bleeding disorders in adolescents. *Obstet Gynecol Clin North Am* **36**(1): 153–162.

Monagle P, Barnes C, Ignjatovic V, Furmedge J, Newall F, Chan A, De Rosa L, Hamilton S, Ragg P, Robinson S, Auldist A, Crock C, Roy N, Rowlands S. (2006) Developmental haemostasis. Impact for clinical haemostasis laboratories. *Thromb Haemost* **95**(2): 362–372.

Petrini P, Seuser A. (2009) Haemophilia care in adolescents-compliance and lifestyle issues. *Haemophilia* **15**(1): 15–19.

Treadwell M, Telfair J, Gibson RW, Johnson S, Osunkwo I. (2011) Transition from pediatric to adult care in sickle cell disease: Establishing evidence-based practice and directions for research. *Am J Hematol* **86**(1): 116–120.

Tussing-Humphreys LM, Nemeth E, Fantuzzi G, Freels S, Guzman G, Holterman AXL & Braunschweig C. (2010) Elevated systemic hepcidin and iron depletion in obese premenopausal females. *Obesity* **18**(7): 1449–1456.

Chapter 42

Allergic and Immunological Disorders in Adolescence

Alyson Kakakios, Dianne Campbell,
Paul Turner and John Tan

1. Introduction

Important allergic or immunological disorders may be first diagnosed in adolescence and bring major new treatment dilemmas to adolescence. In this chapter, we focus upon four such conditions, which in our experience present significant difficulties for our adolescent patients.

2. Food Allergy in Adolescence

Food allergy is a common childhood disorder. Most FA is of the IgE mediated immediate type, but rarer non IgE immunologically mediated FAs such as eosinophilic oesophagitis and food protein enteropathy syndromes also occur. These disorders, with the exception of oral allergy syndrome, are more common in infants and young children than in adolescents and young adults; however their persistence or presentation in adolescence and early adulthood involves specific therapeutic challenges.

2.1. *Prevalence of IgE Mediated Food Allergy*

This has an estimated prevalence of 2% in adolescence. Most FAs in adolescence are a consequence of persistent FAs from childhood rather than new onset, although new sensitisations may occur at this age, particularly with fruits and vegetables as part of the OAS.

2.2. *Symptoms*

Typical symptoms of IgE mediated FA occur within minutes (0–120) of ingestion and include angioedema, urticaria, widespread erythema, rhinitis, throat and mouth tingling, tongue swelling, abdominal pain, vomiting, wheeze, stridor, persistent coughing, hypotension, and cardiovascular collapse. Common food allergens in adolescence are peanuts, treenuts, and seafood. Up to 80% of children outgrow milk, egg, and wheat allergies, but less than 10%–20% of children with peanut, treenuts, and seafood allergies outgrow their sensitisation by adolescence. Adolescents and young adults are at the highest risk of fatal anaphylaxis from FA compared with young children and older adults. Reasons for this are not completely understood, but are likely to include risk-taking behaviour in adolescents with FAs.

2.3. *Factors Increasing Risk in Adolescent Food Allergy*

The increased likelihood of severe allergic reactions and changes in behaviour and risk assessment make adolescence a particularly dangerous period for the food allergic patient. In a highly allergic cohort consisting of adolescents with known FA where 70% had prior anaphylaxis, half of the group admitted to knowingly trying food that contained an allergen to which they were allergic, and 40% did not regularly carry their adrenaline auto injector. Events that were peer group orientated had the lowest reported rates of auto injector carriage. Adolescents reported being most concerned about not being able to eat with their friends and having a limited choice of restaurants.

The relatively high risk of fatal anaphylaxis in this age group is associated with persistent or undertreated asthma, as asthma is an independent risk factor for death from food related anaphylaxis. The adolescent who fails to achieve tolerance to a food in younger childhood represents the more severe end of the FA spectrum, and they may have developed more IgE antibodies to different epitopes of the offending food protein than the child who has attained tolerance.

2.4. *Management*

Current management of FA in adolescence, as for any age group, involves avoidance of offending food proteins and provision of education, dietary advice and an adrenaline auto injector where there is a risk of anaphylaxis. There is currently no widely accepted or safe method of desensitisation to food allergens; however trials using specific oral tolerance induction, anti IgE therapy, and modified immunotherapy are ongoing.

3. Oral Allergy Syndrome

3.1. *Presentation*

OAS is a common allergic manifestation in adolescence and young adulthood, with the majority of cases caused by cross sensitisation to a pre-existing air-borne allergen (aeroallergen) sensitisation as a result of structural homology between pollen and plant proteins. First presentation of OAS in adolescence is common, and is usually predated by childhood perennial or seasonal allergic rhinitis.

Symptoms classically begin within minutes of oral exposure to the offending fruit or vegetable, and comprise itching and/or tingling of the mouth and lips. These may be accompanied by lip angioedema and less commonly gastrointestinal symptoms of cramping, pain, vomiting, or diarrhoea. Anaphylaxis is a rare complication of OAS.

Because the original sensitising aeroallergen in OAS is most frequently pollen, the type of fruits and vegetables responsible for the syndrome vary widely between different geographical locations. In Europe, birch pollen allergen cross reactivity accounts for a significant proportion of OAS with allergy to stone fruit (particularly peach), apple, melon, celery, hazelnut and carrot. Cedar is a significant allergen in Japan and common associated offending foods include apple, cherry, kiwi fruit and tomato. In North America, ragweed and birch are both significant allergens and common associated foods responsible for OAS include banana, cucumber, melons (cantaloupe, watermelon and honeydew) and zucchini. Cross reactive sensitisation with grass and weed pollens in Australia is associated with OAS to melons, kiwi fruit, banana and tomato.

3.2. *Diagnosis*

IgE production to the offending plant allergen and pollen can be demonstrated by allergy skin prick testing or by serum specific allergen IgE assay. Labile plant allergens are responsible for most OAS, and fresh food extracts demonstrate the greatest skin prick sensitivity. This explains why many adolescents with OAS can tolerate the offending fruit and vegetables when cooked, tinned, or preserved but not fresh.

3.3. *Treatment*

Treatment of OAS depends in part upon the discomfort experienced by the adolescent. Avoidance of the allergic food is generally recommended, except with very mild symptoms. Any systemic features of the reaction should prompt suspicion of typical IgE mediated food allergy, and provision of an adrenaline auto injector should be considered in these patients. Immunotherapy with the aeroallergen may have a future therapeutic role.

4. Eosinophilic Oesophagitis

4.1. *Prevalence*

Eosinophilic oesophagitis is an allergic disorder, which in most adolescents is triggered by food allergies and, in some cases, by pollen allergies. Its prevalence has dramatically increased over the last 15 years to about 1 in 11,000.

4.2. *Presentation*

Adolescents with EoE describe intense dysphagia, needing liquids to help swallow. Food impaction requiring endoscopic removal may occur. Other symptoms include heartburn, chest pain, upper abdominal pain and vomiting. Characteristically, teenagers with EoE alter eating habits to control symptoms, chewing carefully, taking longer to eat their food and avoidance of eating in public, in order to prevent the embarrassment of having symptoms. Foods such as meat and bread cause more problems than foods with a softer consistency.

4.3. *Diagnosis*

The only way to diagnose EoE is by endoscopy and biopsy. The diagnostic hallmark of EoE is a marked eosinophilic infiltration in the oesophagus. Teenagers with EoE should also be assessed for food and pollen allergies, because treatment strategies vary according to the underlying pathogenesis.

4.4. *Management*

Treatments include pharmacologic therapy, dietary management and mechanical dilatation. EoE, in contrast to gastro–oesophageal reflux disease, does not typically respond to acid suppression. At present, however, there is no single treatment option which is consistently effective.

5. Allergic Rhinitis in Adolescence

5.1. *Prevalence*

Allergic rhinitis is the most common chronic disease in humans, affecting up to 40% of adolescents and increasing in prevalence. Incidence is greatest in adolescents, in part due to the 'allergic march', where atopic manifestations progress from infantile eczema and FAs through to asthma and AR in later childhood and adolescence.

5.2. *Classification*

AR is classified as either perennial or seasonal. Perennial AR is most commonly caused by sensitisation to house dust mite or other persistent aeroallergens with symptoms occurring throughout the year. Seasonal AR ('hay fever') is usually related to sensitisation to animals, grass, weed

Table 1:   WHO functional classification of allergic rhinitis.

Intermittent	Persistent
• <4 days per week. • OR <4 weeks at a time.	• ≥4 days per week. • AND ≥4 weeks at a time.
Mild • Normal sleep. • Normal daily activities. • Normal work & school. • No troublesome symptoms.	**Moderate–severe** One or more items: • Abnormal sleep. • Impairment of daily activities, sport, leisure. • Problems at school/work. • Troublesome symptoms.

and/or tree pollen. Such a classification can be unhelpful and The World Health Organization recommends an alternative scheme (Table 1).

Table 2 summarises the differences between house dust mite-induced AR and pollen-induced AR. Other relevant symptoms include mouth breathing, snoring, learning/attention problems, and disturbed sleep. The impact of these symptoms on the patient's quality of life should be determined. In the adolescent, with many other potential causes for sleep disturbance and school inattention, a careful history and examination are required to identify the nasal obstruction of AR as a possibility. Otoscopy is useful to exclude other causes of nasal obstruction, such as polyps. Allergy skin prick or allergen specific IgE serum testing is useful when immunotherapy is being considered.

5.3. *Treatment*

Treatment of AR remains challenging, in part due to under-diagnosis but also as a consequence of inadequate management, often using non-prescription medications in a suboptimal manner. Intranasal medications used with optimal technique will achieve reasonable symptom control in almost all cases, but patients often prefer oral medications which may not provide adequate symptom control. Allergen avoidance is difficult and for most individuals, is not practical. Treatment of AR often improves airway symptoms in patients with concomitant asthma.

Table 2: Features of AR caused by house dust mite compared to pollen.

Feature	HDM-induced AR	Pollen-induced AR
Nasal symptoms	Obstruction prominent.	Nasal pruritus and sneezing, obstruction less predominant.
Eye symptoms	Infrequent	Common
Temporality	Perennial	Typically seasonal, though symptoms can persist throughout the year.
Mediators involved	Kinins > histamine	Predominantly histamine
Response to oral antihistamine	Poor	Good
Response to intranasal steroid	Good	Good

5.3.1. *Topical medication*

Intranasal steroids are the most effective treatment available for AR, improving both nasal and ocular symptoms and are recommended as first-line agents in patients with moderate to severe symptoms. A number of preparations are available, many of which can be purchased without prescription. However, poor technique of administration frequently results in treatment failure. Compliance with topical medications can be problematic in adolescents. Once-daily preparations such as fluticasone are recommended, and training in the correct use of nasal sprays may further improve compliance, probably by minimising delivery of the medication to the pharynx where it can cause an unpleasant taste. Intranasal steroids may be effective when used 'as needed', rather than on a regular basis. Combined use with an intranasal antihistamine, such as azelastine, may offer improved symptom relief in aldolescents with histamine-mediated symptoms. Addition of topical ocular therapies can be used to reduce ocular itch.

5.3.2. *Oral medication*

Antihistamines can be very effective against mild-moderate pollen-induced AR, but are generally of little benefit in HDM-induced AR. Leukotriene antagonists, the most common being montelukast, are less effective than antihistamines and do not improve symptoms beyond that which can be achieved with intranasal steroids, however compliance may be higher with oral medications compared to the intranasal route.

5.3.3. *Immunotherapy*

Subcutaneous immunotherapy using small amounts of allergen is an effective treatment for AR in adolescents. This requires monthly maintenance injections over 3–5 years, and has been associated with life-threatening reactions in patients with significant asthma. Sublingual immunotherapy, where the allergen is administered through a pump-dosimeter under the tongue or sublingual tablet, is an effective alternative. Efficacy requires appropriate identification of the causative allergen(s) and compliance on the part of the patient as it typically takes 6–9 months before any benefit is seen. In a grass pollen allergy study, 95% of adolescents complied, despite over 80% of participants experiencing at least mild side effects. This therapy is currently reserved for patients with significant symptoms which do not respond to first line treatment, and should be managed through a specialist allergy service.

6. Common Variable Immune Deficiency in Adolescence

6.1. *Prevalence*

Common variable immune deficiency is the second most common primary immune deficiency after selective IgA deficiency, with a prevalence of 1:25,000. 'Variable' refers to its wide phenotypic variation and clinical manifestations. There are two peak incidences: 1–5 years and 16–25 years, with males and female equally affected. CVID involves multiple organ systems and diagnosis is often delayed. Adolescents with CVID struggle with issues of treatment compliance and disease complications.

6.2. *Presentation*

Adolescents with CVID often present with recurrent sino–pulmonary infections such as pneumonia, sinusitis, conjunctivitis and perforated otitis media. Bronchiectasis and signs of suppurative lung disease may be present at diagnosis. Common causative bacterial organisms include pneumococcus, moraxella, and mycoplasma species. Adolescent CVID may also present with recurrent viral and fungal infections such as cryptosporidia, pneumocystis pneumonia, and herpes. Recurrent infections may result in poor growth and in severe cases, delayed puberty. Chronic gastrointestinal infection, with giardia or campylobacter, is not uncommon. This in turn results in chronic diarrhoea and malabsorption which further exacerbate maturational delay. There are no pathognomonic clinical findings for CVID.

6.3. *Diagnosis*

The presence of maturational delay, thrush, gingivitis, cobblestoning of the posterior pharynx (chronic sinusitis), poor dentition, scarring of the tympanic membranes, digital clubbing, and evidence of chronic suppurative lung disease should alert the clinician to the possible diagnosis. Lymphadenopathy, splenomegaly, arthritis, and rash may also be present, signifying associated autoimmune disease.

Low serum IgG levels accompanied by a low IgA and/or low IgM level (2SD below mean) are the hallmark of CVID, although some patients present with marginally low IgG and borderline IgA/IgM. These patients require monitoring, as this can reflect evolving CVID. Poor or absent response to immunisation with polysaccharide and protein-based vaccines such as pneumococcal, haemophilus influenza type B, tetanus and diphtheria are typical. Full blood count, electrolytes and liver function tests are usually normal. Over time, decreases in lymphocyte counts and a reduced CD4 count can be seen. Most CVID patients will have normal circulating B and T cells. Reduced numbers of circulating memory B cells (CD27+B cells) and switched memory B cells (CD27+IgD–IgM–) can occur. Abnormalities in T cell function can develop over time.

Autoimmune disorders occur in 25% of adolescent CVID. The most common are haematological, with over 10% of CVID patients having an immune thrombocytopaenia, autoimmune haemolytic anaemia, or pernicious anaemia. Autoimmune arthritides also occur. Enteropathy, most commonly manifested as inflammatory bowel disease, occurs in 20% of

CVID patients. CVID is associated with allergic disease especially asthma (50%) and AR. CVID has an increased rate of malignancy especially Non-Hodgkin's lymphoma (8% lifetime incidence) and gastric cancers.

6.4. *Management*

The treatment of CVID is dependent upon severity at presentation and includes the subcutaneous or intravenous infusion of human immuno-globulin, antibiotic prophylaxis and immunosuppressive therapy for those with autoimmunity. Oral antimicrobial therapy with trimethoprim/sulphamethoxazole with regular medical reviews can be instigated if CVID is detected early in the absence of any complications. IVIG is typically administered monthly as an intravenous infusion over 4–5 hours. Regular follow up is the cornerstone of management of patients with CVID, optimally within a multidisciplinary team.

The impact of CVID and its complications on patients' lives can be significant. Adolescents with CVID have to deal with the extra burden of a chronic disease regimen. Poor compliance may lead to recurrent infections, troublesome autoimmunity, inflammatory bowel disease, and suppurative lung disease. Depression and issues with self-esteem can occur and must always be considered in the adolescent who has poor compliance, multiple school absences, and failure to present for follow up appointments. With transition to adult care, multidisciplinary care may be lost. Ideally the immunology team should co-ordinate care of the young adult and organise visits to other specialists as required.

References

Bonilla FA, Geha RS. (2009) Common variable immunodeficiency. *Pediatr Res* **65**(5): 13R–19R.

Busse PJ, Farzan S, Cunningham-Rundles C. (2007) Pulmonary complications of common variable immunodeficiency. *Ann Allergy Asthma Immunol* **98**(1): 1–8; quiz 8–11, 43.

Di Lorenzo G, Pacor ML, Pellitteri ME, Morici G, Di Gregoli A, Lo Bianco C, Ditta V, Martinelli N, Candore G, Mansueto P, Rini GB, Corrocher R, Caruso C. (2004) Randomized placebo-controlled trial comparing fluticasone aqueous nasal spray in mono-therapy, fluticasone plus cetirizine, fluticasone plus montelukast and cetirizine plus montelukast for seasonal allergic rhinitis. *Clin Exp Allergy* **34**(2): 259–267.

Katelaris CH. (2010) Food allergy and oral allergy or pollen-food syndrome. *Curr Opin Allergy Clin Immunol* **10**(3): 246–251.

Monks H, Gowland MH, Mackenzie H, Erlewyn-Lajeunesse M, King R, Lucas JS, Roberts G. (2010) How do teenagers manage their food allergies? *Clin Exp Allergy* **40**(10): 1533–1540.

Radulovic S, Calderon MA, Wilson D, Durham S. (2010) Sublingual immunotherapy for allergic rhinitis. *Cochrane Database of Systematic Reviews*; *Reviews 2010*. John Wiley & Sons, Ltd, Chichester, UK.

Schroeder S, Atkins D, Furuta GT. (2010) Recent advances in the treatment of eosinophilic esophagitis. *Expert Rev Clin Immunol* **6**(6): 929–937.

Webber CM, England RW. (2010) Oral allergy syndrome: A clinical, diagnostic, and therapeutic challenge. *Ann Allergy Asthma Immunol* **104**(2): 101–8; quiz 109–10, 117.

Yun J, Katelaris CH. (2009) Food allergy in adolescents and adults. *Intern Med J* **39**(7): 475–478.

Chapter 43

Cancer in Adolescents and Young Adults

Bhavna Padhye and Melissa Gabriel

1. Introduction

Cancer in adolescents and young adults presents a unique set of challenges as they have a distribution frequency of tumour types that differ from the paediatric population. They also have unique psychosocial, behavioural, and developmental issues, which must be sensitively and adequately addressed during therapy. The literature suggests that access of adolescents to clinical trials, and therefore to acceptable standard of care, is significantly inferior to the experience of younger children. There is growing momentum internationally for greater attention to be given to the treatment and support provided for AYA with cancer.

2. Patterns and Incidence of Cancer in AYA

There are several subgroups to consider within the AYA population. AYA is defined variably as a group aged between 15–40 years, although many AYA programs focus on 15–25 year olds.

Cancer in adolescents (15–19 years of age) occurs at nearly twice the rate observed in 5–14 year olds. However, many of the common malignancies in children younger than five years are virtually absent in AYA. Similarly, those cancers that predominate in adults, such as carcinomas of

569

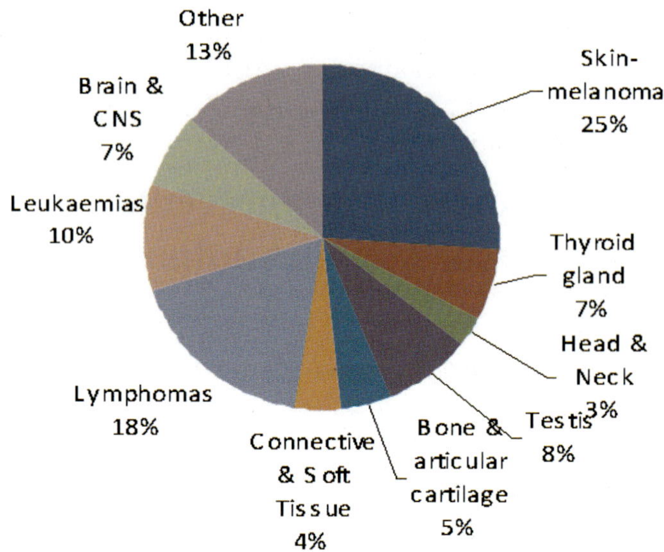

Fig. 1: Cancer types in adolescents and young adults (15–29 years) in Australia.

Source: Australian Institute of Health and Welfare national statistics clearing house data.

the breast, gastro–intestinal and genitourinary tracts are unusual among adolescents. Common malignancies in AYA include melanoma, leukaemia and lymphoma, bone and soft tissue sarcomas, testicular tumours, thyroid cancers and brain tumours.

The type of STS that occurs in AYA is distinct from that of younger patients. Rhabdomyosarcoma, the most common type of sarcoma in childhood, accounts for only 25% of the STS in AYA. The other 75% of STS include synovial sarcoma, liposarcoma, malignant fibrous histiocytoma and malignant peripheral nerve sheath tumours. Osteosarcoma, the incidence of which is extremely low before five years of age and infrequent up to age of 10 years, peaks during teenage years. Ewing sarcoma typically arises in the second decade, with a median presentation age of 15 years.

The incidence of acute lymphoblastic leukaemia declines steadily with age such that by age 15 to 19 years, ALL accounts for only 6% of the cancers. Acute myeloid leukaemia is nearly as common as ALL in 15–19 year olds and more common than ALL in 20–29 year olds.

Chronic myeloid leukaemia increases steadily with age from birth onwards, but it is not as common as either ALL or AML in the 15–29 year age range. The incidence of non-Hodgkin's lymphoma also increases with age and peaks during adolescence, but the sub-type distribution changes.

The incidence of germ cell tumours peaks during adolescence making these the classic adolescent brain tumour. Adult CNS tumours including meningioma, astrocytoma, oligodendrogliomas and oligoastrocytomas begin rising in incidence after adolescence. The classical adult, high grade glioma is relatively rare in adolescence.

3. Specific AYA Issues in Cancer Management

In developed countries, cancer is the leading cause of non-accidental deaths among AYA. More than 80% of cancer mortality burden among 15–19 year olds is due to four malignancy groups: sarcomas, leukaemia/ lymphomas, CNS tumours and germ cell tumours, with leukaemia being the primary contributor. Although thyroid carcinoma and melanoma are among the more common cancers in this age group, they contribute little to the overall cancer mortality burden because of high cure rates. Leukaemia and sarcomas, particularly RMS, ES and OS in AYAs, are associated with a lower five year survival rate compared to younger patients. The reasons for this survival gap are unique.

3.1. *Different Biology*

Very few cancers in the AYA age group are attributable to single environmental or inherited factors. An exception is clear-cell adenocarcinoma of the vagina or cervix, with most cases caused by diethylstilboestrol taken prenatally by their mothers in an attempt to prevent pregnancy loss. Secondary malignancies can appear during adolescence in children who were treated with chemotherapy and/or radiotherapy for a primary cancer.

Those cancers that have a worse outcome in adolescents than in children may not be the same disease, and may therefore need different therapeutic approaches. Two important examples are ES and ALL. The prognosis for AYA with ES has repeatedly been reported to be inferior to paediatric outcomes. The following reasons are proposed.

- Different biological behaviour of ES is seen in AYA with more central axis lesions, larger tumours, and increased resistance to chemotherapy.
- Patient-related covariables, such as comorbidities, decreased treatment tolerance including decreased drug metabolism (altered pharmacokinetics), increased toxicity from similar drug exposure (altered pharmacodynamics) and poor treatment compliance are all cited.
- Treatment-related or iatrogenic factors including differences between paediatric and adult treatment regimens may play a role.

Contemporary clinical trials for ALL have produced five year survival rates of more than 85% for children. Specific treatment outcome data for older adolescents aged 15–19 years are limited because ALL is relatively uncommon in this age group and because such patients are grouped with either adult or paediatric data, depending on referral patterns. Historically, older adolescents have had a much worse prognosis than younger patients, which is explained, in part, by an increased prevalence of high-risk leukaemia and a poorer tolerance and adherence to therapy. Older adolescents with ALL treated in paediatric clinical trials have consistently fared better than those enrolled on adult trials, perhaps because of the more intensive treatment and the more stringent compliance as a result of parental involvement. The poor treatment outcomes obtained with adult regimens have led some oncologists to recommend matched-sibling allogeneic transplantation in first remission in older adolescents. With effective, risk-directed chemotherapy older adolescents can achieve an excellent treatment outcome, similar to the best results reported to date for younger children with ALL.

3.2. *Delay in Diagnosis*

For all solid tumours except Hodgkin lymphoma, as age is increased, the lag time for diagnosis is also increased in AYA. The reasons for delay in seeking medical care and obtaining a diagnosis are multiple.

- AYA have the lowest rates of primary care use.
- With a strong sense of invincibility they may ignore symptoms and delay seeking medical attention.
- Adolescents may be embarrassed about admitting symptoms and sharing personal concerns.
- Physicians and other members of health care teams do not recognise signs and symptoms of cancer, as AYA are not 'supposed' to have cancer. Hence clinical suspicion is low, and symptoms are often attributed to physical exertion, fatigue, and the stress of normal growth and development.

3.3. *Choice of Treatment Setting and Specialist*

AYA patients tend to occupy a no-man's land in health care delivery. Paediatric oncology and adult medical oncology services are driven by different organisational models, particularly around interaction with the patient. The paediatric model of care is based on a complex, sometimes dualistic, relationship between the child, the parents, and the professional, with routine management by an integrated multidisciplinary team.

Compared with the centralisation of paediatric oncology at major academic centres, much of adult oncology care is provided in community private practice settings by individual oncologists who refer to specialists as needed. In the adult model of care, treatment still tends to focus on direct interaction between a lead doctor and the patient, and patient autonomy is assumed in the therapeutic relationship. Hence the patient is expected to capably navigate the medical system, request supportive care consults as desired, and be responsible for appointments and medications. The majority of 15–19 year olds diagnosed with cancer are treated in adult facilities.

Neither a paediatric nor an adult model is ideally suited to provide care for AYA. AYA should be cared for in a unique space with specially trained providers within a culture that recognises *varying levels of developmental maturity* and independent decision making, but *acknowledges the need for navigation and support*, especially around the psychosocial issues of emerging adulthood. Numerous programs are emerging worldwide, in both paediatric and adult oncology settings, which provide comprehensive care to AYA patients. In Melbourne, Australia, recognising that 90% of the 15–25 year old oncology population is treated in adult institutions, the ONTrac@PeterMac program was established entirely within an adult comprehensive cancer centre and has provided dedicated AYA care to more than 500 patients since 2004. This model combines both adult and paediatric expertise, with the integration of research and clinical service development and psychosocial and emotional support.

3.4. *Decreased Participation in Clinical Trials*

Cancer patients aged 15–35 years make up the lowest proportion of patients accrued to clinical trials. Only 20%–35% of 15–19 year olds with cancer are seen in institutions that participate in National Cancer Institute-sponsored clinical trials and only 10% are entered into a clinical trial. In comparison more than 90% of children younger than age 15 years with cancer are managed at such institutions and most are entered into clinical trials. The consistently high proportion of older AYA patients in developed countries who are not entered into clinical trials is referred to as the *AYA gap*. The reasons for this finding are numerous and include a lack of available trials, provision of inadequate or inappropriate information to AYA about clinical trials and inability or reluctance of the patient to participate in the trial. The issue of access to relevant clinical trials is complicated by separate institutional review boards and low accrual targets.

3.5. *Psychosocial Issues and Supportive Care*

For AYA patients normal developmental tasks are paramount, intense and often competing with the requirements of cancer treatment. AYA patients are often on the cusp of autonomy and starting to make more independent decisions, when the diagnosis of cancer renders them 'out of control' and throws them back to being dependent on their parents or guardians.

AYA patients, who are developmentally dependent on peer group approval, often feel isolated from peers by their experience. In addition, many of the adverse effects of therapy can be overwhelming to an adolescent's self-image, which may be fragile under the best of circumstances.

Self-image is compromised by many of the adverse effects of therapy, such as alopecia, weight gain or loss, mucositis and dermatitis (acne, mouth sores), bleeding, infection and susceptibility to infection and need for isolation, impaired sexuality (intimacy, impotency, teratogenicity risk) and mutilating surgery.

Other challenges include the time away from school, work and community that therapy requires. Partner relationships are tested by the strain of the cancer diagnosis and its therapy. Whether a partner stays in the relationship is challenged by fear of relapse or infertility and may be influenced unduly in either direction by guilt or sympathy.

Because of the complex issues of dependence, decision-making during cancer therapy is different for the patient, family, and physician of an AYA than for either younger patients (which is more paternalistic) or for the older adult (which is more patient-centred). The young adult patient may wish to make his or her own decisions, but his or her understanding of the illness may be incomplete or flawed. The provider must be sensitive to this ambiguity.

3.6. *Treatment Adherence*

Adherence to therapeutic regimens, particularly oral chemotherapy, is more problematic in AYAs than in younger and older patients. Adolescents with cancer face many of the factors associated with non-adherence which include complex regimens, a need for substantial behavioural change, problems with therapy supervision as the young person and parents try to negotiate rules, a poor understanding of the seriousness of the condition and beliefs about cancer that favour non-adherence such as denial, invincibility, or fatalism. As an example, the fear of hair loss may override the importance of chemotherapy. Variable adherence should be actively identified and acknowledged. Engagement of the young person in problem-solving, rather than focussing on blame, is the best approach. Reminder systems should be set in place, using reminders that the young person chooses. A discussion with the young person alone and together with their parents to clarify who is responsible for what aspects of the medication schedule must take place.

3.7. *Fertility Preservation*

The treatment of cancer often poses a threat to fertility. Many AYA cancer survivors cite fertility as a primary concern that impacts the quality of their life. Rates of infertility are hard to predict for an individual and depend on gender, age, radiation dose and schedule and chemotherapeutic agent and dose. The oncologist must consider the estimated risk of infertility, the patient's maturity, and the need to initiate therapy immediately when framing the conversation about infertility and the options of germ cell preservation. The gesture of fertility preservation may be of great comfort for patients and their families and may assist them in managing the emotional trauma of the cancer diagnosis and treatment, although the offer may also raise expectations.

4. Summary

In contrast with progress made in all aspects of the management of childhood cancer over the past 40 years, cancer in AYAs has lost out. Medically, their care is complicated by a delay in diagnosis, an uncertainty over the specialty centre and therapy best suited to the patient, a lack of available clinical trials and poor compliance. The care is further complicated by the complex psychological mindset of the adolescent, with issues of dependence, self-image, and relationships with peers and parents. Efforts on many fronts are required to improve AYA outcomes, and include ongoing education of providers regarding issues central to the management of AYA patients, reorganisation of the system to optimise AYA care and increasing participation in clinical trials. An International Working Group has been created under the auspices of the International Society of Paediatric Oncology to help advance the cause of young people with cancer.

References

Albritton K, Bleyer WA. (2003) The management of cancer in the older adolescent. *Eur J Cancer* **39**(18): 2584–2599.

Butow P, Palmer S, Pai A, Goodenough B, Luckett T, King M. (2010) Review of adherence-related issues in adolescents and young adults with cancer. *J Clin Oncol* **28**(32): 4800–4809.

De Bont JM, Van Der Holt B, Dekker AW, Sonneveld P, Pieters R. (2004) Significant difference in outcome for adolescents with acute lymphoblastic leukemia treated on pediatric vs adult protocols in the Netherlands. *Leukemia* **18**(12): 2032–2035.

Ferrari A, Thomas D, Franklin ARK, Hayes-Lattin BM, Mascarin M, Van Der Graaf W, Albritton KH. (2010) Starting an adolescent and young adult program: Some success stories and some obstacles to overcome. *J Clin Oncol* **28**(32): 4850–4857.

Kieran MW, Walker D, Frappaz D, Prados M. (2010) Brain tumors: From childhood through adolescence into adulthood. *J Clin Oncol* **28**(32): 4783–4789.

Lee SJ, Schover LR, Partridge AH, Patrizio P, Wallace WH, Hagerty K, Beck LN, Brennan LV, Oktay K, American Society of Clinical Oncology (2006) American society of clinical oncology recommendations on fertility preservation in cancer patients. *J Clin Oncol* **24**(18): 2917–2731.

Lewis I, Morgan S. (2007) Models of care and specialized units. In: Bleyer A, Barr R, Albritton K (eds) *Cancer in Older Adolescents and Young Adults*, pp. 341–352. Springer Verlag, Heidelberg, Germany.

Pollock BH, Krischer JP, Vietti TJ. (1991) Interval between symptom onset and diagnosis of pediatric solid tumors. *J Pediatr* **119**(5): 725–732.

Pui CH, Pei D, Campana D, Bowman WP, Sandlund JT, Kaste SC, Ribeiro RC, Rubnitz JE, Coustan-Smith E, Jeha S, Cheng C, Metzger ML, Bhojwani D, Inaba H, Raimondi SC, Onciu M, Howard SC, Leung W, Downing JR, Evans WE, Relling MV. (2011) Improved prognosis for older adolescents with acute lymphoblastic leukemia. *J Clin Oncol* **29**(4): 386–391.

Stock W, La M, Sanford B, Bloomfield CD, Vardiman JW, Gaynon P, Larson RA, Nachman J. (2008) What determines the outcomes for adolescents and young adults with acute lymphoblastic leukemia treated on cooperative group protocols? A comparison of children's cancer group and cancer and leukemia group B studies. *Blood* **112**(5): 1646–1654.

Chapter 44

Late Effects of Childhood Cancer Therapy

Helena Gleeson

1. Introduction

Approximately 75% of children and adolescents with a cancer diagnosis are now considered cured. The consequences of successful cancer therapy can manifest either soon after the completion of therapy or many years later. Consequences are defined as 'symptoms and/or changes in function which develop following apparently successful treatment for cancer'. These consequences can be physical, psychological, or social. The Childhood Cancer Survivor Study in the US reported that 42% of survivors 30 years after diagnosis were affected by severe, disabling or life-threatening conditions, or had died due to a chronic condition. The risk was estimated at eight times higher than their healthy siblings. With radiation therapy the health burden starts early. Survivors of bone tumours were most affected (64%), and survivors of leukaemia and nephroblastoma/Wilm tumours were least affected (12% each). Survivors rate their mental health as similar to their peers but their physical health as much reduced. All these young people require some form of long term follow up but less than half receive such follow up. Adolescents who are survivors of childhood cancer may present with a range of issues to healthcare professionals in a range of settings and such professionals need a broad understanding of the management that may be required.

2. Cancer Diagnoses

The incidence of different types of cancer changes with age. The most frequently diagnosed malignancy in childhood is leukaemia (31%), then brain and CNS tumours (25%) and lymphomas (10%). Other tumours occur in much lower frequencies: soft tissue sarcoma such as rhabdomyosarcoma 7%; sympathetic nervous system tumours such as neuroblastoma 6%; renal tumours 6%; bone tumours such as osteosarcoma 4%; melanomas 3%; gonadal & germ cell tumours 3%; and retinoblastoma 3%. From the age of 15 the most frequently diagnosed malignancies in males are — testicular 28%, Hodgkin lymphoma 14%, leukaemia 12%; and in females — melanoma 17%, Hodgkin lymphoma 16%, and ovarian 9%.

3. Cancer Therapies

Different modalities of cancer therapy, including surgery, chemotherapy or radiotherapy, are used alone or in combination depending on the cancer and its staging. Other strategies include bone marrow transplant following preconditioning with total body irradiation or high dose chemotherapy. Accurate past medical history including details of cancer therapy is essential.

4. Consequences and Management

Consequences are dependent on the type of cancer and cancer therapy and the age at which cancer therapy is given. All tissues and systems are potentially affected by cancer treatment. The adverse effects of each therapy are too extensive to cover in detail. Lesser known chemotherapeutic effects include: auditory dysfunction with carbo- and cisplatin; dental caries with all chemotherapy; restrictive lung disease with busulphan, bis-chloroethylnitrosourea, 1-2-chloroethyl-3-cyclohexyl-1 nitrosourea, and bleomycin; renal dysfunction with ifosfamide, carbo- and cisplatin, BCNU and CCNU, and bladder dysfunction with cyclophosphamide and ifosfamide; peripheral neuropathy with vincristine and cisplatin.

5. Consequences from the Perspective of the Adolescent

5.1. *Quality of Life and Neuropsychological Functioning*

QOL can be affected in all childhood cancer survivors, and is multi-factorial with psychological, social, and physical factors. Reduced QOL affects a young person's approach to health care and may result in poor compliance with treatment or appointments. Neuropsychological dysfunction occurs in brain tumour survivors, particularly following cranial irradiation and in other cancers requiring CI, and the risk is higher if given at a younger age. The use of intrathecal chemotherapy (cytarabine, methotrexate) may also have an effect on neurological function. BMT recipients are affected whether or not they have received TBI. Typically young people or their parents will report difficulties at school or work. Psychosocial assessment will identify factors that may be affecting or are being affected by reduced QOL. Psychometric assessment is useful, as is counselling and specific school or workplace support.

5.2. *Appearance*

5.2.1. *Growth*

Growth may be poor around the time of diagnosis and during cancer therapy. After cancer therapy, poor growth occurs because of recurrence, nutritional factors, endocrine consequences following CI, and in BMT recipients, particularly if there are problems with chronic graft versus host disease which may require treatment with steroids. Growth should be monitored in all childhood cancer survivors six monthly through adolescence. If poor growth continues after recurrence and nutritional factors have been excluded, referral to an endocrinologist is essential.

Reduced spinal growth is more obvious during the pubertal growth spurt and is affected by spinal irradiation and chemotherapy. Greater height losses in the spine occur with a younger age at XRT resulting in disproportion: 9 cm reduction in sitting height if SI at one year; 7 cm at five years; 5.5 cm at 10 years. XRT to the spine can also cause kyphosis or scoliosis. Referral to a spinal surgeon may be required.

5.2.2. *Puberty*

Early puberty may occur following CI. Pubertal onset may be delayed or puberty may become arrested because of gonadotropin deficiency secondary to a brain tumour or CI, or gonadal damage following XRT or chemotherapy. Despite normal or assisted progression through puberty, breast hypoplasia following XRT to the breast area may occur. Testicular size can be reduced by gonadotoxic cancer therapy or local irradiation. Breast augmentation or testicular implants may need to be considered if distress persists.

5.2.3. *Obesity*

Obesity and insulin resistance are common in childhood cancer survivors. The aetiology is multifactorial: nutritional; reduced physical exercise; glucocorticoid use; neuro-endocrine consequences of CI with hypothalamic damage and abnormalities of appetite control; growth hormone and sex steroid deficiency.

5.2.4. *Other*

Surgery clearly affects appearance, particularly if the surgery involves the face or spine, or if limb amputation or other mutilating surgery is required. XRT affects the skin and soft tissue causing pigmented skin lesions, atrophy, hypoplasia, and alopecia. XRT of bone causes hypoplasia (particularly noticeable if the mandible is in the XRT field) and deformity, avascular necrosis and fracture. Referral to a dermatologist or surgeon may be required to determine if cosmetic improvements are possible. Healing of XRT damaged tissue is often compromised. Adolescents must be advised to take appropriate precautions to reduce sun exposure in order to reduce the likelihood of skin cancer.

5.3. *Fertility*

Many young people are fertile following cancer therapy and reassurance may be all that is required. Those who have received more gonadotoxic therapy, such as XRT or alkylating agents, particularly recipients of BMT or in the treatment of Hodgkin's lymphoma, require more careful evaluation. Infertility should never be assumed, and advice on contraception should be provided. Referral to a reproductive gynaecologist/andrologist/endocrinologist may be required.

5.4. *Living Life to the Full*

Adolescent survivors of childhood cancer are young people first and it is essential that their survivorship is viewed in the wider context of growing up.

5.4.1. *Education and vocation*

Childhood cancer survivors may fail to achieve their educational and vocational potential due to interruptions in learning, reduced societal expectations, and neurological damage (Section 5.1). This situation may affect independence, and young people may need support and direction to appropriate services.

5.4.2. *Healthy living*

Childhood cancer survivors are as likely or even more likely to explore adverse health behaviours than their healthy peers. Counselling young people on healthy living — diet, exercise, smoking, alcohol, drugs, sex, and sun exposure — forms part of the consultation. This is particularly relevant because of the increased risk of subsequent malignant neoplasms and premature cardiovascular disease.

5.4.3. *Travel*

Advise the young person to be honest and approach larger travel companies and provide them with a letter of support for travel insurance. There are no restrictions on travel or vaccinations if the young person has not had a BMT and has not had their spleen removed. If the young person has had a BMT, travel to North Western Europe, the Northern Mediterranean, North America, and Australasia is safe, but other areas of the world would need careful consideration as travel requires live vaccinations that they cannot have. Endemic malarial areas are particularly dangerous and should be avoided if the young person has had a BMT or their spleen removed. The young person may also require a letter for customs if they need to carry needles and syringes.

6. Consequences from the Perspective of the Healthcare Professional

6.1. *Subsequent Malignant Neoplasms*

Even in their adolescent years, survivors are at increased risk of developing subsequent malignant neoplasms, with about 1 in 25 developing a SMN, a six fold risk compared to the general population. Secondary solid tumours occur in 4% of survivors and secondary leukaemia in 0.2%. SMNs also account for increased mortality. The level of risk and type of SMN depend on the primary cancer diagnosis and type of cancer therapy.

6.1.1. *Cancer therapy*

XRT increases the risk of secondary solid tumours in all tissues in the radiation field. Following chest wall XRT, as used in Hodgkin's lymphoma, there is a 13 times higher risk of breast cancer in females but there is also the potential of increased risk of breast cancer following spinal, flank, and total body irradiation. Chemotherapy increases the risk of secondary acute myeloid leukaemia or myelodysplastic syndrome particularly following the administration of epipodophyllotoxins and alkylating agents. BMT with TBI increases the risk of SMN of the brain, thyroid, oral cavity, and skin 4–8 years post transplant. BMT (usually autologous) with chemotherapy preconditioning, increases the risk of AML/MDS 2.5 years post transplant. Immunosuppressive treatment following transplant may also increase the risk of SMNs.

6.1.2. *Other potential influences on the development of SMN*

Chronic GvHD following BMT increases the risk of SMN of the oral cavity or skin. Familial cancer syndromes such as neurofibromatosis type 1,

Fanconi anaemia and Li–Fraumeni are also associated with SMN, as are hereditary breast cancer families.

Management includes patient education, regular follow-up with a list of symptoms and signs to be checked, advice about healthy living and a warning to seek medical advice for worrying symptoms or signs. There should be a low threshold for imaging with a previous history of CI. For patients at increased risk of breast cancer, patient education and advice about regular self-examination and professional breast examination are essential. For those at particularly high risk from chest wall XRT or familial genetic syndromes, imaging surveillance may be necessary after the age of 25 depending on local protocols. Breast ultrasound is the safest, but this may be limited by the density of breast tissue in young women.

6.2 Cardiovascular Consequences

Cardiovascular consequences are a common cause of increased morbidity and mortality in childhood cancer survivors. Anthracycline therapy, which includes danorubicin, doxorubicin, epirubicin, mitoxantrone, idarubicin, and amsacrine, increases the risk of impaired cardiac function, particularly at doses ≥ 250 mg/m^2 and if thoracic XRT has also been administered. XRT to the thoracic region increases the risk of coronary atherosclerosis and ischaemia. XRT, depending on the field of exposure, can also cause arterial stenosis and early atherosclerosis of the aorta, carotids, and intracranial and renal arteries. Vascular disease may be exacerbated by the increased prevalence of obesity and metabolic syndrome in cancer survivors, particularly in those who have undergone TBI or CI. Symptoms such as impaired exercise tolerance, shortness of breath, palpitations, and chest pain should be sought at each routine review. Any symptoms suggestive of arterial stenosis or atherosclerosis require prompt evaluation and referral to a cardiologist or vascular surgeon, irrespective of age.

Examination should include measurement of BMI, waist, and waist to height ratio (safe level is <0.5), and blood pressure. Measurement of fasting lipid profile and glucose, as well as HbA1c, should also be performed in those with obesity or at risk of the metabolic syndrome or with symptoms of cardiovascular disease. An OGTT may be indicated, particularly if there is a family history of type 2 diabetes. Cardiovascular risk factors should be aggressively treated (Chapter 52), even though the empirical evidence to support this is not yet available.

All patients who have had anthracyclines should have an echocardiogram within 1–3 months of completion of the last dose of anthracyclines, and then repeated 3–5 yearly if normal, particularly at the end of puberty. Increased surveillance is required if a high dose of anthracyclines was administered, if there was also thoracic XRT, if the young person is committed to doing strenuous exercise such as weight lifting, although ideally they should be advised to avoid this, and if the young person is considering pregnancy or is pregnant. A cardiologist must be involved in the monitoring of pregnancy as *labour has been associated with acute cardiac decompensation and death.*

6.3. *Endocrine Consequences*

Endocrine consequences (hypothalamic pituitary axis, thyroid gland and gonads) are common. These are particularly relevant during adolescent years as they may affect quality of life, puberty, growth, bone health and cardiovascular risk and risk of obesity.

6.3.1. *Hypothalamic–pituitary axis*

Patients who have received CI require lifelong endocrine surveillance of pituitary function. The prevalence, speed of onset, severity, and extent of hypopituitarism depends on dose and schedule of XRT and time lapsed following XRT and, for the timing of puberty, the age at CI. The likelihood of hypopituitarism increases if the tumour has affected the hypothalamic–pituitary region. After higher doses of XRT (30+Gy), the onset of hypopituitarism can be within two years of completion of cancer therapy. Table 1 summarises the risk of pituitary hormone deficiencies following XRT. Some patients develop hyperprolactinaemia although this is rarely clinically significant. There have been no reports of diabetes insipidus secondary to XRT, so its appearance is due to tumour regrowth or surgery. Despite some reports there is no clear evidence that chemotherapy damages the hypothalamic–pituitary axis.

Table 1: Risk of hypopituitarism following cranial irradiation.

Dose (Gy) (tumour type)	Pituitary hormone abnormality			
	GH	LH/FSH	TSH	ACTH
7–12 (haematological)	Mild			
18–24 (haematological)	<30%	Early puberty		
30–50 (brain tumours)	50%–100%	Infrequent	3%–6%	3%
50–70 (nasopharyngeal cancers)	100%	20%–50%	60%	27%–35%

In patients with confirmed pituitary hormone deficits, hormonal replacement is usually required lifelong, except GH therapy which may be discontinued at the end of growth or in adulthood if not clinically indicated. All patients diagnosed with GHD require reassessment of pituitary function and particularly GH status at the end of growth, as they will not necessarily have persistent GHD in late adolescence. There is no evidence of increased cancer recurrence on GH, but a potential small increased risk of SMN (relative risk 2.15), particularly meningiomas following CI for a brain tumour, and osteogenic sarcoma in leukaemia patients. The risk is small in comparison to the benefits for most patients and this risk diminishes with time.

6.3.2. *Thyroid gland*

Thyroid dysfunction is common following XRT directly or close to the thyroid gland (including scatter from CI). Thyroid dysfunction may occur following BMT with preconditioning with busulphan. Thyroid dysfunction may also occur secondary to immune dysregulation following BMT. Hypothyroidism occurs frequently (30%) following CI/craniospinal irradiation for brain tumours, TBI and mantle XRT for Hodgkin's lymphoma. Hypothyroidism is more likely at higher doses of XRT.

Thyroid nodules are more frequent following XRT, 5% of which are malignant and thus an increased risk of 6 to 16 times above nodules in non-irradiated thyroids. The risk of nodules and therefore malignancy steadily increases from low doses of XRT up to 30 Gy after which the risk declines. The risk is increased if the patient had XRT before the age of 10, is female, or has an elevated TSH over a period of time (latency 5 to 25 years). The type of thyroid malignancy and natural history does not differ from thyroid malignancy occurring de novo and the treatment approach is the same. Screening guidelines vary. Screening with palpation is more likely to detect clinically significant thyroid nodules (>1 cm) and may reduce unnecessary further investigation and surgery that would not influence the clinical outcome. Ultrasound is recommended by others because of experience that clinically significant thyroid malignancy will be missed.

All patients who are at risk of thyroid dysfunction need annual thyroid function tests. If there is a persistent elevation of TSH, thyroxine therapy should be commenced. A mildly elevated TSH and a low/low to normal FT4 in a patient who has received CI may signify TSH deficiency rather than primary thyroid dysfunction. In this setting, ensure that the ACTH axis is normal before starting thyroxine.

6.4. *Fertility and Pregnancy*

It is during adolescence that concerns about fertility and future pregnancy may become an issue. The detailed discussion may have been had with their parents at the time of diagnosis, but the young person may have been given very little information. Some young people who were scheduled to have gonadotoxic cancer therapy may have undergone a procedure to potentially preserve fertility. Some young people who have evidence of potential fertility, but who are at risk of early gonadal failure, could be offered fertility preservation post therapy.

All patients should receive counselling about the possible implications of their cancer therapy on fertility. XRT, including TBI, may damage the gonads. Chemotherapeutic agents which include alkylating agents, cisplatin, cytarabine, dacarbazine, and procarbazine, particularly in the treatment of Hodgkin's lymphoma, and chemotherapy preconditioning for BMT are all gonadotoxic. Sometimes ovarian damage may result in premature menopause, reducing the window of opportunity to achieve fertility. The older the patient's age at the time of cancer therapy, the more likely that ovarian failure will occur. If the XRT field included the uterus, there may be a reduction in uterine size and blood flow, muscle fibres, and distensibility affecting pregnancy outcome. In those who have had abdominal XRT there is a three fold increased risk of premature birth, a two fold increased risk of delivering low-birth weight offspring and an increased risk of miscarriage. With the exception of familial cancer syndromes, offspring do not appear to have an increased cancer risk.

7. Delivery of Care

Ideally, care for childhood cancer survivors is provided by a multidisciplinary team that is capable of providing long term management through adolescence into adulthood. Existing services are generally located in paediatric centres, despite the fact that many of the patients are adults. It is hoped that this situation will change so that adult survivors can access adult services. Individuals require provision of accurate information about their previous cancer therapy, the potential consequences that should be screened for and how often this screening should take place. This information should be in a transportable format and the young person's family doctor supplied with identical information. The young person should have an opportunity to discuss the information and demonstrate that they understand what is needed. The young person should also be provided with the necessary psychosocial support from professionals and peers through one to one consultations, groups and social networking so that they have every opportunity to successfully enter adulthood.

References

Brabant G, Toogood AA, Shalet SM, Frobisher C, Lancashire ER, Reulen RC, Winter DL, Hawkins MM. (2012) Hypothyroidism following childhood cancer therapy — an under diagnosed complication. *Int J Cancer* **130**(5): 1145–1150.

Darzy KH. (2009) Radiation-induced hypopituitarism after cancer therapy: Who, how and when to test. *Nat Clin Pract End Met* **5**(2): 88–99.

Ergun-Longmire B, Mertens AC, Mitby P, Qin J, Heller G, Shi W, Yasui Y, Robison LL, Sklar CA. (2006) Growth hormone treatment and risk of second neoplasms in the childhood cancer survivor. *J. Clin. Endocrinol. Metab* **91**(9): 3494–3498.

Geenen MM, Cardous-Ubbink MC, Kremer LCM, Van Den Bos C, Van Der Pal HJH, Heinen RC, Jaspers MWM, Koning CCE, Oldenburger F, Langeveld NE, Hart AM, Bakker PJM, Caron HN, Van Leeuwen FE. (2007) Medical assessment of adverse health outcomes in long-term survivors of childhood cancer. *JAMA* **297**(24): 2705–2715.

Jenkinson HC, Hawkins MM, Stiller CA, Winter DL, Marsden HB, Stevens MCG. (2004) Long-term population-based risks of second malignant neoplasms after childhood cancer in Britain. *Br J Cancer* **91**(11): 1905–1910.

Neglia JP, Friedman DL, Yasui Y, Mertens AC, Hammond S, Stovall M, Donaldson SS, Meadows AT, Robison LL. (2001) Second malignant neoplasms in five-year survivors of childhood cancer: Childhood cancer survivor study. *J Natl Cancer Inst* **93**(8): 618–629.

Oeffinger KC, Mertens AC, Sklar CA, Kawashima T, Hudson MM, Meadows AT, Friedman DL, Marina N, Hobbie W, Kadan-Lottick NS, Schwartz CL, Leisenring W, Robison LL, Childhood Cancer Survivor, S. (2006) Chronic health conditions in adult survivors of childhood cancer. *N Engl J Med* **355**(15): 1572–1582.

Reulen RC, Winter DL, Lancashire ER, Zeegers MP, Jenney ME, Walters SJ, Jenkinson C, Hawkins MM. (2007) Health-status of adult survivors of childhood cancer: A large-scale population-based study from the British childhood cancer survivor study. *Int J Cancer* **121**(3): 633–640.

Shalet SM, Gibson B, Swindell R, Pearson D. (1987) Effect of spinal irradiation on growth. *Arch Dis Child* **62**(5): 461–464.

Sigurdson AJ, Ronckers CM, Mertens AC, Stovall M, Smith SA, Liu Y, Berkow RL, Hammond S, Neglia JP, Meadows AT, Sklar CA, Robison LL, Inskip PD. (2005) Primary thyroid cancer after a first tumour in childhood (the childhood cancer survivor study): A nested case-control study. *Lancet* **365**(9476): 2014–2023.

Sklar C, Whitton J, Mertens A, Stovall M, Green D, Marina N, Greffe B, Wolden S, Robison L. (2000) Abnormalities of the thyroid in survivors of Hodgkin's disease: Data from the childhood cancer survivor study. *J Clin Endocrinol Metab* **85**(9): 3227–3232.

US Children's Oncology Group (2008) Long term follow up guidelines for survivors of childhood, adolescent and young adult cancers. Version 3.0. Arcadia, CA: Children's Oncology Group. Available online at: www.survivor shipguidelines.org. (Accessed September 25, 2012.)

Chapter 45

Common Cardiology Problems
in Adolescence

Mugur Nicloae and Dorothy Radford

1. Introduction

Most adolescents with heart disease have congenital heart lesions, diagnosed and treated in infancy and childhood (Table 1). However, long term follow-up after surgery is required. Occasionally, a congenital lesion remains undiagnosed and is found in the young adult. Rheumatic heart disease is now uncommon, except in indigenous populations. Presentations with tachyarrhythmias in patients with both structurally normal hearts and in those who have had surgery are frequent. Psychosocial factors and pregnancy considerations assume growing importance.

2. Congenital Heart Lesions

2.1. *Atrial Septal Defect*

ASD is one of the most common congenital heart defects. There is a 2:1 female predominance.

Table 1:	Classification of congenital heart disease.

Shunts	**Stenotic**	**Cyanotic**
Atrial septal defect.	Pulmonary stenosis.	Tetralogy of Fallot.
Ventricular septal defect.	Aortic stenosis.	Transposition.
Patent ductus arteriosus.	Coarctation of aorta.	Truncus arteriosus.
Atrio–ventricular canal.	Mitral stenosis.	Univentricular heart.

2.1.1. *Classification*

An ASD represents a persistent inter-atrial communication. There are four types of ASD: *ostium secundum ASD* localised in the fossa ovalis, and accounting for 75% of all ASD cases; *ostium primum ASD* is localised inferiorly near the crux of the heart. There is invariably an association with a cleft in the anterior leaflet of the mitral valve. It is commonly encountered in Down syndrome and accounts for 15%–20% of cases; *sinus venosus ASD* is less common (5%–10%) and is always associated with anomalous pulmonary venous drainage; a *patent foramen ovale* is part of the foetal circulation and usually closes soon after birth.

2.1.2. *Presentation*

An ASD may present in adolescence as a new diagnosis. Symptoms can be subtle or absent. There may be tiredness, dyspnoea, or palpitations from atrial arrhythmias due to right heart volume overload. Usually there is a soft systolic pulmonary flow murmur. Rarely, the ASD is diagnosed after the occurrence of paradoxical emboli or TIA.

2.1.3. *Diagnosis*

Clinical examination may reveal no physical signs with a small ASD. With a large defect, an ejection systolic pulmonary flow murmur, a mid-diastolic tricuspid flow murmur, and a widely split, fixed second heart sound can be heard. Cyanosis in the presence of ASD is rare, unless there is severe pulmonary hypertension or co-existent pulmonary stenosis with right-left shunt. The chest X-ray shows cardiomegaly due to right heart enlargement, prominent pulmonary arteries and increased pulmonary vascularity. The electrocardiograph may show right axis deviation in ostium secundum ASD or left axis deviation with an ostium primum ASD. There is usually incomplete right bundle branch block. *The presence of atrial arrhythmias in an adolescent should raise the suspicion of structural heart disease.* The echocardiogram is the investigation of choice for identifying an ASD. MRI is the gold standard in assessing the right ventricular size and function and can also identify anomalous pulmonary veins or other associated congenital heart defects.

2.1.4. *Management*

An ASD should always be closed when there is right heart enlargement, either via surgery or percutaneous devices if smaller. Small ASDs and PFOs in totally asymptomatic patients can be left alone and monitored. The presence of pulmonary arterial hypertension requires further careful assessment. The adolescent who underwent closure of a secundum ASD in childhood is usually well and asymptomatic. There is only a small potential for the development of late complications, such as atrial arrhythmias or PAH. Percutaneous device closure requires surveillance, as a few cases of erosion of the device with pericardial tamponade have occurred, as has device thrombus formation with embolism. The adolescent who underwent surgical closure of an ostium primum ASD or sinus venosus defect, has more potential for late complications. Mitral valve regurgitation can progress, due to failed or incomplete repair of the cleft in the anterior leaflet, with mitral valve replacement required. Narrowing or obstruction of the superior vena cava or of the redirected pulmonary veins can occur after sinus venosus ASD closure.

2.2. *Ventricular Septal Defect*

VSD is the most common congenital heart defect, with a high rate of spontaneous closure in infancy and childhood. VSDs are frequently associated with other congenital heart defects.

2.2.1. *Classification*

There are four types of VSDs: muscular, membranous, outlet VSD and inlet VSD. Spontaneous closure is common in the muscular form. Membranous is the most frequent un-operated defect seen in adolescents. Prolapse of the aortic cusp into an outlet defect is important and spontaneous closure is uncommon. Inlet defect is commonly seen in Down syndrome patients.

2.2.2. *Presentation*

The adolescent with an unrepaired VSD is likely to be asymptomatic.

2.2.3. *Diagnosis*

The predominant clinical finding is the presence of a harsh, loud, pan systolic murmur maximal at the left sternal edge. The CXR will be normal in small defects. It may show cardiomegaly from left ventricular dilatation and increased vascularity with a moderate shunt. Prominent proximal pulmonary arteries with peripheral cut-off occur with severe PAH. The ECG is usually non-diagnostic in small defects, but will show right ventricular hypertrophy if there is PAH. Echocardiography provides the basic diagnostic tool. The presence of aortic regurgitation should always be defined as this will require intervention.

2.2.4. *Management*

VSD closure should be considered when there is LV volume overload or a history of endocarditis. If PAH has occurred, further careful assessment is necessary to define its degree and potential reversibility. The adolescent with VSD may be more suitable for percutaneous closure than a child due to better size ratio between the VSD and the anatomical structures of the heart. Ongoing surveillance is important to assess for LV dilatation, evidence of PAH or of aortic incompetence from cusp prolapse.

The patient who underwent closure in childhood can present in adolescence with signs of endocarditis (additional vigilance in IV drug use), aortic regurgitation, complete heart block, LV dysfunction, ventricular arrhythmias, PAH or residual VSD.

2.3. *Patent Ductus Arteriosus*

The ductus arteriosus is an obligatory communication between the aorta and pulmonary artery in the foetal circulation. It should close shortly after birth. A persistent duct accounts for about 10% of all CHD.

2.3.1. *Presentation*

The clinical presentation varies according to the size of the duct. There may be an innocent sounding systolic murmur or the classic continuous machinery-like murmur of a moderate to large duct. The latter is associated with a collapsing pulse from the wide pulse pressure.

2.3.2. *Diagnosis*

The ECG is normal with a small PDA. With a large PDA with significant left–right shunt, it may show left atrial enlargement or LV hypertrophy. The CXR may show cardiomegaly due to left atrial and LV enlargement. Echocardiography is the diagnostic imaging mode. Careful and thorough assessment should be performed when PAH is present or suspected. An aortogram is always performed prior to percutaneous device closure, for precise measurements and to assess the shape of the PDA.

2.3.3. *Management*

A small, silent PDA without left heart volume overload can be left alone. When a duct causes LV dilatation with a significant left to right shunt, closure is indicated. An episode of endocarditis, after appropriate antibiotic treatment, also triggers the need for PDA closure. Severe irreversible PAH is a contraindication to closure. The adolescent with a PDA requiring closure is likely to be amenable to percutaneous device closure. Surgical closure is indicated when the size of duct is too large for the devices. Antibiotic prophylaxis is only indicated for six months after closure if there is no residual shunt. A young person with a previous surgical repair of a PDA is usually asymptomatic with no significant sequelae. Complications of closure can include phrenic or recurrent laryngeal nerve palsy, thoracic duct injury, or re-canalisation.

2.4. *Bicuspid Aortic Valve*

The bicuspid aortic valve is the most common congenital cardiac abnormality and is found in 1%–2% of the population. There is a male predominance and some cases are familial. It may be found in adolescents with an incidental murmur or by chance finding on echocardiography. A bicuspid aortic valve is also the most common cause of aortic stenosis in later life, now that rheumatic valve disease is diminishing. Thus, life-long follow-up is indicated once the lesion is found. The valve may become incompetent or develop endocarditis. It can be associated with an aortopathy resulting in aortic root dilatation and the risk of dissection. There is a frequent association with coarctation of the aorta, a PDA and Turner syndrome.

2.5. *Coarctation of the Aorta*

Coarctation is a congenital narrowing of the thoracic aorta around the site of the insertion of the ductus arteriosus. Most cases are diagnosed and treated in infancy and childhood. However, the condition can be missed and found subsequently in association with hypertension, a murmur, or a bicuspid aortic valve.

2.5.1. *Clinical features*

Palpation of the femoral pulses is the key to diagnosis. These pulses are weak and delayed in comparison to the radial and brachial pulses. The blood pressure in the upper limb will be significantly higher than in the lower limb. A bruit is usually heard in the inter-scapular area, over the site of coarctation.

2.5.2. *Diagnosis*

The CXR may show *the three sign* where the aortic arch is seen, then an indentation, then a bulge from post-coarctation dilatation. Notching of the inferior borders of the ribs occurs when large intercostal collaterals develop. The ECG may show LV hypertrophy.

Imaging with echocardiography, MRI, or aortography will delineate the lesion and associated abnormalities.

2.5.3. *Management*

Coarctation of the aorta should be repaired unless the gradient across the defect is minor. Long term follow-up is essential and on-going therapy for hypertension may be indicated. Complications such as re-coarctation, or aneurysmal formation at the repair site can occur. Other potential events include aortic dissection, endocarditis, premature coronary artery disease, cerebral berry aneurysm rupture, and complications from a bicuspid aortic valve.

2.6. *Tetralogy of Fallot*

Tetralogy of Fallot is the most common cyanotic CHD. Approximately 12% of patients with tetralogy have 22q11 chromosome deletion syndrome. Tetralogy includes pulmonary stenosis, VSD, overriding aorta which straddles the VSD, and RV hypertrophy. Early complete repair is usually achieved in the first year of life. Pulmonary valve replacement will become necessary, and is commonly required in young adults. It is rare these days to find a patient with unoperated tetralogy. Such a patient will show cyanosis, finger clubbing, an RV lift, and a harsh ejection systolic murmur from the pulmonary stenosis.

Adolescents who have had a successful surgical repair are usually asymptomatic and may become lost to follow up. They come to medical attention when complications such as endocarditis or arrhythmias occur. Significant pulmonary regurgitation is the most common complication of tetralogy repair. It may be well tolerated for years, but progressive dilatation and dysfunction of the right ventricle occur. This can result in right heart failure, ventricular arrhythmias and sudden death. Often there is a repairable abnormality such as the need for pulmonary valve replacement.

ECG usually shows right bundle branch block. A Holter monitor should be performed regularly to rule out arrhythmias. Exercise stress testing can be used to monitor for deterioration in exercise capacity.

Echocardiography is invaluable in assessing the adolescent with tetralogy repair and can identify the numerous complications. The presence of severe pulmonary regurgitation with RV dilatation should be treated with a pulmonary valve replacement. Such tissue valves still require follow-up as they deteriorate with time needing further replacement. Some tetralogy patients need electrophysiological studies, radiofrequency ablation of arrhythmias or cardiac pacemakers and implantable defibrillators.

2.7. *Transposition of the Great Arteries*

In complete transposition of the great arteries, the aorta is anterior and arises from the right ventricle while the pulmonary artery is posterior and arises from the left ventricle. Deoxygenated blood from the body flows out the aorta, and oxygenated blood from the pulmonary veins recirculates to the pulmonary artery. Surgical correction is done in infancy or death ensues. Older operations involved an atrial switch or baffle. Many young adults followed in cardiac clinics have had these procedures. Atrial arrhythmias and obstruction are frequent sequelae.

2.8. *Other Complex Congenital Heart Defects*

The Fontan procedure is performed for defects which have only one effective ventricle such as single ventricle and hypoplastic left ventricle. The operation must still be regarded as palliative. These patients have disastrous sequelae if they lose blood volume. They can also be susceptible to many complications, including thromboembolism, ventricular dysfunction, valve regurgitation, arrhythmias, endocarditis, hepatic dysfunction from chronic congestion and protein-losing enteropathy. The adolescent growing up after this procedure may present acutely, and it is important that doctors have an understanding of the problems.

3. Tachyarrhythmias

3.1. *Paroxysmal Supraventricular Tachycardia*

This presents commonly in adolescents. The episodes may be brief and self-terminating, or can be more prolonged. Any precipitating factor should be sought. These include caffeine drinks, alcohol, smoking, drug abuse, emotion, hyperthyroidism or underlying heart disease. Initial therapy is to try vagal manoeuvres such as Valsalva or carotid sinus stimulation. Intravenous adenosine can be given for rapid termination. Regular antiarrhythmic drug therapy with flecainide or sotolol needs consideration. Electrical cardioversion is appropriate for prolonged and resistant bouts causing haemodynamic compromise. Electrophysiological study with a view to radiofrequency ablation may be curative. *Tachyarrhythmias associated with post-operative CHDs are common, and can be life threatening.* The incidence increases with increasing age. When tachyarrhythmias occur, these should be treated promptly and then the underlying cardiac haemodynamics reassessed for developing problems which might require intervention. Chamber dilatation, hypertrophy, and myocardial scarring can all contribute to the occurrence of arrhythmias.

3.2. *Atrial Flutter*

This also occurs in adolescents and young adults who have had previous surgery for CHD. They will not always complain of palpitations, but will notice fatigue, dyspnoea, dizziness, and other non-specific symptoms. The ECG needs to be carefully analysed for flutter waves and increased ventricular rate (Fig. 1). Atrial flutter responds to low energy electrical cardioversion.

3.3. *Atrial Fibrillation*

This tachyarrhythmia similarly occurs in post-operative CHD patients. It may respond to pharmacological cardioversion with flecainide or amiodarone. There is always concern about the possibility of embolism from atrial thrombi if the arrhythmia has been present for more than a couple of days and electrical cardioversion is usually done in association with transoesophageal echocardiography to detect any thrombus. If found, anticoagulation with warfarin for several weeks, and drug control of heart rate will be necessary, before cardioversion is done. Sometimes, re-repair of heart lesions, reduction of atrial size, and surgical cryoablation will eliminate the problem.

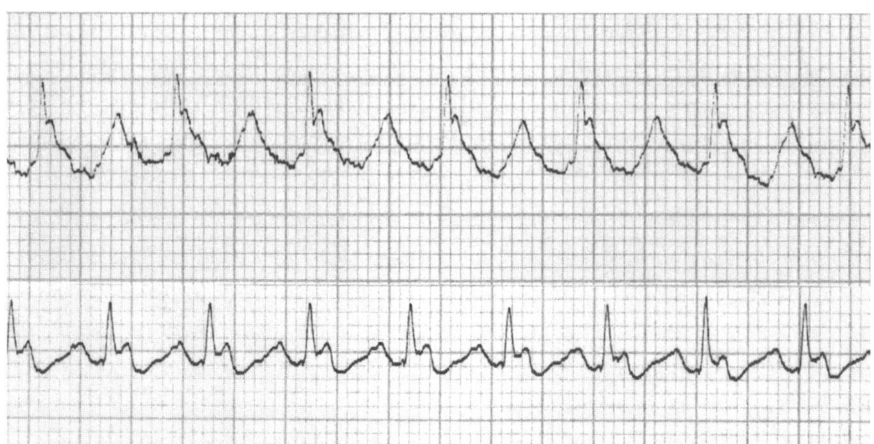

Fig. 1: Shows two strips of ECG lead 2 from the same patient. Both show atrial flutter. The saw-tooth waves in the top tracing are easily recognised. The lower tracing is less easily seen and can be misdiagnosed.

3.4. *Ventricular Tachycardia*

This can herald sudden cardiac death. It occurs after operations requiring ventriculotomy and patch insertion such as tetralogy repair. The development of severe pulmonary incompetence with RV dilatation can be the cause, and then a pulmonary valve replacement is indicated.

4. Sudden Cardiac Death in Adolescents and Young Adults

The most common disorder accounting for this devastating event, which often occurs on the sporting field, is a structural abnormality of the heart, including hypertrophic cardiomyopathy. Conduction abnormalities such as Wolf–Parkinson–White and long-QT syndrome are responsible for about 10%, along with a severe blow to the chest, asthma, and substance abuse. HCM has a prevalence of 1 in 500 and a number of genetic abnormalities affecting the sarcomere (cardiac contractile unit) have been identified. The known risk factors include family history of sudden death, family history of an inherited cardiac defect, previous cardiac arrest, recurrent syncope or tachyarrythmia or abnormally thick left ventricle on

ECG. Cardiology referral is essential for formal screening. HCM is best treated by an implantable cardioverter-defibrillator.

5. Bacterial Endocarditis

Endocarditis is a serious and debilitating illness which can result in severe haemodynamic compromise to the patient with structural heart disease. Prevention is important, but cannot always be achieved. Then, early diagnosis and treatment become essential. The adolescent needs to be made aware of the importance of seeking medical attention if there are prolonged fevers associated with malaise and constitutional symptoms. Education on endocarditis prophylaxis is also necessary.

The American Heart Association has published revised guidelines for prophylaxis for dental work. The therapeutic regimen of administering two grams of amoxicillin one hour before a dental procedure involving trauma to the oral mucosa and gums (or other procedures where acute bacteraemia might occur) stands. However, it is recommended only for patients with:

- Prosthetic heart valves.
- Previous endocarditis.
- Cyanotic CHD — unrepaired or palliated.
- Repaired CHD with prosthetic material.
- Repaired CHD with residual defects.
- Cardiac transplants with valvulopathy.

6. Psychosocial Aspects of Congenital Heart Disease

Only the most simple congenital heart lesions are cured by cardiac surgery. The majority of operations must still be considered palliative. Complications can be expected and lifelong follow-up is required. Repeat operations are necessary to replace valves and upgrade conduits. Events such as arrhythmias and endocarditis occur. These result in hospitalisations, need for medications and interruption of the normal routines of life. Pacemakers and implantable defibrillators make the patient constantly aware of their condition and of the fact that they are different from their peers. There will be times of absence from school or work, limitations in exercise capacity and inability to be involved in some sporting activities.

Adolescents begin to perceive that they have a life-threatening condition. At the same time they are going through the normal physical and emotional changes of growing up, trying to complete their education, making future plans, establishing relationships and becoming independent from their parents. Some try to cope by ignoring their heart problem and dropping out of follow-up clinics.

7. Transition to Adult Care

The transition clinic is important where there is an organised and supervised changeover from paediatric to adult follow-up. Such clinics aim to educate the young adult about his or her own heart, give advice on coping strategies, and provide contacts to telephone when there are health concerns or psychological problems. Young adults are taught to take responsibility for their own health, medications and appointments. Pleasant contact is essential and reminder phone calls about missed appointments will be necessary.

7.1. *Psychological Counselling*

Psychological counselling about coping strategies can be helpful. These patients often have low self esteem and can be prone to anxiety and depression. Because of peri-operative problems they may be left with cognitive defects which involve memory, attention, concentration, reasoning, and learning. These and their physical problems may make it difficult to obtain satisfying employment.

7.2. *General Health*

Adolescents should be counselled about general good health measures including diet, exercise appropriate for their condition, and the risks of smoking and recreational drugs. Sexual health, contraception, and pregnancy need to be raised in an age appropriate way. Sexual activity may uncommonly precipitate cardiac symptoms. What is more likely is that the young person may be worried that this might occur but be too embarrassed to ask.

7.3. *Pregnancy*

Young women with cardiac lesions should receive early age appropriate advice about contraception and their personal risk. The cardiac conditions which are associated with high risk pregnancies are:

- Eisenmenger syndrome — 40%–50% risk of death.
- Mechanical heart valves with warfarin therapy.
- Impaired ventricular function with ejection fraction <40%.
- Fontan circulation.
- Marfan syndrome with aortic root diameter >40 mm.
- Persistently cyanosed CHD.
- Obstructive lesions — significant aortic & mitral stenosis.

References

Brickner ME, Hillis LD, Lange RA. (2000) Congenital heart disease in adults. First of two parts. *N Engl J Med* **342**(4): 256–263.

Gersony WM, Rosenbaum MS. (2002) *Congenital heart disease in the adult.* McGraw-Hill, New York, London.

Shephard R, Semsarian C. (2009) Advances in the prevention of sudden cardiac death in the young. *Ther Adv Cardiovasc Dis* **3**(2): 145–155.

Thorne S, Clift P. eds. (2009) *Adult congenital heart disease.* Oxford University Press, UK.

Warnes CA. ed. (2009) *Adult congenital heart disease.* Wiley-Blackwell, USA.

Wilson W, Taubert KA, Gewitz M, Lockhart PB, Baddour LM, Levison M, Bolger A, Cabell CH, Takahashi M, Baltimore RS, Newburger JW, Strom BL, Tani LY, Gerber M, Bonow RO, Pallasch T, Shulman ST, Rowley AH, Burns JC, Ferrieri P, Gardner T, Goff D, Durack DT, American Heart Association Rheumatic Fever, Endocarditis, and Kawasaki Disease Committee; American Heart Association Council for Cardiovascular Disease in the Young; American Heart Association Council on Clinical Cardiology; American Heart Association Council on Cardiovascular Surgery and

Anesthesia, Quality of Care and Outcomes Research Interdisciplinary Working Group. (2007) Prevention of infective endocarditis: Guidelines from the American Heart Association: A guideline from the American Heart Association rheumatic fever, endocarditis, and Kawasaki Disease Committee, Council on cardiovascular disease in the young, and the Council on clinical cardiology, Council on cardiovascular surgery and anesthesia, and the quality of care and outcomes research interdisciplinary working group. *Circulation* **116**(15): 1736–1754.

<h1 style="text-align:center">Chapter 46</h1>

<h1 style="text-align:center">Adolescent Renal Medicine</h1>

Siah Kim and Deirdre Hahn

1. Introduction

Adolescent and young adult renal medicine presents a challenge to the physician. Clinical presentations of renal disease during this period reflect the adult spectrum of disease, yet survival with renal replacement therapy currently extends well into the second decade such that a strong knowledge of the common childhood and congenital conditions is also essential. In Australia, survival of renal replacement therapy (transplant, dialysis) in the paediatric population is currently at 79% at 10 years, and at 20 years it is 66%. The antecedents of adult chronic kidney disease and its risk factors, namely hypertension, obesity and Type 2 diabetes mellitus, are also emerging during adolescence and young adulthood.

The aim of this chapter is to detail the common clinical presentations in adolescents (Table 1) and discuss the key issues relevant to the management of chronic kidney disease and transplantation.

2. Renal Conditions in Adolescents

2.1. *Haematuria*

Transient microscopic haematuria in the absence of proteinuria or hypertension is commonly caused by the benign condition, thin basement

605

Table 1:   Common clinical presentations during adolescence and their causes.

Clinical presentation	Causes
Haematuria	Thin GBM disease
	Renal cysts or stones
	Cystitis
	Henoch–Schönlein Pupura
	Alport disease
	IgA nephropathy
	Autosomal dominant polycystic kidney disease
Nephritic Syndrome	Post-streptococcal GN
	IgA nephropathy
	Mesangiocapillary GN
Proteinuria +/− Nephrotic Syndrome	Orthostatic proteinuria
	Transient
	Focal segmental glomerulosclerosis
	Lupus nephritis
	Minimal change disease
	Membranous GN
Raised Creatinine	Tubulointerstitial nephritis
	Acute tubular necrosis
	Nephronophthisis
	Medullary cystic kidney disease

membrane disease, in both adolescents and adults. Isolated haematuria can often be observed, with further investigations indicated as per Table 2.

2.2. *Nephritic Syndrome*

Nephritic syndrome is defined by haematuria, oedema, and hypertension and is classically associated with post streptococcal glomerulonephritis. This presents typically two weeks post Group A Strep skin infection or pharyngitis, with an older age of presentation from mid childhood noted recently. The prognosis for PSGN remains excellent, with complete remission typical. In Australia, the incidence is significantly higher amongst Indigenous populations.

Table 2: When to further investigate haematuria and how?

Associated symptoms	Suggested diagnoses	Investigations
Proteinuria	IgA nephropathy	FBE/UEC/CMP/Albumin
Hypertension	HSP nephritis	Urine microscopy looking
+/− elevated	Alport disease	for dysmorphic RBCs
creatinine	PSGN	C3/C4
	Wegener's/Goodpasture's	ASOT/Anti DNase B
	(rare)	cANCA and Anti GBM Ab
Pain	ADPKD	Consider renal biopsy
	Renal calculi	Renal ultrasound, CT
		kidney/ureters/bladder

Forms of malignant glomerulonephritis can present during adolescence
in a similar manner, with associated elevated creatinine. These include IgA
nephropathy, mesangiocapillary glomerulonephritis, and rarely Wegener's
glomerulonephritis and Goodpasture's Syndrome.

2.3. *IgA Nephropathy*

IgA nephropathy is caused by IgA deposition in the glomerulus and secondary immune related damage. Haematuria is commonly seen, with
associated proteinuria and hypertension. Transient gross haematuria may
be precipitated with upper respiratory tract infections. Progression to end
stage kidney disease occurs in 15% to 20% in 10 years and 30% to 40% in
20 years. Nephrotic range proteinuria, hypertension, and elevated creatinine are poor prognostic indicators.

2.4. *Alport Syndrome*

Alport syndrome is caused by a mutation in genes coding for Type IV collagen, leading to a progressive degeneration of the basement membrane. It
presents as renal impairment and high frequency sensorineural hearing loss.
The most common form is X-linked, with adolescent males presenting with
haematuria with or without proteinuria, *and* a family history of chronic kidney disease and/or hearing loss. Female carriers of the X-linked form often
have microscopic haematuria. The syndrome occurs in 1:50,000 births.

2.5. *Autosomal Dominant Polycystic Kidney Disease*

The prevalence of ADPKD is estimated between 1:400 to 1:1,000 people. In ADPKD the cystic structures are present throughout the tubular system, with multiple cysts found bilaterally. The clinical presentation varies and adolescents are often asymptomatic. They may present with haematuria without proteinuria, associated hypertension and/or loin pain with palpable kidneys on examination. The associated extra-renal hepatic cysts and cerebral aneurysms are uncommon during adolescence, but screening imaging may be warranted in the context of a positive family history of cerebral aneurysms.

2.6. *Henoch–Schönlein Pupura*

HSP is a small vessel vasculitis more commonly seen in children, but which is also seen in adolescents. HSP typically presents with a pupuric rash on the extremities, subcutaneous oedema, abdominal pain and arthralgia. Renal manifestations are seen in 30% to 50% of patients, usually in the form of isolated microscopic haematuria. Nephrotic range proteinuria and nephritic-nephrotic syndromes are seen in around 20% and 1% respectively. Renal manifestations are more common in older children and adolescents, and in patients with associated abdominal pain. Disease recurrence is seen in approximately 25% of patients, more commonly in older children and adolescents and in those who present with nephritis. Follow up of patients with renal manifestations should continue for six months to ensure resolution.

2.7. *Proteinuria*

Transient proteinuria is seen in the setting of acute febrile illness and exercise but is typically no greater than 2+ on urine dipstick. The most common cause of proteinuria in adolescents is orthostatic proteinuria which is characterised by less than 25 mg protein/mmol creatinine on first void urine in the morning, and less than 1 g/day urinary protein excretion. The incidence of orthostatic proteinuria increases with age and it is considered benign.

2.8. *Nephrotic Syndrome*

Nephrotic syndrome is characterised by oedema, proteinuria and hyperlipidaemia. Nephrotic range proteinuria is defined as >50 mg/kg/day or 1.7 g/day in adolescents, which is equivalent to a spot urinary protein to creatinine ratio of 200–250 mg/mmol creatinine. Adolescents with nephrotic range proteinuria are much less likely than children to have minimal change disease — only 30%–40%. Hence, renal biopsy is indicated in adolescents who present with nephrotic range proteinuria.

Table 3 lists possible diagnoses and suggested investigations in the setting of proteinuria. HIV, hepatitis B and hepatitis C can all cause nephropathy, which typically present as proteinuria. Screening adolescents for these blood borne viruses should be considered.

2.9. *Focal Segmental Glomerulosclerosis*

In adolescents, steroid resistant nephrotic syndrome correlates with FSGS on biopsy. This carries a much poorer prognosis than the steroid sensitive nephrotic syndrome of children with gradual progression to end stage renal failure. Treatment options include combination therapies of steroids with cyclosporine, mycophenolate, and monoclonal antibodies, which have a variable efficacy including a partial or complete remission. Disease recurrence of FSGS is high following transplantation.

2.10. *Lupus Nephropathy and Membranous Nephropathy*

Systemic lupus erythematosus typically presents as a multi-system disorder. However, it can present as isolated renal disease. The presentation and

Table 3: When to investigate proteinuria and how?

Associated features	Suggested diagnoses	Suggested investigations
Proteinuria <1 g/day	Orthostatic proteinuria	First void protein creatinine ratio
Proteinuria >1.5 g/day	FSGS Minimal change disease Membranoproliferative GN	Screen for blood borne viruses Renal biopsy
Systemic symptoms in adolescent female	Lupus nephritis	C3/C4 ANA/ds DNA Renal biopsy

histopathology are highly variable, with microscopic haematuria and proteinuria alone (<1 g total protein/day) at the benign end of the spectrum. Membranous nephropathy is rare in adolescence, but lupus nephritis may present as such.

2.11. *Membranoproliferative Glomerulonephritis*

Primary MPGN predominates in adolescence and typically presents as nephrotic range proteinuria with hypertension and renal impairment. Secondary MPGN develops in association with disorders such as hepatitis B, SLE, and cancer. Complement levels are typically low. Approximately 50% of patients progress to end stage renal failure within 10 years of the initial presentation, with alternate day prednisolone seen to stabilise the clinical course.

3. Other Causes of Renal Impairment in Adolescents

Tubulointerstitial nephritis is an important cause of renal impairment in adolescence. The classical presentation of acute TIN is with elevated creatinine, rash and fever. TIN is commonly secondary to drugs such as NSAIDs and antibiotics. Microscopic haematuria, urinary eosinophils, and granular or hyaline casts are often present, but significant proteinuria and haematuria are uncommon. Renal function generally improves with the removal of the triggering agent.

Chronic TIN is associated with the chronic renal impairment seen in obstructive uropathy or vesico-uretic reflux. However, juvenile nephron–ophthisis can also present in adolescence with chronic TIN with growth failure, anaemia, polyuria, and renal impairment.

Acute tubular necrosis is seen in the setting of critical illness and also with nephrotoxic agents such as gentamicin and the calcineurin inhibitors, tacrolimus and cyclosporine.

4. Management of the Adolescent with Chronic and End Stage Kidney Disease

There are specific nuances in the management of CKD in the adolescent, with paediatric and adult perspectives meeting, and sometimes in conflict.

The causes of CKD in adolescence are often found in infancy and childhood, and involve renal hypoplasia/dysplasia and posterior urethral valves, reflux nephropathy, HSP nephritis, and post residual haemolytic uraemic syndrome. Progression to ESKD is influenced by a number of modifiable factors. However, primary disease and age of onset also significantly influence progression to ESKD, with the glomerulonephropathies showing a more rapid course compared to hypoplasia/dysplasia.

4.1. *Growth and Nutrition*

The negative impact of CKD on growth is particularly noted in adolescence. Puberty is delayed by about 2.5 years, and the growth spurt is reduced. The causes of growth disturbance and principles of managment are highlighted in Table 4. Final adult height is improved by growth

Table 4: Contributing factors to sub-optimal growth in adolescents with chronic kidney disease. Data from CARI guidelines unless otherwise stated.

Causes	Management principles
Renal osteodystrophy	
Low Ca/High PO$_4$	Ca supplementation and PO$_4$ binders
High PTH	Consider use of cinacalcet in dialysis patients for secondary hyperparathyroidism prevention
	Calcitriol to prevent pain and deformity
	Benefits in linear growth unclear
	Maintain PTH under twice normal for age
Chronic acidosis	Oral sodium bicarbonate to maintain HCO$_3$ > 22 mmol/L
GH-IGF-1 axis suppression	GH replacement at doses of 28 units/m^2/week improves final adult height
Poor caloric intake	Assess intake with assistance of renal dietician
	Maintain recommended energy intake for age
	May need enteral feeding
	Protein at or above FAO-WHO-UNU recommendations
Steroids	Consider use of steroid sparing regimens, dependent on underlying disease condition

hormone therapy and transplantation. Pubertal growth post-transplantation is of the same velocity as healthy peers, but no catch-up growth occurs.

4.2. *Anaemia*

Anaemia is an independent risk factor for mortality. Anaemia has also been linked to LV hypertrophy and reduced exercise capacity in adolescents with ESKD, and is associated with poorer quality of life. Some adult studies have shown that a higher Hb (>130 g/L) is associated with an increased risk of access thrombosis, stroke, and higher rates of dialysis initiation, and so the current recommendation is to maintain Hb between 100–115 g/L. This is achieved through the use of erythropoietin and darbepoietin injections, and administration of iron to maintain ferritin >100 µg/L and transferrin saturation >20%.

4.3. *Hypertension and Proteinuria*

Hypertension has been identified as an independent risk factor for CKD progression in adolescents and young adults. The ESCAPE study showed that aggressive treatment of blood pressure with an aim to be <50th centile for age reduced the rate of decline in eGFR over a five year period, with all subjects in the study receiving an ACE inhibitor with additional agents used if further BP reduction was required. Such aggressive targets are currently not widely used, with the general recommendation to keep SBP and DBP <95th percentile for age and height. Current adult guidelines suggest a target BP <125/75 mmHg, particularly if proteinuria >1 g/day.

Minimising proteinuria is essential to control the progression of CKD. Proteinuria is also an independent risk factor for cardiovascular mortality. ACEIs have a clear benefit in reducing both BP and proteinuria and are first line in the management of hypertension and proteinuria in CKD. ACEIs and angiotensin II receptor blockers can safely be used in combination. Beta-blockers have been shown to be superior to calcium channel blockers in preventing the progression of CKD. ACEIs and ARBs are associated with foetal renal dysgenesis and third trimester foetal death in utero, and are contraindicated in pregnancy.

4.4. *Cardiovascular Risk*

In adolescents with ESKD, the risk of cardiovascular death is much higher than the general population. Young adults with childhood onset CKD have the same risk of cardiovascular mortality as that of a 75 year old adult. Cardiovascular deaths among adolescents and young adults are most often due to sudden cardiac arrest, arrhythmia, and cardiomyopathy, in contrast to the cardiac death associated with coronary artery disease seen in the adult CKD population.

5. Management of the Adolescent with Renal Transplant

Australian registry data show that adolescents have a high risk for rejection and graft failure, with 5 and 10 year survival rates of 65% and 50% respectively, lower than both younger children and young adults. This trend is also seen in North America, with adolescents having a significantly poorer graft survival. Living related donation and pre-emptive transplant (no dialysis) have been shown to improve graft survival, with a 'therapeutic' wait on dialysis shown to be detrimental to graft survival. Overall mortality following transplantation is lower than on dialysis, with the primary causes of death being cardiovascular disease, infection and malignancy.

5.1. *Medications — See Table 5*

5.2. *Infection*

Infection remains one of the major causes of death post kidney transplantation, with the risk of sepsis increased due to immunosuppression. Risk is reduced through the use of prophylactic co-trimoxazole to prevent pneumocystis pneumonia, and also valganciclovir to prevent primary CMV disease or reactivation during the first 3 to 6 months post-transplantation. Other important infections include BK virus nephropathy, which presents as isolated rising creatinine with detection of BK virus in blood or urine via PCR. EBV related post-transplantation lymphoproliferative disease also has a variable presentation and occurs about 6 months post-transplant. Fever and lymphadenopathy are the most common presentation.

Table 5: Side effects and important interactions of commonly used medications in adolescents and young adults with CKD.

Transplantation	SE	Interactions	Pregnancy category
Tacrolimus *Immunosuppression*	HT, headache, tremor Alopecia and hyperglycaemia Nephrotoxicity	Azoles, omeprazole, simvastatin, clarithromycin/ erythromycin, phenytoin	C
Mycophenolate *Immunosuppression*	GIT disturbance and diarrhoea Bone marrow suppression especially neutropaenia	Other immunosuppressive medications	D
Steroids *Immunosuppression*	Oedema, weight gain with central fat re-distribution, hypertension, acne, fragile skin, inhibits growth, amenorrhoea, mood disturbance	Mifepristone, phenobarbitone/ phenytoin	A Increased oro-facial clefts if used in first trimester
Trimethoprin and sulphamethoxazole *PCP prophylaxis* Valganciclovir *CMV prophylaxis*	Skin sensitivity reactions GIT symptoms Marrow suppression, dermatitis, GIT symptoms	Methotrexate	C D D

Renal disease			
Cyclosporin *Nephrotic syndrome*	Hirsutism, gingival hyperplasia, nephrotoxicity, tremor, headache	Carbamazepine, fluvoxamine, amlodipine, azoles	C
Cyclophosphamide *Nephrotic syndrome*	Myelosuppression, infertility, alopecia, GIT upset	Other cytotoxic agents	D

(Continued)

Table 5: *(Continued)*

Risk factors		Interactions	
ACEI/ARB	Hypotension, cough, high K/creatinine	NSAIDs, loop diuretics	D
Statins	Deranged LFTs, myalgia, GIT symptoms	Fibrates increase risk of myopathy, cyclosporin	D
Beta-blockers	Wheeze, respiratory symptoms, insomnia, nightmares, depression, poor concentration	Clonidine, ergot alkaloids, sympathomimetics	C
CCB	Oedema, rash, fatigue, dizziness, gingival hyperplasia	Other antihypertensives	C

Source: Australian Medicines Handbook 2011.

5.3. *Rejection*

The primary cause of graft failure in adolescents and young adults remains chronic allograft nephropathy (36%), however non-compliance accounts for approximately 20%. Table 5 contains the commonly used medications and their side effects, with particular focus on those which may interfere with adherence in adolescents.

5.4. *Malignancy*

Death rates from malignancy increase steadily from the time of transplant, accounting for 2% 4 to 9 years post-transplant and increasing to 17% 15 years post-transplant. Hence many malignancies do not appear until adolescents have been transferred to adult services. The most common cancers are skin cancers, accounting for 60%, with minimal contribution to mortality. Non-Hodgkin's lymphoma accounts for 25% and is the most common cancer to cause death.

5.5. *Cardiovascular Risk*

The leading cause of death in the adolescent and young adult age group is cardiovascular disease, accounting for around 50% of all deaths in those on dialysis. Amongst transplanted patients, the risk is smaller, with cardiac causes accounting for 11% of all deaths. Post-transplantation, many cardiovascular risk factors, including hypertension, impaired glucose tolerance and hyperlipidaemia are still prevalent, and represent both pre-existing underlying disease and side effects from medication. It is important to monitor for these and treat as required.

5.6. *Pregnancy and the Kidney Transplant Recipient*

Pregnancy is now common post-transplantation, but carries a significantly increased risk of pre-ecplampsia for the mother, and of IUGR and prematurity for the baby. Current registry data does not show a higher incidence of congenital abnomalies associated with the use of calcineurin inhibitors, azathioprine or steroids, but there have been some reported abnormalities with mycophenolate mofetil. There are few safety data on other agents including therapeutic antibodies and MTOR inhibitors.

6. Other Issues in Adolescents with Chronic Kidney Disease

6.1. *Quality of Life*

Some adolescents and young adults with CKD, including those with ESKD (and on dialysis) rate their quality of life the same as the general population. Others show significantly reduced QOL particularly those on dialysis. It is important to be aware that clinicians have consistently been shown to under rate their patients' QOL.

6.2. *Education and Employment*

Formal IQ testing has found that adolescents and young adults with ESKD have an IQ significantly lower than sibling controls, falling within the low average range. There was no difference in memory, behaviour and self esteem. Higher rates of unemployment have been reported in adults with childhood onset ESKD but significantly lower than those with adult onset ESKD.

7. Emerging Risk Factors for Adult Onset CKD During Adolescence

7.1. *Hypertension*

Hypertension in adolescents is defined as an average systolic or diastolic BP >95th centile for height, age and gender on three occasions. As isolated hypertension is sometimes seen in the clinical setting in this age group, 24 hour ambulatory BP monitoring is often required to clarify the diagnosis. Primary hypertension increases in adolescence, and it is strongly associated with overweight and obesity, with 30% of overweight or obese adolescents hypertensive. Investigations include urine dipstick, UEC, lipid profile, fasting glucose, TFTs, LFTs, and an ECG to detect evidence of LVH. Paired plasma renin/aldosterone, urinary catecholamines, and imaging studies are indicated if there is a suspected underlying associated medical cause. Lifestyle changes such as increased physical activity, reduced dietary salt and increased potassium (if renal function normal), and weight reduction are currently recommended. ACEIs/ARBs and calcium channel blockers are first line therapy.

7.2. *Other Risk Factors*

Diabetes related kidney disease is the leading cause of ESKD in Australia and many other countries, with an increasing incidence. Impaired glucose tolerance and early onset Type 2 diabetes is associated with obesity. Annual screening for all adolescents with Type 1 or Type 2 diabetes with urine ACR is currently recommended.

7.3. *High Risk Groups: Indigenous Australians*

Within the 14–24 year old age group, the incidence of ESKD is four times higher amongst Indigenous Australians than the non-Indigenous population. The incidence of both micro-albuminuria and macro-albuminuria is also significantly higher in the 15–24 year old Indigenous age group and screening for albuminuria is currently suggested in the Indigenous adolescent. A similar situation holds true for many other indigenous and First Nation populations.

8. Transition to Adult Care: Specific Issues for the Renal Patient

Transition to adult services represents a significant rite of passage for many adolescents with CKD and has been identified as a time when non-compliance increases. Home dialysis services become available which are associated with better outcomes, particularly for those with other cardiovascular risk factors. Combined oral contraceptives may exacerbate underlying hypertension and should be used with caution. Adolescents and young adults should also be made aware of their increased cardiovascular risk and smoking should be discouraged and a healthy lifestyle promoted.

References

Bawden HN, Acott P, Carter J, Lirenman D, Macdonald GW, McAllister M, McDonnell MC, Shea S, Crocker J. (2004) Neuropsychological functioning in end-stage renal disease. *Arch Dis Child* **89**(7): 644–647.

Beier UH, Green C, Meyers KE. (2010) Caring for adolescent renal patients. *Kidney Int* **77**(4): 285–291.

Brandt JR, Jacobs A, Raissy HH, Kelly FM, Staples AO, Kaufman E, Wong CS. (2010) Orthostatic proteinuria and the spectrum of diurnal variability of urinary protein excretion in healthy children. *Pediatr Nephrol* **25**(6): 1131–1137.

Caring for Australasians with Renal Impairment (2011) *CARI guidelines.* Available online at: http://www.cari.org.au/guidelines.php. (Accessed 1 August 2011.)

Fine RN, Martz K, Stablein D. (2010) What have 20 years of data from the North American Pediatric Renal Transplant Cooperative Study taught us about growth following renal transplantation in infants, children, and adolescents with end-stage renal disease? *Pediatr Nephrol* **25**(4): 739–746.

Groothoff JW, Grootenhuis MA, Offringa M, Stronks K, Hutten GJ, Heymans HSA. (2005) Social consequences in adult life of end-stage renal disease in childhood. *J Pediatr* **146**(4): 512–517.

Escape Trial Group., Wuhl E, Trivelli A, Picca S, Litwin M, Peco-Antic A, Zurowska A, Testa S, Jankauskiene A, Emre S, Caldas-Afonso A, Anarat A, Niaudet P, Mir S, Bakkaloglu A, Enke B, Montini G, Wingen AM, Sallay P,

Jeck N, Berg U, Caliskan S, Wygoda S, Hohbach-Hohenfellner K, Dusek J, Urasinski T, Arbeiter K, Neuhaus T, Gellermann J, Drozdz D, Fischbach M, Moller K, Wigger M, Peruzzi L, Mehls O, Schaefer F. (2009) Strict blood-pressure control and progression of renal failure in children. *N Engl J Med* **361**(17): 1639–1650.

Kennedy SE, Mackie FE, Rosenberg AR, McDonald SP. (2006) Waiting time and outcome of kidney transplantation in adolescents. *Transplantation* **82**(8): 1046–1050.

McDonald SP, Craig JC, Australian & New Zealand Paediatric Nephrology Association. (2004) Long-term survival of children with end-stage renal disease. *N Engl J Med* **350**(26): 2654–2662.

McKay DB, Josephson MA, Armenti VT, August P, Coscia LA, Davis CL, Davison JM, Easterling T, Friedman JE, Hou S, Karlix J, Lake KD, Lindheimer M, Matas AJ, Moritz MJ, Riely CA, Ross LF, Scott JR, Wagoner LE, Wrenshall L, Adams PL, Bumgardner GL, Fine RN, Goral S, Krams SM, Martinez OM, Tolkoff-Rubin N, Pavlakis M, Scantlebury V, Women's Health Committee of the American Society Of Transplantation. (2005) Reproduction and transplantation: Report on the AST Consensus Conference on Reproductive Issues and Transplantation. *Am J Transplant* **5**(7): 1592–1599.

Rees L. (2009) Long-term outcome after renal transplantation in childhood. *Pediatr Nephrol* **24**(3): 475–484.

Shroff R, Ledermann S. (2009) Long-term outcome of chronic dialysis in children. *Pediatr Nephrol* **24**(3): 463–474.

Staples AO, Greenbaum LA, Smith JM, Gipson DS, Filler G, Warady BA, Martz K, Wong CS. (2010) Association between clinical risk factors and progression of chronic kidney disease in children. *CJASN* **5**(12): 2172–2179.

Van Husen M, Kemper MJ. (2011) New therapies in steroid-sensitive and steroid-resistant idiopathic nephrotic syndrome. *Pediatr Nephrol* **26**(6): 881–892.

White A, Wong W, Sureshkumur P, Singh G. (2010) The burden of kidney disease in indigenous children of Australia and New Zealand, epidemiology, antecedent factors and progression to chronic kidney disease. *J Paediatr Child Health* **46**(9): 504–509.

Chapter 47

Common Rheumatological Conditions in Adolescence

Davinder Singh-Grewal

1. Introduction

Both childhood and adult type rheumatic diseases are present in adolescence. Musculoskeletal complaints are the third commonest reason for adolescents presenting to primary care. About 1 in every 100 young people, between the ages of 12 and 19 years, suffers rheumatic symptoms which persist more than six months. One third of children with arthritis will continue to have active disease into adulthood. Approximately 20% of systemic lupus erythematosus and a significant proportion of idiopathic Raynaud disease develop prior to adulthood, with the largest pre-adult peak in the peri-pubescent period. Non-inflammatory diseases including idiopathic pain syndromes and spondylolisthesis are characteristically encountered in the adolescent years.

2. Arthritis

2.1. *Juvenile Idiopathic Arthritis and Its Subtypes*

JIA is the commonest rheumatic disease of adolescence and young adulthood with a prevalence of 58/100,000 in 15 to 24 year olds. The aetiology of JIA is unknown but it is likely to have a strong genetic basis

621

with as yet unidentified infectious or environmental triggers. There are six subtypes: oligoarticular, polyarticular, systemic, enthesistic, psoriatic, and other.

2.1.1. *Oligoarticular arthritis*

It is the commonest form of JIA, usually involves the large joints of the lower limbs and is predominant in childhood.

2.1.2. *Polyarticular arthritis*

This type affects five or more joints at disease onset and is sub-divided into two groups, depending on the presence or absence of rheumatoid factor. Up to 25% of polyarticular JIA is associated with a positive RF and teenage girls are at particularly high risk from this combination. Polyarticular arthritis with RF positivity probably represents early onset adult seropositive rheumatoid arthritis and is likely to be a destructive and rapidly progressive disease requiring aggressive treatment. As in adults, positive anti-cyclic citrullinated peptide antibodies are associated with more aggressive disease. Patients with RF-positive polyarticular JIA usually have symmetrical involvement of large and small joints, including hands and wrists. Rheumatoid nodules and vasculitis may be present, as in adults. Adolescents with RF negative polyarticular JIA with a positive ANA are still at risk of uveitis but have a significantly better long term prognosis than those with a positive RF.

2.1.3. *Systemic arthritis*

The fevers, rash, serositis, hepatosplenomegaly, and adenopathy may present before the arthritis becomes apparent. The fever is quotidian, spiking once or twice a day and returning to baseline or below baseline. Raised inflammatory markers, a leucoytosis and a thrombocytosis are characteristically seen. Systemic JIA presents prior to adolescence and 50% continue to have disease into adolescence, and are at risk of significant joint damage.

2.1.4. *Enthesitis related arthritis*

Enthesitis related arthritis, previously known as juvenile ankylosing spondylitis, predominantly affects males with an onset in adolescence. Less than 25% of adolescents with ERA have inflammatory back pain as seen in adults, whereas enthesitis or inflammation of points of insertion of tendons and ligaments into bone is common, along with asymmetrical peripheral large joint arthritis. Older adolescents and young adults may present with typical AS symptoms. HLA-B27 is positive in 80% to 90% of patients with ERA and there is often a family or personal history of other HLA-B27 related illness, including acute painful anterior uveitis and inflammatory bowel disease. Adolescents with ERA are likely to have ongoing disease and develop more typical features of the disease, including spondylitis, into adulthood.

2.1.5. *Psoriatic arthritis*

The arthritis may develop prior to psoriasis and often presents with asymmetrical large joint arthritis in adolescents. A family or personal history of psoriasis or the presence of nail pitting, or dactylitis (inflammation of an entire digit including the small joints and tendon sheaths) is required to confirm the diagnosis. Around 50% of patients will be HLA-B27 positive and a proportion will also be ANA positive and thus at risk of asymptomatic uveitis.

2.2. *Complications of Juvenile Idiopathic Arthritis*

Complications of JIA are disease related and treatment related. The most significant long term physical complication is permanent joint damage and is predominant in severe JIA resistant to treatment, RF positive polyarticular arthritis or those with other forms of JIA which have not been treated early or aggressively enough. Even the mildest forms of JIA including oligarticular disease may develop significant complications in skeletal growth if disease is inadequately treated, resulting in leg length discrepancy with postural scoliosis, and micrognathia in adolescence.

Uveitis develops in 20% to 30% of ANA positive disease, and 10% of these will have impaired vision. Uveitis is asymptomatic and without regular slit lamp examination may be missed until the patient develops glaucoma, cataracts, and/or keratopathy.

2.3. *Treatment of Juvenile Idiopathic Arthritis*

Current treatment approaches are aggressive and aim for complete disease remission to prevent long term damage and disability.

2.3.1. *Pharmacological therapies for juvenile idiopathic arthritis*

Local therapy with intra-articular steroid injections is favoured in oligoarticular disease and is successful in 90% of patients. Traditional systemic therapies such as methotrexate, sulphasalazine, and newer biologic agents such as the monoclonal anti-tissue necrosis factor agents are needed in only a small proportion. Systemic therapies, including corticosteroids, are commonly used in those with systemic and polyarticular disease and should be introduced early on in the disease course if there is inadequate response to other therapies. Weight gain and metabolic abnormalities with high dose corticosteroid therapy, the potentially hazardous drug interaction of methotrexate with alcohol, the infectious and teratogen risk of immunosuppressive agents and the potential long term malignancy risk with biologic agents are all significant for adolescents and young adults, and often reduce compliance.

2.3.2. *Non-pharmacological therapies for juvenile idiopathic arthritis*

Physical therapies ensure maintenance of a range of motion of affected joints, and of the strength and function of adjacent muscle groups. Physiotherapy concentrates on gross motor function, particularly locomotion, and occupational therapy on hand function.

2.4. *Prognosis and Outcome*

In most forms of JIA long term outcomes are strongly related to the duration of active disease and consequent joint damage, making early aggressive management a key to improved outcomes. Complications of the disease include those directly due to the pathological process itself, and those due to the therapies used such as osteoporosis and changes in physical appearance secondary to corticosteroids. Severe disease is also associated with delayed growth and pubertal development. Females with JIA have higher rates of menorrhagia, difficulty conceiving and premature ovarian failure. Psychological morbidity is common, with higher rates of anxiety and depression than the general population. Educational and employment achievement are also significantly impaired in JIA, with unemployment rates as high as 30%.

3. Systemic Lupus Erythematosus

3.1. *Aetiology and Epidemiology*

SLE is a chronic, relapsing and remitting multi-organ inflammatory disease that affects 8 per 100,000 children and adolescents. Autoantibodies, including the anti-double stranded DNA antibodies which correlate with disease activity, are diagnostic. Up to 20% of patients with SLE have an onset of disease in late childhood or adolescence with the median age of onset of juvenile SLE being 12 to 14 years. The female to male ratio is 5:1 (lower than in adult populations), and prevalence and severity are higher in Asian, black and Hispanic populations.

3.2. *Clinical Presentation*

Patients usually present with constitutional symptoms such as fever, fatigue, weight loss, and anorexia. The classic clinical features are a malar or discoid rash, arthritis, alopecia, and palatal ulceration, accompanied by thrombocytopaenia and/or lymphopaenia. SLE is a life-threatening disease characterised by periods of remission and relapse. Each flare of disease activity is associated with the accrual of end organ damage and worsened long term outcome. Adolescent patients with SLE have a very high risk of renal and central nervous system involvement, both of which are associated with significant morbidity and mortality.

3.3. *Treatment*

Most patients will require prolonged treatment with systemic corticosteroids and immunosuppressive agents to induce and maintain remission. Immunosuppressive agents including methotrexate are used for limited skin and joint disease. Azathioprine, mycophenolate, cyclophosphamide and rituximab are required for nephritis or CNS disease. All patients without a contraindication (including retinal or hepatic disease) should be treated with hydroxychloroquine as an adjunctive therapy since it has been shown to reduce relapse rates. This treatment exposes patients to the rare risk of retinopathy and regular ophthalmological assessment, including formal visual fields, will be required. Excessive UVB exposure from sunlight can result in an increase in SLE activity, so high sun protection factor sunscreen and avoiding high exposure to sunlight are essential. Compliance failure is a major cause of flare in the adolescent age group.

3.4. *Outcomes*

The long term outcome for SLE has improved over the past three decades from around 40% ten year survival to up to 95%. Nonetheless, long term disease remission is rare in patients with early onset SLE. Adolescents with SLE have been shown to suffer greater cumulative damage from chronic disease and treatment associated adverse effects. Patients with SLE have an increased risk of severe infection, due to the inherent immune dysregulation, compounded by treatment with immunosuppressive medications. Young women with SLE have a 50-fold increase in myocardial infarction when compared to healthy controls, a common cause of death in patients with SLE who survive adolescence. Every attempt should be made to control known cardiovascular risk factors in adolescent patients (Chapter 52).

4. Musculoskeletal Pain Syndromes (Pain Amplification Syndromes)

Chronic pain syndromes are well recognised in adults. Adolescents also suffer from these conditions and pain without an organic cause is under recognised in young people. They may present with a number of clinical manifestations including headache, abdominal pain, and musculoskeletal pain. The consistent hallmark of these conditions is subjective symptoms and disability greatly in excess of any objective findings. Failure to recognise the potentiating physical and psychological factors of the pain may prolong suffering and disability.

4.1. *Classification*

4.1.1. *Diffuse idiopathic pain*

DIP describes a pattern of generalised pain often associated with fatigue, school absence, and sleep disturbance. In some instances, a preceding infection or illness can be identified, with a slow recovery and the development of DIP. The adult counterpart of DIP is fibromyalgia that, unlike DIP, has defined diagnostic criteria including the presence of tender points. Fibromyalgia is associated with a very poor functional prognosis, while DIP is felt to have a better long term outcome. There is significant overlap between DIP and other described conditions such as myofibrositis, myofascial pain syndrome, nonarticular rheumatism, and rheumatic pain modulation disorder. Rather than debate the terminology or speculate on the specific cause of the symptoms, an approach which tackles the dysfunction and the psychology of the symptoms is a more prudent one.

4.1.2. *Localised pain syndromes*

These are limited to one area — usually a limb in the case of musculoskeletal pain — and previously classified as reflex sympathetic dystrophy but more recently reclassified as complex regional pain syndrome. Common triggers include minor injury followed by a period of prolonged immobilisation. Physical examination reveals painful hypersensitivity of the skin to even mild stimulus such as soft touch (allodynia), vascular and temperature changes on the affected limb and in severe long-standing cases, contracture and trophic changes. As for DIP a preceding illness, psychological stressors or a family history of chronic pain are often identified.

4.2. *Diagnosis*

Diagnosis relies on recognition of the possibility of DIP or CRPS and judicious investigation to exclude other plausible organic causes. Patients with pain syndromes and their families commonly consult multiple physicians in different subspecialty fields in the search for a treatable organic cause. When multiple investigations have failed to elicit this and the patient shows the classical clinical features of pain amplification, the clinician should address the possibility of a pain syndrome with the patient and their family and progress with an appropriate treatment plan.

4.3. *Treatment*

A multidisciplinary rehabilitation program is the most effective management strategy. Pharmacological therapies for pain are ineffective on their own and require concurrent physical and psychological approaches. Nonsteroidal anti-inflammatory medications, simple analgesics, opioid drugs, anticonvulsants (particularly gabapentin) and anti-depressants have all been used without the benefit of any randomised controlled trials. Physical therapy and occupational therapy to provide somatic desensitisation of allodynia, treatment of contracture, muscle wasting, and immobility are an essential part of CRPS management. Both DIP and CRPS will benefit from a general mobility and fitness plan to improve aerobic fitness, but also as a means to develop a regular routine for patients who will have often long departed from regular school, social, and home routines. A graded approach is usually the most effective and may comprise psychological support and intervention in patients with mood or anxiety disorders. Patient education around the neurobiology of pain and the somatic responses to pain has an important role in initial recovery, and in the development of future self management skills. It is important to engage both the patient and their family in the therapy program to ensure compliance and success.

4.4. *Outcomes*

With the institution of an appropriate multidisciplinary treatment program, the outcome of DIP and CRPS is generally positive, with high rates of return to school, social, and family routines. Young people with delayed diagnosis or prolonged symptoms are thought to have the poorest outcomes. While relapse is quite common, patient education regarding symptoms and early re-engagement with therapy can reduce the impact of relapse.

5. Back Pain

Back pain is relatively common in young people, with the lifetime prevalence below the age of 20 years between 70% and 80%. Examination of the back is an essential part of the rheumatic examination of the young person.

5.1. *Aetiology*

There are many causes of back pain. Lumbar disc protrusion, apophyseal injury, and apophyseal ring fractures should be considered when nerve root pain and persistent pain after trauma are present.

5.1.1. *Mechanical causes of back pain*

This group includes a number of separate conditions and non-specific back pain constitutes the largest component of this group in adolescence and young adults.

Scoliosis occurs in up to 3% of adolescent patients. Most are right sided, idiopathic, asymptomatic, and evident on examination with asymmetry on forward bending. Severe scoliosis may cause pain, but this is rare. Thus the presence of pain should alert the physician to the possibility of a more significant underlying pathology, such as tumour or infection. Other signs that indicate a serious underlying cause include a left sided scoliosis, rapid progression of scoliosis, neurological symptoms, or an abnormal neurological examination. Scoliosis warrants radiological investigation in most cases and forms an important part of surveillance of even idiopathic scoliosis as a small proportion (<10%) will require orthopaedic intervention in the form of bracing or surgery.

Hyperlordotic back pain, also known as lumbosacral strain, spondylogenic back pain or lumbar facet syndrome, is essentially an overuse syndrome involving the posterior elements of the spine including muscles, tendons, and facet joints. It is more common in athletes and has many of the symptoms and signs of spondylolysis or spondylolisthesis, requiring these conditions to be excluded. Treatment involves improving core strength and hamstring flexibility. *Spondylolysis, spondylolisthesis*, and *Scheuermann disease* are discussed in Chapter 26.

5.1.2. *Inflammatory causes of back pain*

Inflammation of the sacroiliac joints or spine may cause back pain and is usually associated with the ERA or psoriatric arthritis forms of JIA (Section 2.1.4). Pain, sometimes with radiation into the buttocks, and morning stiffness are the hallmarks of inflammatory back pain. Clinical findings include tenderness over the sacroiliac joints or pain on stressing the sacroiliac joints by manoeuvres such as compression of the pelvis or flexion, abduction and external rotation of the hip, and reduced lumbar spine mobility. Plain radiographs may be normal early in the disease but later show clear changes of sclerosis and fusion of the joints. Bone scan or MRI may identify abnormalities much earlier in the disease process.

6. Rarer Rheumatic Conditions in Adolescents and Young Adults

6.1. *Juvenile Dermatomyositis*

JDM is an idiopathic inflammatory myopathy that also affects the skin in 95% of cases. Patients usually present with proximal muscle weakness and rash. Muscle enzymes, including creatine kinase and transaminases are elevated. Diagnostic muscle biopsy has been largely replaced by MRI. Treatment involves high dose steroids in combination with immunosuppressive agents similar to SLE. As the onset of JDM is uncommon in the adolescent age group one must be wary of alternate diagnoses such as inherited myopathy, infection, particularly parasitic infections, or malignancy related myopathy. Half of all patients with JDM will be in remission within four to five years, and half will still have active disease through adolescence.

6.2. *Systemic Vasculitides*

These are characterised by the presence of inflammation and necrosis of blood vessel walls. Henoch–Schönlein Purpura, Kawasaki disease, Wegener's vasculitis, Churg-Strauss Syndrome, Takayasu arteritis, polyarteritis nodosa, microscopic polyangiitis, sarcoidosis and Bechet syndrome are all systemic vasculitides. Each has a unique clinical profile. It is prudent when confronted by unusual, systemic symptoms to consider a broad differential diagnosis that includes these conditions.

6.3. *Periodic Fever Syndromes (Auto-Inflammatory Syndromes)*

These conditions are characterised by recurrent self-limited episodes of fever and associated inflammatory symptoms including abdominal pain from peritonitis, headache from aseptic meningitis, chest pain from pericarditis or pleuritis, skin rashes and arthritis. During episodes, patients will have elevated inflammatory markers and neutrophil counts. Episodes are not due to infection, and patients are clinically and biochemically well between episodes. The underlying abnormality is genetic and lies in the regulation of the inflammatory process. Often there is a positive family history of similar symptoms. Genetic testing is available for most forms. Familial Mediterranean fever is the commonest of these conditions and while onset is during the first decade of life in 50% of patients, a diagnosis is frequently not made until adolescence. Treatment with non-steroidal anti-inflammatories or corticosteroids can ameliorate symptoms during an attack, but will not prevent further attacks. Daily colchicine is successful in preventing episodes and has been shown to prevent amyloidosis. Treatment is lifelong.

6.4. *Raynaud's Disease and Phenomenon*

Raynaud's sign describes a sequence of blanching, cyanosis, and erythema seen as the typical white, blue, and red colour change of the peripheries, particularly the fingers or toes. The aetiology is arterial constriction initially resulting in blanching, followed by tissue hypoxia and finally reflex hyperaemia. Raynaud's phenomenon describes these findings when there is an underlying connective tissue disorder. Raynaud's disease describes the symptoms if there is no underlying cause found. Triggers include cold and physical or emotional stress. Raynaud's disease may develop in the adolescent years. Raynaud's phenomenon is far less frequent. Treatment of Raynaud's disease usually requires only environmental measures including maintaining core temperature through appropriate clothing, while more severe symptoms can be treated with calcium channel blockers or vasodilators.

6.5. *Scleroderma*

Scleroderma is a general term for hardening and thickening of the skin. There are two subgroups of scleroderma, localised or systemic.

Limited systemic disease is described by the CREST syndrome: calcinosis, Raynaud's syndrome, oesophageal dysmotility, sclerodactyly, and telangiectasia. Pulmonary fibrosis, constrictive pericarditis, pulmonary hypertension, systemic hypertension, and generalised gut dysmotility occur in the more severe systemic disease. Treatment involves corticosteroids (be wary of the possibility of hypertensive crisis with high doses) and immunosuppression.

6.6. *Overlap Syndromes*

Many of the systemic inflammatory conditions described above share a number of clinical and serological features. Overlap or undifferentiated systemic inflammatory disease are terms used to describe patients who possess features of more than one condition and thus do not fit easily into a single diagnosis. A larger proportion of adolescents and young adults, when compared to older adults, fall into this overlap group at initial presentation. With time many develop features most consistent with a single diagnosis. Treatment is initially targeted to the specific pathological process observed rather than the presumed diagnosis.

References

Adam V, St-Pierre Y, Fautrel B, Clarke AE, Duffy CM, Penrod JR. (2005) What is the impact of adolescent arthritis and rheumatism? Evidence from a national sample of Canadians. *J Rheumatol* **32**(2): 354–361.

Hiraki LT, Benseler SM, Tyrrell PN, Hebert D, Harvey E, Silverman ED. (2008) Clinical and laboratory characteristics and long-term outcome of pediatric systemic lupus erythematosus: A longitudinal study. *J Pediatr* **152**(4): 550–556.

Jones GT, Macfarlane GJ. (2005) Epidemiology of low back pain in children and adolescents. *Arch Dis Child* **90**(3): 312–316.

Maillard SM, Davies K, Khubchandani R, Woo PM, Murray KJ. (2004) Reflex sympathetic dystrophy: A multidisciplinary approach. *Arthritis Rheum* **51**(2): 284–290.

McDonagh JE, White PH. eds. (2005) *Adolescent Rheumatology*. Informa Healthcare USA Inc, New York.

Petty RE, Southwood TR, Manners P, Baum J, Glass DN, Goldenberg J, He X, Maldonado-Cocco J, Orozco-Alcala J, Prieur AM, Suarez-Almazor ME, Woo P, International League of Associations for Rheumatology. (2004) International League of Associations for Rheumatology classification of juvenile idiopathic arthritis. *J Rheumatol* **31**(2): 390–392.

Purcell L, Micheli L. (2009) Low back pain in young athletes. *Sports Health: A Multidisciplinary Approach* **1**(3): 212–222.

Schanberg LE, Sandborg C, Barnhart HX, Ardoin SP, Yow E, Evans GW, Mieszkalski KL, Ilowite NT, Eberhard A, Levy DM, Kimura Y, Von Scheven E, Silverman E, Bowyer SL, Punaro L, Singer NG, Sherry DD, McCurdy D, Klein-Gitelman M, Wallace C, Silver R, Wagner-Weiner L, Higgins GC, Brunner HI, Jung L, Soep JB, Reed A, Atherosclerosis Prevention in Pediatric Lupus Erythematosus, I. (2009) Premature atherosclerosis in pediatric systemic lupus erythematosus: Risk factors for increased carotid intima-media thickness in the atherosclerosis prevention in pediatric lupus erythematosus cohort. *Arthritis Rheum* **60**(5): 1496–1507.

Shenoi S, Wallace CA. (2010) Tumor necrosis factor inhibitors in the management of juvenile idiopathic arthritis: An evidence-based review. *Paediatr Drugs* **12**(6): 367–377.

Chapter 48

Genetics and Adolescents

David Sillence

1. Introduction

A thorough understanding of the psychosocial impact of genetic disorders
in adolescents is central to both translating the modern advances in
genetic medicine into practical and positive health benefits for young
people, and improving understanding. Some heritable disorders have or
have had a profound impact on the psychosocial functioning of adolescents. First, there are disorders such as cystic fibrosis, the thalassaemias,
and the muscular dystrophies in which morbidity and mortality, while
high in adolescent years, are gradually changing in developed countries.
Increased life expectancy brings a new set of morbidities.

Adolescents are keenly aware and often depressed by the death or
increasing illness of close friends whom they have regarded as just one of
their 'well' friends.

What is more alarming for teenagers is watching friends manifest
symptoms of major psychiatric illness with genetic aetiology, coupled
with their own feelings of powerlessness to help a friend. Bipolar affective disorder, obsessive compulsive disorder and panic disorder are just a
few of the disorders with high heritability and which have major disrupting effects on school performance and relationships.

Adolescent distress will also be high where a parent develops symptoms of Huntington disease (a progressive neurodegenerative disorder

with late onset dementia), or familial cancers such as ovary and breast. In this scenario, adolescents are often the silent and forgotten witnesses who need reassurance and clear explanation of what is happening and of their own genetic risk.

Adolescents have become a target group for screening programs for a range of disorders. There is evidence that for integrated community genetic programs in which both education and consent are included, there is a high uptake of screening. However there are psychosocial hazards.

2. Talking with Adolescents About Heritability

Teenagers often become aware, through their enquiries (but frequently not because of parental transparency), that there is a heritable disorder in the family which might affect them or their reproductive choices. This is particularly the case where they have an increased chance of being a non-manifesting carrier or being affected with a disorder that is not penetrant until later in life. Young people have access to almost unlimited information resources and these may reassure or further add to their anxiety.

There are several sources of information about adolescents and their response to the prospect of screening for carrier status or pre-symptomatic genetic diagnosis. These derive from psychosocial studies of the outcomes of:

- Adolescent carrier screening programs.
- Pre-symptomatic testing for late onset disorders with delayed adolescent or young adult penetrance.

2.1. *Genetic Testing and Screening in Adolescents*

Heterozygote screening programs for specific genetic disorders were introduced in the 1960s. Mandated heterozygote screening programs in many states of the US, such as the Sickle Cell Screening program, although implemented by well-meaning professionals, inevitably stigmatised populations and were met with considerable opposition. Mandated screening was perceived by predominantly African Americans as a further program for discrimination. The screening was confused at best, as guidelines for heterozygous carriers were confused with risks for homozygous carriers.

Kaback and colleagues in the early 1970s, noting the higher frequency of Tay–Sachs disease in the Ashkenazi Jewish population, introduced voluntary screening programs for young adults in the Jewish population. This was a remarkable program in that its implementation followed extensive consultation with religious and community leaders, accompanied by community education, and group and personal counselling. In a further visionary program, Kaback and colleagues developed college student screening programs. Subsequently other young adult, and even high school student screening programs for heterozygous carrier status have been piloted and evaluated.

As early as 1996, Mitchell and colleagues had reported on a schools carrier screening program for Tay–Sachs and beta-thalassaemia. Testing occurred one week following an educational activity with an in-school informational exchange and discussion about genetic disorders. Barlow-Stewart and colleagues describe the evolution of a genetic screening program for Tay-Sachs disease and cystic fibrosis with Australian Jewish high school students. The program comprised an onsite education session followed by carrier testing. Only students who attended the educational program were offered testing. When evaluated 3 to 6 years later, there was a high retention of knowledge about the genetics of these disorders, no evidence of stigmatisation of carriers and low concern. Moreover 96% of students who had testing were positive about the testing procedure. The 11 carriers detected in the program indicated that they would inform a future partner about their result.

2.2. *Presymptomatic and Predictive Testing of Young Adults for Late Onset Genetic Disorders*

There is an extensive literature dealing with the outcomes of pre-symptomatic and predictive testing of young adults for late onset disorders such as Huntington disease and familial cancers. The policy statement of the Human Genetics Society of Australasia in 2008 provides an excellent summary of the current professional views of highly experienced experts in the field. Genetics and counselling professionals now have some 30 years experience arising out of studies of the psychosocial impact of pre-symptomatic testing for Huntington Disease. It is clear that this type of testing is best undertaken by teams in settings with access to skilled counselling and psychosocial assistance. There is also consensus that the process should involve:

- Pre-test and post-test counselling.
- A period between pre-test counselling and giving results in which there is opportunity for further discussion or even for a pause to reconsider whether it is the appropriate time to proceed.
- The presence of a support person, a family member or friend, who can provide constant support through the process of testing which might take several months by the time a result is delivered.

There is further consensus that while an absolute age cut-off need not apply, an age of 18 years and above corresponds to a level of psychosocial maturity which is necessary to assimilate the myriad of consequences arising from a diagnosis.

3. Where Teenagers Can Go for Information

Current studies of adolescent learning indicate that adolescents and young adults in particular are far more likely to go to the worldwide web for information. In addition social networking has become an important space for sharing information and obtaining support. None of these sources are particularly focused on providing professional support and sensitively explained information either about heritability or genetic disorders. One risk for adolescents trawling the internet is that they might be attracted to sites which offer personalised medicine which for a fee will provide probabilistic information about common medical conditions or risk without a contextual explanation.

3.1. *Genetics on the Web*

There are several important Web URLs which are clearing houses for genetic information (see Table 1).

- The Centre for Genetic Education site has a comprehensive list of fact sheets, contacts, and guidelines.

Table 1: Important websites.

Centre for Genetic Education	www.genetics.com.au
Human Genetics Society of Australia	www.hgsa.com.au
Orphanet Encyclopaedia	www.orpha.net
EURORDIS	www.eurordis.org
Wikigenetics/Wikipedia	www.wikigenetics.org
	www.wikipedia.org

- On a global basis, Orphanet is the most comprehensive database of information available freely on the web to lay persons and professionals. There is no adolescent targeted portal.

3.2. *Help for Parents in Explaining Genetic Concepts and Disorders*

Skilled professional genetic counsellors are available in most major and many smaller country centres in Australia and this is similar in other parts of the developed world. Genetic counselling is a new profession and in some areas there is inadequate resource allocation. Some counsellors have achieved special proficiency in counselling adolescents but often counselling is best given by a multidisciplinary team comprising an adolescent health worker and genetic counsellor.

3.3. *Direct to Consumer Genetic Testing*

The internet has enormous potential for good. Clearly it empowers everyone including adolescents with knowledge necessary for decision making in life. However the vulnerability of this population could be exploited by 'for profit genetic testing'. While some sites make quite reasonable financial charges for a genomic assessment, it is not always clear that the comparison population genetic testing data, on which their conclusions and predictions are based, come from populations which are sufficiently related to that of the young person making the enquiry.

Teenagers in a multicultural community such as Australia are not necessarily aware that the population studies which are used in estimating probabilities for lifestyle and general health issues from genomic markers used by some direct to consumer genomic testing companies are often completely foreign to their ethnic background and genetic makeup.

3.4. *Transitional Specialty Services for Chronic Genetic Disorders in Young Adults*

Many genetic disorders are both sufficiently frequent and complex to require multidisciplinary services long term for optimum care. While there are excellent models for disease management for the more common genetic disorders, there is a paucity of specialist services for many other disease groups. These include the Neuromuscular group (Neurofibromatosis and the Muscular Dystrophies), Connective Tissue Dysplasia group (Marfan, Ehlers–Danlos and Loeys–Dietz syndromes and some 600 other disorders) and Inborn Errors of Metabolism (Phenylketonuria and several hundred other rare disorders).

3.4.1. *Neuromuscular disorders*

These affect about 1 in 1,000 individuals and are characterised by chronic muscle weakness, loss of ambulation, and in some cases respiratory and cardiac failure leading to early death. The most common neuromuscular disorder is Duchenne muscular dystrophy, a progressive disorder that affects about 1 in 5,000 males and that typically results in death from respiratory or cardiac failure between the ages of 20 and 35 years. Even though there is a lack of specific therapies that address the underlying cause of muscle weakness, major improvements in morbidity and mortality have been achieved through careful management of joint contractures, scoliosis, respiratory and cardiac function, home/school/work environments, and psychosocial well-being. Due to its high incidence in all populations of the world and relatively homogeneous natural history, health outcomes in DMD provide a useful yardstick to assess neuromuscular services between regions.

3.4.2. *Neurofibromatosis*

This is an autosomal dominant condition which has three main types. Neurofobromatosis-1 has a prevalence of 1 in 4,000. There are varying degrees of clinical severity, and learning difficulties are common in childhood. While most cases are mild, ongoing surveillance is required throughout adult life for complications which include plexiform neurofibroma, malignant transformation, and optic gliomas.

The European Organisation for Rare Disorders has drawn attention to the lack of services and continuity of services from paediatric care for these patients. This is an area which urgently needs to be rectified.

4. Principles of Genetics

The principles of genetics are well-covered for lay persons through the fact sheets of the Centre for Genetic Education. What is not understood is that modern genetic diagnosis and counselling is highly sophisticated and ever changing. Wikipedia and Wikigenetics used in a complementary way often have useful monographs and the quality and reliability of these are improving.

Some recent advances in genetic medicine which will impact in the near future on genetic counselling include:

- Array comparative genomic hybridisation.
- High throughput sequencing and the promise of a USD1000 genome sequence of an individual's genome.
- A better understanding of epigenetics and its impact on health.
- Pre-implantation genetic diagnosis and technologies which alter risk and perception of risk as well as possibilities for avoidance of reproductive transmission.

5. A Future for Adolescent Genetic Health

All areas of health information suffer from a burgeoning array of facts and knowledge. Provision of practical and accurate advice to adolescents requires professionals who can integrate insightful counselling with the vast body of specialised genetic knowledge. The challenge for clinicians will be to progressively re-adjust their focus towards understanding adolescents' fears and responses to genetic disorders on one hand and to the adolescent's own personal known or as yet undeclared inherited makeup on the other hand. The website of the Centre for Genetic Education is one of the most useful clearing houses for current information.

References

Barlow-Stewart K, Burnett L, Proos A, Howell V, Huq F, Lazarus R, Aizenberg H. (2003) A genetic screening programme for Tay-Sachs disease and cystic fibrosis for australian Jewish high school students. *J Med Genet* **40**(4): e45.

Burnett L, Barlow-Stewart K, Proos AL, Aizenberg H. (2003) The "Gene Trustee": A universal identification system that ensures privacy and confidentiality for human genetic databases. *J Law Med* **10**(4): 506–513.

Cousens NE, Gaff CL, Metcalfe SA, Delatycki MB. (2010) Carrier screening for beta-thalassaemia: A review of international practice. *Eur J Hum Genet* **18**(10): 1077–1083.

Eagle M, Baudouin SV, Chandler C, Giddings DR, Bullock R, Bushby K. (2002) Survival in Duchenne muscular dystrophy: Improvements in life expectancy since 1967 and the impact of home nocturnal ventilation. *Neuromuscul Disord* **12**(10): 926–929.

Griswold CM, Ashley SS, Dixon SD, Scott JL. (2011) Genetic Counselors' experiences with adolescent patients in prenatal genetic counseling. *J Genet Couns* **20**(2): 178–191.

Human Genetics Society of Australia. (2008) Position statement: Pre-symptomatic and predictive testing in children and young people. http://www.hgsa.org.au/website/wp-content/uploads/2009/12/2008PS02-Pre-symptomatic-predictive-testing-in-children-young-people.pdf. (Accessed 1 March 2012.)

International Huntington Association and World Federation of Neurology Research Group on Huntington's Chorea. (1994) Guidelines for the molecular genetics predictive test for Huntington's disease. *Neurology* **44**: 1533–1536.

Kaback M, Lim-Steele J, Dabholkar D, Brown D, Levy N, Zeiger K. (1993) Tay–Sachs disease — carrier screening, prenatal diagnosis, and the molecular era. An international perspective, 1970 to 1993. The international TSD data collection network. *JAMA* **270**(19): 2307–2315.

Kosky R, O'hanlon A, Martin G, Davis C. (2000) *Clinical Approaches to Early Intervention in Child and Adolescent Mental Health*, vol.5. Adelaide, Australian Early Intervention Network for Mental Health in Young People.

Mitchell JJ, Capua A, Clow C, Scriver CR. (1996) Twenty-year outcome analysis of genetic screening programs for Tay–Sachs and beta-thalassemia disease carriers in high schools. *Am J Hum Genet* **59**(4): 793–798.

Scriver CR. (2006) Community genetics and dignity in diversity in the quebec network of genetic medicine. *Community Genet* **9**(3): 142–152.

Strachan T, Read AP. (2010) *Human Molecular Genetics*, 4th ed. Garland Publishing Inc, UK.

Chapter 49

Urological Problems in Adolescence

Grahame H H Smith

1. Introduction

This chapter covers common clinical urological problems that can present during adolescence. The focus is on presentations and issues that can result in adverse outcomes if not properly managed.

2. Problems of the Penis and Foreskin

In some boys the foreskin is not fully retractile until after puberty. Forceful attempts to retract the foreskin can result in trauma to the foreskin with scar formation and the development of phimosis. Failure of retraction during adolescence requires expert assessment and management.

2.1. *Phimosis*

Prior to puberty, a tight non-retractile foreskin is usually due to a physiological phimosis. Pathological phimosis is generally due to lichen sclerosis (balanitis xerotica obliterans), the aetiology of which is unknown. In most cases the foreskin becomes tight and no longer retractile. Examination reveals thickening of the foreskin around the foreskin opening with white discolouration. Steroid cream will sometimes correct the problem, but usually a circumcision is required.

2.2. *Circumcision*

The pros and cons of circumcision are numerous and a good summary is provided by the Royal Australasian College of Physicians statement on circumcision. Occasionally, complications of circumcision present in early adolescence.

2.2.1. *Meatal stenosis*

This occurs in 2% to 5% of boys who have had a circumcision. The narrowed meatus results in a fine powerful urinary stream, which arcs upwards. The problem can be corrected with a meatotomy under local or general anaesthesia.

2.2.2. *Suture sinuses*

These can develop as epithelial skin grows along sutures from the time of circumcision. The suture material dissolves, leaving a skin tunnel which collects desquamated epithelium. The sinuses appear as small black spots.

2.2.3. *Surgical adhesions*

During a circumcision the foreskin is forcefully peeled back from the glans. This leaves a raw epithelial surface on the glans and occasionally the shaft skin heals to this surface.

2.3. *Fraenulum*

Occasionally teenage boys present complaining of a tight foreskin fraenulum, causing discomfort or ventral tilting of the glans with erection. Usually, with repeated erections, the fraenulum stretches and the problem resolves. If the problem persists after 16 years of age then surgical correction is required.

2.4. *Hypospadias*

2.4.1. *Aetiology and presentation*

Hypospadias is thought to result from incomplete virilisation of the phallus between the 12th and 14th weeks of gestation and is usually an isolated condition. Endocrine investigation may be required if hypospadias is associated with failure of testicular descent or inadequate androgenisation.

2.4.2. *Classification*

Hypospadias can be distal or proximal. Most cases of hypospadias are distal and do not cause significant morbidity. Proximal hypospadias makes up about 20% of cases and if not corrected is often associated with difficulty directing the urinary stream and with ventral chordee.

2.4.3. *Surgical repair*

There are two windows of time when it is ideal to repair hypospadias. The first is between six months and two years of age. The other is when the child/adolescent decides he wants it repaired.

2.4.4. *Post hypospadias surgery problems*

- Circular or retracted meatus: this is a relative indication to re-operate to improve the urinary stream.
- Hair growth in the neourethra: this can result in dysuria, and infection. Depilation techniques can remove hair.
- Abnormal urethral function: post void dribbling, lack of ejaculation or post ejaculation dribbling are best treated by milking the urethra between finger and thumb to empty it. Revision surgery is technically challenging and requires sub-specialist surgery.

2.5. *Chordee*

Chordee can be either congenital, or acquired (secondary to Peyronie disease which is rare before midlife). Congenital chordee is usually associated with hypospadias, but can occur in isolation. If there is more than a 20° bend with erection, then this can interfere with intercourse. It can be surgically corrected.

3. Testicular Conditions

Asymmetric testis growth during puberty is common and it is advisable to observe testicular asymmetry for 1 to 2 years to see if catch up growth occurs.

3.1. *Testis Not in the Scrotum*

3.1.1. *Undescended*

About half of undescended testes at birth spontaneously descend to the scrotum by six months of age. An acquired undescended testis develops because of a persistent fibrous remnant of the processus vaginalis in the spermatic cord which prevents the cord lengthening during height growth. Acquired undescended testes present around seven or eight years of age. Undescended testes carry an increased risk of testicular malignancy, with or without operation. Orchidopexy prior to puberty does decrease this risk. Any male with a history of an undescended testis should be instructed to examine their testes once a month after puberty and report any changes. A visual or palpable change of the testis is an indication for a testicular ultrasound and tumour markers (alpha-foetoprotein and beta human chorionic gonadotropin). Fertility is usually normal when there has been a unilateral undescended testis. Males with spina bifida have an increased incidence of undescended testes, which is due to an abnormality of the L2 spinal segment.

3.1.2. *Retractile testes*

Retractile testes are common and in most cases physiologically normal. The cremasteric reflex elevates the testis into the groin with anxiety or cold. It is uncommon after puberty.

3.1.3. *Ectopic testes*

These are rare and always require surgical correction.

3.1.4. *Impalpable testes*

Over half of these are due to an absent or atrophic testis. A quarter will be intra-abdominal or in the inguinal canal. Bilateral impalpable testes or a unilateral impalpable testis plus hypospadias are indications to investigate for a possible intersex abnormality with laparoscopy or with an inguinal exploration. Testes can only be proven to be absent if blind ending testicular vessels can be identified. Ultrasound, CT scanning and MRI scanning have not been shown to be sensitive enough to exclude an intra-abdominal testis and are generally not indicated.

3.2. *Torsion of the Testis*

The annual incidence of torsion of the testis is 1:4000. The peak incidence occurs around the time of puberty. Torsion is associated with obstruction to blood flow. Most testes do not survive after 12 hours of torsion.

3.2.1. *Presentation*

Patients present with pain in the scrotum associated with a high riding testis. Often there is associated nausea and vomiting, with swelling and erythema as later signs. Adolescents may present with isolated abdominal pain and be too embarrassed to describe the scrotal symptoms. If suspected it is important to ask specifically about scrotal pain and to examine the scrotum. The gold standard for diagnosis and treatment is urgent surgical exploration. Testicular ultrasound is only indicated if the patient is thought not to have a torsion or if a testicular tumour is suspected. The differential diagnosis includes a torsion of the appendix testis, idiopathic scrotal oedema, epididymitis secondary to a urinary tract infection or secondary to a sexually transmitted infection, and idiopathic testicular pain.

3.2.2. *Treatment*

As an urgent first aid measure, it is sometimes possible to manually reduce a torsion by rotating the testis outwards. If the testis is found to be twisted at the time of surgical exploration then it is untwisted and fixed in the scrotum. A clearly necrotic testis is best removed. The opposite testis is also explored and fixed to prevent a torsion on the other side.

3.3. *Varicocoele*

Approximately 10% to 15% of adolescents have a varicocoele. Varicocoeles almost always occur on the left side and are secondary to damaged valves in the testicular vein, which drains to the left renal vein. Varicocoeles can be associated with other venous pathology such as haemorrhoids. Testicular pain or poor growth of the ipsilateral testis are the indications to consider correction. Varicocoeles are best corrected by transvenous embolisation, which has the highest success rate and the lowest complication rate. A recent Cochrane review has not shown any improvement in fertility with varicocoele treatment.

4. Pelviureteric Junction Obstruction

PUJ obstruction occurs in about 2% of the population. It is more common in males. Kinking of the PUJ results from an abnormally high takeoff of the ureter from the renal pelvis. It can also be due to an ectatic ureter folding back on itself at the PUJ. This ectasia is thought to correct itself as the child grows in height. Most adolescents with a PUJ obstruction present with symptoms, including intermittent loin pain, abdominal pain, vomiting, urinary tract infections or haematuria and symptoms almost always require an operation.

The differential diagnosis includes vesicoureteric reflux, a urethral valve or a vesicoureteric junction obstruction. A renal and bladder ultrasound is the initial investigation. A PUJ obstruction can be corrected with a pyeloplasty (open or laparoscopic), which is successful in 95% of cases. Following a satisfactory initial post-operative assessment with ultrasound or diuretic renography, patients should be reviewed at 12 months with a further ultrasound. If there is significantly reduced function in the affected kidney then a yearly blood pressure check following puberty is recommended. Renal obstruction can result in renal scarring which increases the risk of hypertension in later life.

5. Vesicoureteric Reflux

Vesicoureteric reflux can be divided into primary reflux, due to a deficient vesicoureteric valve mechanism, or secondary reflux due to abnormal bladder function. Patients with spina bifida or patients with a posterior urethral valve clearly have abnormal bladder function. In these patients poor bladder emptying compliance and an increased outlet resistance contribute to high bladder pressures which in turn lead to reflux and renal damage. Patients with primary reflux have normal bladder function. Unfortunately the majority of patients lie somewhere between these two extremes.

There is currently a controversy about whether or not medical or operative intervention for primary reflux is worthwhile. Two large randomised studies comparing prophylaxis alone, with prophylaxis and open surgical correction of reflux, failed to show any reduction in the incidence of new renal damage. Alternate surgical therapies include cystoscopic injection of a stable polysaccharide-based gel under the ureteral opening. Treating dysfunctional elimination syndrome with urotherapy (bladder training) has been shown to speed the resolution of reflux. The incidence of urinary tract infections falls with increasing age and by adolescence UTIs are rare in males. The incidence of UTIs in females increases again with the onset of sexual activity. The outcome measures that should be looked at to assess the effectiveness of treatment include the incidence of UTIs (lower and upper), the incidence of new renal injury and the incidence of renal failure and hypertension. There are very few randomised studies that address these outcomes. Renal scarring, rather than the presence or absence of reflux, best predicts morbidity in pregnancy.

6. Neurogenic Bladder — Spina Bifida as an Example

The bladder has two main functions. It stores urine at low-pressure between voiding and empties urine completely with voiding. In spina bifida these two functions can be affected to a different extent. The parasympathetic outflow for the bladder originates from S2 to S4, so even adolescents with low lesions will have abnormal bladder function.

6.1. *Failure to Empty and to Store*

Failure of emptying results from a failure of the external sphincter to relax during voiding, due to an interruption of the spinal pathway that coordinates voiding. Abnormal bladder function is often accompanied by abnormal bowel function. There is a tendency for constipation, and assistance may be required with faecal evacuation.

6.2. *Assessment*

The main urological outcome measures that are assessed in neurogenic bladder are new renal injury and urinary continence. Baseline investigations at the time of diagnosis should include anatomical and functional studies of the urinary tract.

6.3. *Baseline Intervention*

Patients are commenced on regular clean intermittent catheterisation, three to four times daily. The frequency of catheterisation can be reduced if minimal volumes are drained. Patients are commenced on anticholinergic medication to relax the bladder and improve storage capacity.

6.4. *Follow-up*

Patients with a neurogenic bladder are at risk of developing new renal injury due to recurrent UTIs and/or high bladder pressures. Patients need to be carefully followed through adolescence, as often during this period they become poorly compliant with therapy. Catheterisation may not be performed regularly, and medication may not be taken regularly. It is likely (but unproven) that the early introduction of regular, clean intermittent catheterisation and anticholinergics will improve long term bladder function. Patients who continue to be incontinent despite clean intermittent catheterisation four times a day and anticholinergic therapy require further assessment with urodynamics. A detrusor pressure more than 40 cm of water is thought to increase the risk of progressive renal injury.

6.5. *Treatment for Reduced Bladder Capacity*

In patients who have evidence of progressive renal injury despite clean intermittent catheterisation, other therapies should be considered. The next step is to improve bladder drainage with either a urethral dilatation or with a vesicostomy. In older children and adolescents, botulinum toxin can be injected into the bladder which works best where there is minimal fibrosis in the bladder. In the past, an ileal conduit was performed to divert the urine to a stoma, but is now rarely performed.

The most effective treatment to correct the failure of bladder storage is a bladder augmentation, using a segment of intestine or stomach. Most patients who have been augmented require clean intermittent catheterisation in order to empty. Failure to catheterise can result in the bladder becoming overfull with increased pressures, and bladder rupture. This can be a particular problem during adolescence, as adolescents often play down the degree of their disability and fail to catheterise regularly. High alcohol intake can lead to diuresis and to sedation, and a forgotten night catheterisation may end in rupture of the bladder.

Other long-term complications of bladder augmentation include an increased risk of bladder stones, problems with acidosis due to reabsorption of acid from the augmented bowel, recurrent infections due to inadequate bladder emptying, mucus blocking catheters making intermittent catheterisation difficult, B12 deficiency and an increased risk of bladder malignancy. The patient's renal function needs to be kept under close review after surgery.

7. Dysfunctional Elimination Syndrome

Dysfunctional elimination syndrome is also known as dysfunctional voiding syndrome. These patients present with one or more of the following problems:

- Daytime or nighttime incontinence.
- Recurrent UTIs.
- Progressive renal damage.

The patients have abnormal bladder function. They can have a failure of bladder storage due to an overactive bladder or due to reduced bladder compliance. Alternatively failure of bladder emptying due to infrequent voiding or due to failure of the bladder sphincter mechanism to relax during voiding is present. Intercurrently these patients tend to suffer from constipation, which may contribute to their abnormal bladder function and may be due to the same cause as their abnormal bladder function. Dysfunctional voiding may remain a problem in adolescence if specific therapy is not instituted.

The mainstay of treatment is urotherapy, which is retraining to a normal bladder habit by:

- Improved fluid intake.
- Regular timed voiding.
- Treatment of constipation.
- Voiding with a coordinated detrusor contraction and a relaxed external sphincter.

8. Exstrophy and Epispadias

Exstrophy/epispadias occurs in about one in 50,000 children. Males with epispadias have a urethral meatus that is dorsally situated on the penis and in female epispadias, the clitoris is bifid and the external sphincter mechanism is poorly formed. In bladder exstrophy, there is associated epispadias and a bladder which is open on the lower abdominal wall. In cloacal exstrophy, there is epispadias associated with an open bladder and open rectum (and open vagina in females). The aims of surgical treatment are to achieve continence and preserve renal function. There are longer term problems associated with repair which have a high impact in adolescence. Incontinence is common after bladder exstrophy repair. Females with exstrophy/epispadias have normal fertility, but they do have an increased incidence of vaginal prolapse. Males are potentially fertile, since the testes and ejaculatory ducts develop normally, but there may be ductal obstruction after surgery.

9. Renal and Ureteric Calculi

9.1. *Aetiology and Investigation*

Kidney and bladder stones are less common in adolescents than in adults and investigation is more likely to reveal a clear aetiology. Structural abnormalities of the renal tract are more common, as are metabolic abnormalities. The minimum investigations to perform are serum sodium, calcium, creatinine, and uric acid, urine culture, a spot urine calcium to creatinine ratio and a spot urine cystine test to exclude disorders of calcium metabolism (including hyperparathyroidism), renal tubular acidosis and cystinuria, cystinosis and Fanconi syndrome. Uric acid stones may occur with and without demonstrable abnormalities of uric acid metabolism. Recurrent UTIs are associated with triple phosphate stones.

9.2. *Symptoms and Signs*

Stones in adolescents can present with symptoms or be detected incidentally, while investigating other problems. Symptoms include renal colic with classic severe pain radiating from loin to groin, haematuria, and recurrent UTIs.

9.3. *When to Treat*

The management of renal stones in adolescents is similar to that in adults.

9.3.1. *Asymptomatic renal calculi*

These should almost always be treated due to the risk of renal colic and recurrent infection.

9.3.2. *Ureteric colic*

Stones in the ureter up to 6 mm in diameter will often pass spontaneously. The indications for intervention include failure of conservative management, persistent severe pain or problems with renal obstruction. An active increase in fluid intake does not help renal calculi to pass. Alpha blockers and calcium channel blockers have been shown to improve the passage of ureteric calculi. For upper ureteric calculi, extracorporeal shock wave lithotripsy remains an option. For upper or lower ureteric calculi, ureteroscopy is highly effective.

9.3.3. *Renal calculi in association with infection*

This situation can lead to severe sepsis. If ureteric obstruction is present, then this may lead to septicaemia and shock. Most staghorn calculi are associated with chronic infection and the infection cannot be eradicated until the stone is eliminated.

9.3.4. *Adjunctive therapies*

The maintenance of dilute urine by increasing oral fluid intake is to be encouraged, with adolescents aiming to pass two litres of urine a day. This should be particularly encouraged in hotter months. A high calcium intake will bind to oxalate in the gut and has been shown to reduce kidney stones in those people known to be at risk. Avoidance of high dose Vitamin C and foods containing oxalate (green leafy vegetables, rhubarb) have also been suggested, but with limited evidence to support this approach. Alkanisation of urine is effective for uric acid stones. Potassium citrate supplements help reduce the recurrence of calcium oxalate stones.

References

Baillie CT, Fearns G, Kitteringham L, Turnock RR. (1998) Management of the impalpable testis: The role of laparoscopy. *Arch Dis Child* **79**(5): 419–422.

Baird AD. (2011) Exstrophy in the adolescent and young adult population. *Semin Pediatr Surg* **20**(2): 109–112.

Baskin LS, Kogan BA. eds. (2005) *Handbook of pediatric urology.* 2nd ed. Lippincott Williams and Wilkins, Philadelphia.

Baskin LS, Ebbers MB. (2006) Hypospadias: Anatomy, etiology, and technique. *J Pediatr Surg* **41**(3): 463–472.

The Royal Australasian College of Physicians. (2010) *Circumcision of infant males.* Available online at: http://www.racp.edu.au/index.cfm?objectid=65118B16-F145-8B74-236C86100E4E3E8E2010). (Accessed 1 March 2012.)

Evers JHLH, Collins J, Clarke J. (2009) Surgery or embolization for varicoceles in subfertile men. *Cochrane Database Syst Rev*, CD000479.

Hutson JM, Balic A, Nation T, Southwell B. (2010) Cryptorchidism. *Semin Pediatr Surg* **19**(3): 215–224.

Leclair MD, Heloury Y. (2010) Non-neurogenic elimination disorders in children. *J Pediatr Urol* **6**(4): 338–345.

Mansfield JT, Snow BW, Cartwright PC, Wadsworth K. (1995) Complications of pregnancy in women after childhood reimplantation for vesicoureteral reflux: An update with 25 years of followup. *J Urol* **154**(2): 787–790.

Metcalfe PD, Rink RC. (2007) Bladder augmentation: Complications in the pediatric population. *Curr Urol Rep* **8**(2): 152–156.

Nagler EVT, Williams G, Hodson EM, Craig JC. (2011) Interventions for primary vesicoureteric reflux. *Cochrane Database of Syst Rev*, CD001532.

Woodhouse CR. (2001) The fate of the abnormal bladder in adolescence. *J Urol* **166**(6): 2396–2400.

Chapter 50

Common Gynaecological Problems in Adolescence

Kim Matthews and Peter Benny

1. Introduction

Gynaecological issues in adolescence encompass both medical and surgical aspects and range from simple concerns that can be addressed over the phone to those issues that require detailed assessment and management in a tertiary referral clinic. The latter is essential in the care of the complex adolescent, and may require medical, surgical, gynaecological, adolescent, nursing, and psychological services.

2. History and Examination

2.1. *History*

Getting to know the young person first with some general questions before embarking on more sensitive areas is helpful. The history is usually taken with the carer present, but it is also important to give the adolescent some time by themselves where confidential issues related to gynaecological concerns can be discussed.

Stage of pubertal development, whether menarche has been attained and the menstrual cycle pattern need to be determined. The duration of bleeding (which can be as few as 2 to 3 days but often as much as 7 to

10 days), and associated symptoms such as pain and heaviness of flow should be determined. The volume of menstrual loss is often difficult to estimate, but the number of tampons or pads used in 24 hours and the presence of any flooding or significant clotting are a guide. Counting from day one of the cycle (first day of bleeding) to the next cycle's day one should be in the range of 23 to 35 days. Presence of any premenstrual symptoms such as breast tenderness, bloating or mood swings may confirm ovulation is occurring. A menstrual calendar/diary can be very helpful and online versions are easily accessible. Pain at times other than the menses can be related to ovulation or gastroenterological causes. It is also important to establish if the young person is sexually active and if there is a possibility of pregnancy.

Gynaecological history such as surgery and loss of ovarian tissue and a general history including cancer treatment, genetic syndromes, and general debilitating illness needs to be determined. Family history with particular attention to the mother's gynaecological history and age of menarche of mother and sisters is important. Often a family history of difficult periods or endometriosis will be a concern for the young person and their carers. A family history of thrombophilia or a bleeding disorder also needs to be determined, as this can have implications for management.

2.2. *Examination*

Gynaecologic examination needs to be performed in a manner with which the young person is comfortable and with discussion prior as to whether they wish their carer to be present. This usually depends on the age and maturity of the young person. If there are any concerns, then it is prudent to have a chaperone present.

Abdominal examination for assessment of tenderness and the presence of scars is performed, followed by examination of the external genitalia including mons, labia, clitoris, urethral meatus and hymen. Presence of discharge and degree of oestrogen effect is ascertained.

Vaginal examination is not always necessary and should not be performed if the patient refuses or is hesitant. Cultural beliefs also need to be sensitively discussed and acknowledged. When an examination is required with unusual bleeding or discharge, every effort must be made to explain the process and be as gentle as possible. Examination will only be successful with a cooperative relaxed patient. Unless urgent action is required, vaginal examination can be deferred to a later consultation. Reassure the patient that she may stop the examination at any time. Special narrow speculums are utilised, and should be warmed first. Some practitioners recommend insertion of the speculum obliquely then rotating gently to the horizontal position to avoid stimulating the urethra but gentle insertion in the horizontal plane is also possible. A rectal examination can be an alternative, particularly if a mass needs to be excluded.

2.3. *Use of Pelvic Ultrasound*

The trans-abdominal approach is the most common in adolescence. A sexually active adolescent may be comfortable with the trans-vaginal approach. The trans-abdominal ultrasound gives excellent views through a full bladder, particularly in a non-obese patient. It is best performed in the follicular phase, just after the menses, where a thin endometrium and small antral follicles are expected. An ultrasound is an important investigation when pain is present or if blood flow to the ovary also needs to be assessed. A luteal phase ultrasound may be diffcult to assess. Consider deferral unless an ovarian torsion is suspected and urgent intervention required.

3. The Normal Menstrual Cycle

A good understanding of the follicular and luteal phases and the hormonal controls of the menstrual cycle is necessary to recognise when there is significant deviation from normal.

Time discussing the normal menstrual cycle with the patient is often very useful, especially when there is deviation from the normal.

4. Common Medical Issues in Adolescent Gynaecology

4.1. *Dysfunctional Uterine Bleeding*

DUB is common and is often due to the immaturity of the hypothalamic–pituitary–ovarian axis. Other causes may include severe debilitating

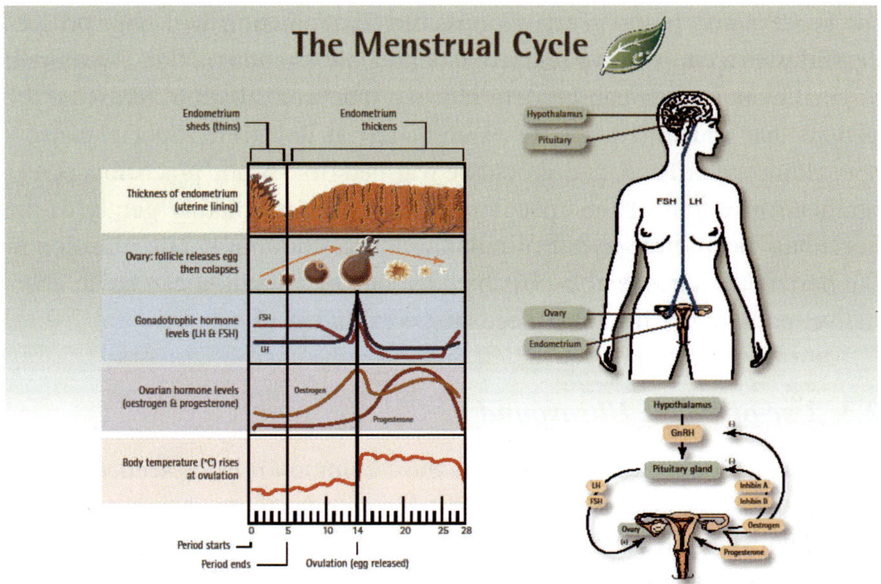

Fig. 1:   Image courtesy of Merck Serono Australia Pty Ltd.

general illness, emotional stress, thyroid and other hormonal disease, ovarian dysgenesis, or body image concerns with disordered eating.

All may be associated with anovulatory cycles, with irregular bleeding and unpredictable shedding of the endometrium. These cycles can be short occurring every 2–3 weeks or can occur with continuous bleeding for over a month after a prolonged period of amenorrhoea. Most cases are self-limiting and resolve within 1–2 years of the onset of menses.

Polymenorrhoea (frequent menses), menorrhagia (excessive amount of menstrual bleeding) and metromenorrhagia (irregular and frequent heavy bleeding) are all common presenting symptoms. In extreme cases, presentation can be to the emergency department with torrential bleeding and haemodynamic compromise. In this situation it is important to rule out pregnancy complications, coagulation defects, local utero–vaginal causes such as trauma or tumours, and rarely hormone secreting ovarian neoplasms.

Investigations should include a full blood count, including platelets, coagulation studies and a pelvic ultrasound. A hormone profile including

HCG, oestradiol and TSH (to exclude the menorrhagia of primary hypothyroidism) may be required. If anovulatory bleeding is determined as the cause, then its severity will determine the treatment plan.

- In *mild cases* with no changes to the full blood count, simple measures such as a menstrual calendar and advice on healthy lifestyle, diet, and use of oral iron and multivitamins are all that is required. Nonsteroidal anti-inflammatory medication can be utilised to help reduce blood loss if menorrhagia is present. Advice on when to contact if further heavy bleeding occurs is also given. Follow up is required.

- In *moderate cases*, where there is some degree of anaemia, iron supplementation and hormonal therapy is usually commenced. This can be as a cyclic gestagen, such as medroxyprogesterone acetate or norethisterone from days 15–28 of the cycle, but may need to be started earlier on day 10–12 if the bleeding pattern occurs by day 14 of the cycle. The use of a monophasic OCP is an alternative. This regimen is used for six months, then it is stopped, and the menstrual pattern again determined. The combined OCP is more effective but if there are parental or patient concerns with using the OCP or a medical contraindication to the OCP such as hypertension or history of thrombotic episodes, then use gestagens alone. Concerns about oestrogen effect on final height in the first 12 months after menarche are generally not warranted as attainment of menarche implies that over 95% of final adult height has been achieved.

- In *severe cases*, hospitalisation is required. Significant anaemia is usually present which requires intravenous fluids and consultation with a haematologist. Transfusion is considered only if acute blood loss is continuing and the haemoglobin is extremely low. Initial hormonal management is with high dosage gestagen. Medroxyprogesterone acetate, 20 to 40 mg every 4 to 6 hours, is better tolerated than other types as it produce less nausea. If bleeding continues add ethinyl oestradiol as the OCP. Antiemetics may help if higher dose oestrogen is required. These high doses are required for a few days, and then a slow weaning regimen is instituted to achieve amenorrhoea and give the young person time to recover from the acute anaemia. High dose iron therapy is commenced and the use of tranexamic acid considered in the short term to further reduce menstrual flow. Follow up and maintenance regimens similar to those for moderate cases are then used. Blind dilatation and curettage is rarely performed because of the risks of damage to the young cervix and the rare occurrence of tumours as the aetiology.

4.2. *Dysmenorrhoea*

Painful periods are common and 15% of young women have severe symptoms that disrupt their life and often their education. The most common cause of dysmenorrhoea is an excess physiologic production of prostaglandins which are released by the endometrium as it is shed. Higher volumes of menstrual flow will also be enough to increase pain, by producing minor dilatation of the cervical canal. Retrograde flow of menses, which stimulates the peritoneal lining, explains the back pain with and immediately prior to menstruation.

Other rare causes of pain with menses such as tumours, congenital anomalies or pelvic inflammatory disease need to be excluded. A full blood count and pelvic ultrasound are initial investigations. If a rare cause is suspected, a pelvo–renal ultrasound and MRI may be performed.

Management includes education regarding the normal cycle and physiologic reasons for the pain, use of NSAIDs at the onset of menstruation or pain, or *preferably* 24 to 48 *hours before the onset of symptoms.*

If these measures are not effective the next line of treatment is the OCP. A family history of thrombophilia needs to be excluded before commencing this medication, and advice given on how to minimise risks when flying long distance or anticipating extended bed rest following major surgery. Which OCP to use will be influenced by cost, side effect profile including androgenic symptoms, and ease of usage. The OCP relieves pain and reduces flow in all but 10% of young women. The role of laparoscopy is limited to these cases with persistent pain despite treatment. Occasionally, the use of gonadotropin releasing hormone analogues to temporarily inhibit cycling is beneficial. GnRH analogue use is limited by the concerns of an extended low oestrogen environment contributing to a reduction in peak bone mass and later risk of osteoporosis.

4.3. *Polycystic Ovarian Syndrome*

PCOS is a heterogeneous syndrome with multiple and variable features and definitions. The most common features are those of hyperandrogenism, including acne, hirsutism and rarely alopecia, and ovulatory dysfunction including irregular menstruation. The appearance of polycystic ovaries on ultrasound can occur *without* the clinical features described above. Obesity can be both a contributing factor to the development of and a consequence of PCOS. Distinction needs to be made between PCOS (10% of women of reproductive age) and the more common finding of polycystic change (22% of women) on ultrasound.

4.3.1. *Symptoms*

These can commence from the time of entering puberty but reliance on menstrual irregularity can be misleading, due to the variation in cyclicity in the early post-menarchal years and the fact that women with PCOS can also have regular cycles. Even the symptoms of hyperandrogenism may be hard to distinguish from acne, seborrhoea and normal increase in body hair during normal adolescence.

4.3.2. *Criteria for diagnosis*

Three main consensus groups have defined criteria for the diagnosis of PCOS in adulthood and adolescence. The *National Institute of Health* (1990) define PCOS as clinical hyperandrogenism and/or hyperadrogenaemia, oligo-ovulation, and exclusion of other known disorders. The *Rotterdam criteria* (2003) define PCOS, after exclusion of other disorders causing menstrual irregularity and androgen excess, as two of the three following features: oligo-ovulation or anovulation; clinical and/or biochemical signs of hyperandrogenism; PCO on ultrasound with 12 peripheral cysts and increased ovarian volume. The *Androgen Excess Society* (2006, revised 2009) recognises that the definition will evolve but currently uses hyperandrogenism (hirsutism and/or hyperandrogenaemia), ovarian dysfunction (oligo-ovulation and/or PCOS), and the exclusion of other androgen excess or related disorders.

4.3.3. *Diagnosis of polycystic ovaries in adolescence*

This presents difficulties due to the high incidence of anovulation that is common after menarche, and the normal multifollicular ovaries containing up to 12 follicles per ovary seen in this age group. The use of each consensus group's PCOS diagnostic criteria will produce different PCOS prevalence in an adolescent population. There is always a concern about incorrect diagnosis of a condition which has long term health risks. It may be more beneficial to discuss the features suggestive of the diagnosis, and consider ways to minimise future risks. Thus the main objective in adolescence is to identify an 'at-risk' population that may have longer term health issues such as diabetes, hypercholesterolaemia, and heart disease. The emergence and persistence of the common diagnostic features, insulin resistance in a young woman with obesity or a strong family history of diabetes, and the specific developmental history of small for gestational age, rapid weight gain and overshoot in infancy, and premature pubarche would indicate risk.

The investigations performed to make the diagnosis of PCOS are ultrasound (limited if trans-abdominal in an obese adolescent), FSH, LH, testosterone, SHBG, free androgen index, prolactin to exclude prolactinoma, 17 hydroxyprogesterone (morning sample) to exclude congenital adrenal hyperplasia, DHEAS as a measure of adrenal androgen production, and morning and evening cortisol levels to exclude Cushing syndrome. If there is a history of insulin resistance or obesity, a glucose tolerance test and fasting lipids should also be performed.

4.3.4. *Management of PCOS*

The treatments goals are to reduce the secretion and bioavailability of ovarian androgens, minimise anovulation to reduce the risks of DUB, endometrial hyperplasia and later fertility issues, and the control or reversal of insulin resistance and associated metabolic disturbance. The most important aspect is attention to lifestyle issues and weight loss.

Metformin is a useful drug. It is an insulin sensitiser which reduces insulin levels and the associated stimulation of androgens, thereby increasingly SHBG production and reducing the levels of available or free testosterone. Metformin improves glucose uptake and the metabolic derangements seen in PCOS. Daily doses of 1,500–2,000 mg are used, which are often limited by gastrointestinal side effects. As metformin will induce ovulation, the young woman must be counselled about adequate contraception. The OCP is useful for treating irregular cycles and hirsutism. The gestagens that are used in combination with oestrogen are variably androgenic. Desogestrel and gestodene tend to be less androgenic.

Anti-androgens may be used in conjunction with the OCP. The most common is the aldosterone antagonist, *spironolactone* (100–200 mg daily). It may alter liver function and increase potassium levels (monitor after initiation), and may induce cycle irregularity if used alone. *Cyproterone acetate* can be used as the gestagen in a combined OCP. The dose is low and generally it is effective for acne, but not for hirsutism. Higher doses, 50–100 mg may be used in combination with a standard OCP. Flutamide and finasteride have been used, but availability will vary from country to country. Their effect on the terminal hair follicle is slow, and as with other anti-androgen therapy, 6 to 12 months is required before their effect on hirsutism can be assessed. Discussion of possible fertility issues in later life can be a good motivator for some adolescents with PCOS, but be mindful of overburdening the young person. Identify that there are many ways that their fertility can be assisted in the future.

4.4. *Oligomenorrhea and Secondary Amenorrhoea*

These symptoms indicate possible pathology either centrally (hypothalamus or pituitary) or in the end organs (ovary or uterus). Exclusion of pregnancy is imperative. Central causes are associated with an abnormal pulsation of GnRH. Pituitary disorders leading to panhypopituitary function or specific reduced secretion of gonadotropins are associated with amenorrhoea. Hyperprolactinaemia and thyroid dysfunction are also important causes. Investigation and management are the same as for primary amenorrhoea (Chapter 20).

Ovarian dysgenesis leading to premature ovarian failure occurs in 1% of females less than 40 years of age, with an incidence of one in 10,000 by 20 years of age. Mosaic Turner syndrome and autoimmune diseases are the most common diagnoses. The thin patient with multifollicular ovaries, raised LH and oligomenorrhoea, is a particular sub-group that requires attention. They will often exhibit some minor central components, as well as ovarian pathology. Adequate treatment of this entire group with oestrogen/progesterone to maintain peak bone mass is required and careful follow up into the early adult years is advised. They will often have ongoing fertility issues.

4.5. *Vulval and Vaginal Issues*

4.5.1. *Vulvovaginitis*

This is the most common non-specific presentation to adolescent gynaecology. Hygiene associated vulvovaginitis can occur in adolescents with a low oestrogen environment. There is often associated pruritis and discharge. In adolescence, candidiasis is the more common cause of vulvovaginitis as it prefers an oestrogenic environment. The decision to perform a vaginal swab will depend on the clinical setting. Vaginoscopy is only required if there is vaginal bleeding, suspicion of a foreign body or neoplasm, or persistent vulvovaginitis. Treatment consists of attention to hygiene, keeping the vulva cool, clean, and dry, and avoiding tight clothing and wool, bubble baths and all but the mildest of soaps. Topical corticosteroids are reserved for severe cases.

4.5.2. *Vulvodynia*

A painful vulva occurs from ongoing irritation where the nerve endings have been sensitised. Analgesia, as well as treating the underlying irritant is required.

4.5.3. *Swelling of the vulva and labia*

These can occur in various clinical settings and are usually due to dependent oedema. Symptomatic treatment is the mainstay. Trauma to the area needs careful evaluation, injuries to the rectum and urethra need exclusion, and management may be medical or surgical.

4.5.4. *Labial inequality*

Normal development can be asymmetric, particularly of the labia minora. Reassurance is generally all that is required as adequate symmetry is usually achieved by the end of puberty. Labioplasty may be requested when there is excessive tissue. Deferral of a decision to late adolescence is ideal, and consultation with a plastic surgeon may be appropriate. Labial agglutination is a condition of a low oestrogen environment and is treated with short term use of topical oestrogen and emollients.

5. Common Surgical Issues in Adolescent Gynaecology

5.1. *Endometriosis and Pelvic Pain, Including Chronic Pelvic Pain*

The gynaecologic causes of pelvic pain include pelvic inflammatory disease, adhesions, fibroids, outflow tract obstruction, dysmenorrhoea and importantly, endometriosis. The adolescent with chronic pelvic pain has often seen several practitioners and missed a lot of school, but may still remain undiagnosed. Psychological support and assessment along with pain management services are important in this scenario.

5.1.1. *Endometriosis*

This is an important cause of pelvic pain to exclude and is assessed by laparoscopy. A pre-operative ultrasound is important, but Ca125 levels are not always helpful in this age group. The decision to perform laparoscopy usually occurs if medical therapy has not relieved the pain. The incidence of endometriosis in adolescence is debated, and there may be a genetic predisposition. The incidence may be higher in those patients with an obstructive anomaly of the genital tract. The appearance of endometriosis at laparoscopy in the adolescent differs from the adult, with early lesions consisting of more red and clear lesions, rather than the classic 'powder burn' lesions. Combination treatment with surgical treatment of visible lesions, together with pre- and post-operative hormonal manipulation (including suppression with continuous OCPs or GnRH agonists), along with psychological support offer the best long-term outcomes. Young women should also be counselled about the recurrent nature of endometriosis.

5.2. *Ovarian Cysts Including Ovarian Torsion*

The most common diagnosis will be a *functional* ovarian cyst. This may be asymptomatic and diagnosed incidentally, or present with a mass effect. Those that are 5 cm or less generally resolve spontaneously; between 5 and 10 cm can resolve or may require surgery; above 10 cm require surgical intervention because of the high risk of torsion. The decision is also influenced by AFP, Ca125 and beta hCG levels which, if elevated, may indicate an underlying neoplasm.

The most common benign *non-functional* ovarian cysts will be mucinous cystadenomas and mature teratomas (dermoids) and paraovarian cysts. These require removal and a laparoscopic approach is preferred, with the aim to conserve ovarian tissue. Mature teratomas are bilateral in 15% of cases, and further teratomas may develop.

Adnexal torsion requires prompt diagnosis and urgent laparoscopy and detorsion. Torsion may be idiopathic or occur with underlying ovarian pathology. Ultrasound with Doppler flow gives both false positives and negatives. A later ultrasound is required to detect any underlying pathology when the tissues are less oedematous. The role of oophoropexy is debated but may be beneficial if the torsion is idiopathic or recurrent.

5.3. *Congenital Anomalies of the Reproductive Tract*

5.3.1. *Imperforate hymen (or low vaginal atresia)*

This is the most common anomaly presenting in early puberty with pain and a bulging hymen. The degree of haematocolpos will be evident on ultrasound. More complex cases of higher transverse septums and obstructed hemi vaginas associated with a didelphic uterus (double uterus and cervix) need to be excluded prior to surgery as these cases require expert surgery. Surgery for imperforate hymen involves drainage and resection of a central portion of the hymen to prevent recurrence and infection. Surgery for the more complex cases involves marsupialisation of the obstructed vaginal septum.

5.3.2. *Müllerian agenesis*

This occurs in 1 in 5,000 births and usually presents in adolescence with primary amenorrhoea. Psychosocial support at the time of diagnosis is imperative. Creation of an adequate vagina is only attempted when the young person is emotionally prepared, and usually coincides when sexual activity is contemplated. The initial approach is always vaginal dilatation therapy. In an expert service and with adequate support, dilatation is successful in creating a functional vagina in the majority of patients. There are various surgical procedures for creation of a neovagina, but none are ideal.

5.4. *Solid Tumours of the Reproductive Tract in Adolescence*

These are rare and require involvement of a gynaecologic oncologist. Germ cell tumours form the majority and include dysgerminomas, immature teratomas, yolk sac tumours, and gonadoblastomas (in XY dysgenetic gonads). Stromal cell tumours include granulosa cell and Sertoli–Leydig tumours. Both groups have a favourable prognosis and respond to minimally invasive surgery, tailored radiotherapy, and targeted chemotherapy.

5.5. *Laparoscopy in the Adolescent*

The surgical management of many gynaecologic conditions is similar in adulthood and adolescence. The main difference is that in the adolescent population, preserving ovarian tissue is paramount, unless ovarian malignancy is present. Techniques for entry into the abdomen need to be carefully thought through, as the distance between umbilicus and the aortic bifurcation is usually reduced in this age group. If any concerns, Palmer's point (left sub-costal, para-rectus) can be utilised where previous abdominal surgery, large pelvic masses, or obesity are a concern.

6. Menstrual Management in the Developmentally Delayed Patient

Menstrual hygiene, DUB, premenstrual behavioural disorders, and pain can all be significant issues requiring medical support.

6.1. *Oral Therapy*

Minimising menstruation with the use of cyclical gestagens or back to back packets of the OCP are the mainstays of treatment. Most young women can manage the OCP for the school term, allowing menses to occur during school holidays, with 3–4 menses per year. Breakthrough bleeding and side effects will limit the use of this regimen. OCPs are also utilised in the management of premenstrual behavioural disorders, usually giving 2–3 packets in a row to avoid the fluctuation in hormone levels. Always consider analgesia for associated dysmenorrhoea.

6.2. *The Levonorgestrel IUS*

This is also very effective in minimising the number of bleeding days and has very few side effects due to its local activity and minimal blood hormone levels. It can be utilised if the OCP is contraindicated or not working effectively. It requires general anaesthetic for insertion.

6.3. *Endometrial Ablation or Hysterectomy*

Very rarely a surgical option is required if all other measures fail. This approach is usually in the setting of an underlying condition such as a bleeding disorder or in conditions which do not respond to adequate hormonal therapy. In most countries there are legal requirements which must be met when seeking treatment with surgical options.

7. Fertility Preservation in Patients with Significant Childhood Illness

Cytotoxic therapy (malignancy and severe autoimmune disease), surgery or radiation can all reduce the ovarian follicle pool. In the adolescent patient with no partner, the only available current options are:

- Ovarian tissue cryopreservation: this is only for those tumours without a high risk of ovarian involvement, as autotransplantation can be associated with the reintroduction of tumour cells.
- Oophoropexy to remove the ovary from the radiation field.

- Oocyte cryopreservation is a viable option for post menarchal girls with no partner.
- GnRH agonists (and potentially the newer antagonists) aim to produce a low gonadotropin and low oestradiol state and may have an independent suppressive effect on the ovary by upregulating sphingosine-1-phosphate inhibition of somatic cell apoptosis.
- Embryo cryopreservation may be suitable for the older adolescent with a long term partner, after full discussion and counselling.

Most of the interventions are still in their infancy and no clear guidelines exist at this stage. These techniques require referral to specialised centres and/or a cycle of oocyte stimulation and collection, which can delay the start of chemotherapy. The number of successful pregnancies from these methods is increasing although success rate remains low. Discussion is the most important component of management so that these patients and their families can make decisions for their future.

8. Transition to Adult Care

Many adolescent issues in gynaecology are self limiting, as the impact of hormonal change diminishes and progression to adulthood results in improved regularity of menstrual cycles. Adolescents with PCOS, those who require hormone replacement therapy (gonadal dysgenesis and those affected by the long-term issues of cancer therapy) and those with structural anomalies will all require transition. Many of these patients will also require assistance with fertility issues. The role of anti-müllerian hormone as a test of ovarian reserve is emerging. AMH levels are still only a guide and need to be interpreted in the context of both the individual's menstrual cycle and the limited data in younger age groups. AMH may also reflect the severity of PCOS, with the same caveats. The patient with complex developmental delay will also need ongoing gynaecologic management as well as an identified care coordinator.

References

Altcheck A, Deligdisch L. eds. (2009) *Pediatric, adolescent & young adult gynecology.* Wiley-Blackwell, Oxford, UK.

Azziz R, Carmina E, Dewailly D, Diamanti-Kandarakis E, Escobar-Morreale HF, Futterweit W, Janssen OE, Legro RS, Norman RJ, Taylor AE, Witchel SF, Task Force on the Phenotype of the Polycystic Ovary Syndrome of the Androgen, Excess and PCOS Society. (2009) The Androgen Excess and PCOS Society criteria for the polycystic ovary syndrome: The complete task force report. *Ferti Steril* **91**(2): 456–488.

Carpenter SEK, Rock JA. (1992) *Pediatric and adolescent gynecology*. Raven Press, New York.

Domingues TS, Rocha AM, Serafini PC. (2010) Tests for ovarian reserve: Reliability and utility. *Curr Opin Obstet Gynecol* **22**(4): 271–276.

Emans SJH, Goldstein DP. eds. (1990) *Pediatric & adolescent gynecology*, 3rd ed. Boston (MA): Little, Brown and Company.

Greydanus DE, Bricker LA, Feucht C. (2011) Pharmacotherapy for obese adolescents. *Pediatr Clin North Am* **58**(1): 139–153.

Grover S. (2007) Bleeding disorders and heavy menses in adolescents. *Curr Opin Obstet Gynecol* **19**(5): 415–419.

Hickey M, Doherty DA, Atkinson H, Sloboda DM, Franks S, Norman RJ, Hart R. (2011) Clinical, ultrasound and biochemical features of polycystic ovary syndrome in adolescents: Implications for diagnosis. *Hum Reprod* **26**(6): 1469–1477.

Strauss JF, Barbieri RL. eds. (2009) *Yen and Jaffe's reproductive endocrinology physiology, pathophysiology and clinical management*, 6th ed. Elsevier, Saunders, Philadelphia.

Chapter 51

The Andrology of Adolescence

David J Handelsman

1. Introduction

Andrology is the study of male reproductive health, medicine, and biology. Intersecting with men's somatic health, andrology has three major domains — fertility, androgenisation (the attainment of male secondary sexual characteristics), and sexuality (Fig. 1). Each function is subserved by the *testis* which, under tight neuroendocrine control by the hypothalamus and pituitary, displays a unique ontogeny developing in *two distinct temporal phases*. Prenatal sexual differentiation culminates in development of a foetal testis, which then remains dormant postnatally for more than a decade before puberty.

During puberty, the testis undergoes its final growth and maturation to support the achievement of sexual and reproductive competence. During a few years of the adolescent decade, male puberty is a dramatic physiological process which involves a 30-fold increase in testosterone production leading to the maturation of androgen target tissues while the testis increases 15-fold in size due to the initiation of spermatogenesis.

Natural male fertility requires both the production and delivery of spermatozoa into the female reproductive tract by a sexual act timed to fertilise an ovulated oocyte. The testis fulfils the dual functional roles of spermatogenesis and steroidogenesis to achieve respectively the twin goals of fertility and virilisation (acquiring full adult male secondary

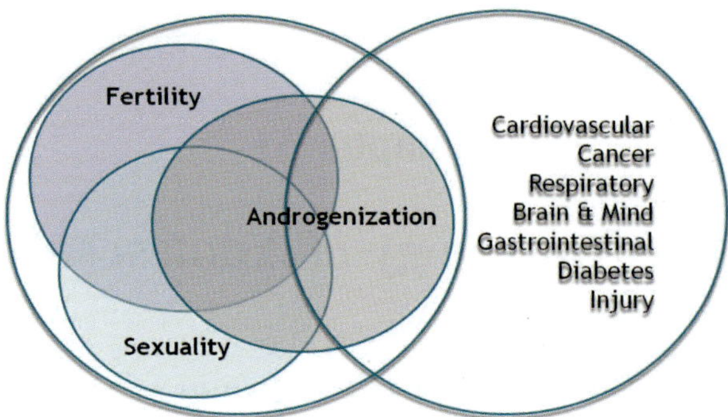

Fig. 1:   Reproductive Health, General Health

sexual characteristics). The germinal epithelium lining the seminiferous tubules produces structurally specialised spermatozoa that undergo functional maturation during their storage in the epididymis prior to ejaculation. Testosterone secretion has both local androgenic effects on spermatogenesis and accessory glands, as well as extra-testicular effects on reproductive and somatic tissues. Among its extra-testicular actions, testosterone secretion also completes the development of the reproductive system including catalysing the unfolding of mature male sexuality as well as exerting anabolic effects on androgen target tissues.

2. Puberty

Towards the end of childhood, puberty is initiated by a neuroendocrine mechanism which lifts the cerebral restraint exerted throughout infancy on episodic hypothalamic gonadotropin releasing hormone secretion. Recent clinical studies are identifying an increasing array of intermediate regulators including KAL1, GP54 (kisspeptin), FGFR1, DAX1, GnRHR, prokineticin2 and its receptor, NELF, and CHD7 all discerned from molecular genetic studies of rare, familial mutations resulting in pubertal failure. Nevertheless, the trigger of the neuro-endocrine cascade that culminates in puberty remains elusive.

Puberty is a dynamic, developmentally-timed, brain-driven process of reproductive maturation that transforms an immature boy into a sexually competent and fertile man. The dramatic increase in testosterone secretion at puberty provides a sharp increase in androgen exposure for all tissues, as virtually all express the androgen receptor. Androgen effects are most evident in classical androgen target tissues including both reproductive (testis, accessory glands) and somatic (muscle, bone, brain, liver, kidney, skin, hair) organs, but androgenic effects are manifest in most tissues. The precipitate onset of physical and reproductive maturity precedes by years the development of gender role and identity as well as emotional maturity, social restraint and executive judgement, features of brain development that characteristically lag behind puberty.

3. Disorders of Male Puberty

3.1. *Normal Puberty*

Male puberty is first evident clinically between the ages of 10–14 years with precocious or delayed puberty defined by its appearance outside these limits. The most objective and reliable sentinel feature heralding onset of puberty is testis growth. The hormonal cascade of puberty triggers the most intense physical and mental changes a healthy body ever experiences between birth and death. Timely completion of puberty has a major impact on a man's self-image and niche in society, forming the basis of lifelong personal identity through successful integration into domestic, social, and occupational networks. Consequently, however well nascent young men usually surmount this chronological disjunction between physical and emotional maturation, mistiming of sexual maturation strains their ability to smoothly bridge into a well adjusted manhood.

3.2. *Precocious Puberty*

Precocious male puberty is the appearance of virilisation prior to the age of 10 years. The clinical presenting features of premature virilisation reflect androgen exposure, regardless of whether the androgens are of exogenous or endogenous origin. It is necessary to distinguish between true premature, centrally mediated puberty of early onset but otherwise normal sequence from pseudo-puberty due to virilisation from androgen exposure without central activation of authentic puberty. The distinction can be verified by measuring testis size and serum LH, FSH and testosterone levels. In true central puberty, the testis increases in size and serum LH, FSH and testosterone are detectable above pre-pubertal levels. In pseudo-puberty, testis volume and serum LH and FSH remain at pre-pubertal levels. Serum testosterone is also suppressed if androgen exposure is due to exogenous synthetic androgens. However testosterone will be increased if due to exogenous testosterone, or endogenous testosterone and/or its precursors as a result of adrenal (congenital adrenal hyperplasia) or testicular (Leydig cell tumours, hCG-secreting teratoma) origin.

3.3. *Delayed Puberty*

The long term impact of delayed puberty is often overlooked, yet it has subtle but profound and enduring consequences on a man's ultimate psychosocial adaptation. A significant lag in attaining the visible signs of manhood may leave a deleterious legacy of faulty integration into micro- and macro-societal networks. Insidiously, this may impoverish socialisation due to hindered development of secure, intimate partnerships, and family formation.

Most boys with a delayed puberty have a slower tempo but otherwise normal puberty — known as constitutional delay of puberty — often conforming to a familial pattern ('late bloomer'). Functionally, this represents an abnormal prolongation of the reproductively immature, gonadotropin deficient pre-pubertal state. Boys with CDP ultimately complete puberty untreated although, in a minority, the time taken and consequential lag in maturation relative to peers is sufficiently troublesome to require short-term androgen treatment for primarily psychosocial reasons. Mildly delayed male puberty represents a spectrum overlapping the timing of normal male puberty.

Treatment replicating pubertal virilisation may be warranted not only to ameliorate the impact of the developmental mistiming relative to peers in psychosocial adjustment, but also to avert the physical consequences of delayed puberty such as the compromise of peak bone mass attained in early adulthood. Treatment requires use of testosterone, which exhibits the full spectrum of androgen action, rather than synthetic androgens which are usually not aromatisable and/or hepatotoxic. Although clinical experience indicates a significant long term toll in psychosocial functioning in some boys with CDP, there is only limited evidence from the few available studies confirming impaired quality of life, body image or social adjustment in adulthood. Most studies have focused primarily on final height, peak bone mass, and skeletal phenotype or the psychological effects of short stature, all of which can be adversely affected. Unfortunately the impact of delayed male puberty on psychosocial adjustment including establishment of a social niche and identity have been little studied. Delayed puberty is often undertreated with the concerns of parents and patients reassured and treatment deferred by exaggerated concerns about testosterone treatment relative to the insidious but profound and progressive impact of delayed virilisation on social integration.

4. Male Reproductive Health Disorders in Adolescence

4.1. *Klinefelter Syndrome*

The testis is the body's most accessible internal organ to clinical examination, yet it is among the least scrutinised medically. One unfortunate consequence is the severe under-diagnosis of Klinefelter syndrome, the most consistent feature of which is small, firm testes of <4 mL in volume. Although KS is present in 1:600 male births and the most frequent single cause of androgen deficiency or azoospermia, it is diagnosed in only ~25% of cases during lifetime (and only ~10% before puberty) indicating that most men go through life without a single pelvic examination by a medical professional, a striking contrast with women.

4.2. *Fertility*

The bulk of testis volume is occupied by the seminiferous tubules so that the health of spermatogenesis is readily apparent by measuring testis size and consistency. While accurate, objective measurement of testis volume by MRI is relatively expensive, office ultrasound (if available) or orchidometry are practical alternatives for clinical use. Orchidometers (obtainable from Andrology Australia at www.andrologyaustralia.org) should be available to anyone evaluating the reproductive health of adolescent males.

4.2.1. *Vulnerability of seminiferous tubules*

The intensely proliferative germinal epithelium of the seminiferous tubules makes spermatogenesis highly vulnerable to irradiation or chemical cytotoxins. Hence, cancer treatment is among the most frequent causes of damage to spermatogenesis leading to male subfertility. Both therapeutic ionising irradiation and chemotherapy drugs, notably alkylating agents, are damaging to spermatogenesis. The spermatogenic damage caused by such treatments show some dose dependency and recovery over years following completion of cancer treatment. Infertility due to impaired spermatogenesis can occur with relative preservation of testosterone production, although some mild lowering of serum testosterone and elevation of serum LH, a pattern termed compensated primary hypogonadisn, is often present but has no clear clinical significance. By contrast, after completion of puberty, spermatogenesis is relatively insensitive to non-cytotoxic chemical environmental impacts.

4.2.2. *Causes of male subfertility*

Many disorders causing lifelong male infertility have their origins in early life. Although these may be present from birth or before puberty, the asymptomatic manifestations of male subfertility will only be evident in adult life after completion of testis growth at puberty. Such disorders include genetic defects in spermatogenesis and testicular pathologies (cryptorchidism, testicular torsion, orchitis, varicocoele). Each of the testicular pathologies can be unilateral so that if the contralateral testis remains unaffected sperm output from a single healthy testis is usually sufficient to preserve fertility. While cryptorchidism and torsion may be diagnosed and treated by orchiopexy from infancy onwards, the long term beneficial effects of early surgery remain difficult to verify. Bilateral cryptorchidism carries a higher risk of testicular tumours and this risk is not necessarily rectified by scrotal placement, presumably because developmental defects of testis formation are more important than the extra-scrotal location.

4.2.3. *Prevention of subfertility*

Prevention of testicular damage is feasible in some circumstances. Mumps vaccination is effective in preventing post-pubertal orchitis, which often causes long-term testis damage. Early surgical correction of varicocoele, which produces progressive unilateral damage to spermatogenesis in the left testis, remains unproven and cannot be recommended given the uncertain evidence of detrimental effects of varicocoele on male fertility. Barrier protection from sexually transmitted infections, involving overt symptomatic as well as subclinical organisms (as examples chlamydia and gonorrhoea), is another form of at least partially effective protection.

4.2.4. *Preservation of fertility in the adolescent cancer patient*

In young men with cancer, fertility preservation is feasible and has a high likelihood of success if required; however, usage is infrequent so sperm cryopreservation is best considered a form of fertility insurance. Sperm cryopreservation should be offered to all sexually mature men who have not completed their families. Sperm collection is feasible for adolescents as young as 12 to 13 years but depends on the maturity of the adolescent and his family and management requires experience, sensitivity, and reassurance in an atmosphere of urgency. Semen is collected via masturbation, and invasive procedures (epididymal aspiration, testicular biopsy) should be avoided with their proper role being harvesting sperm for *in vitro* fertilisation fertility treatment if sperm output has not recovered after cancer treatment. With intracytoplasmic sperm injection, a low sperm output which would limit natural fertility, may be effectively used in conjunction with IVF. For pre-pubertal boys, fertility preservation methods such as testicular biopsy for germ cell transplantation remain experimental.

4.3. *Virilisation*

Adequate virilisation is essential for maintenance of male reproductive health throughout life. Virilisation requires Leydig cell secretion of testosterone which occurs at adult male levels at three periods: during foetal, early postnatal, and post-pubertal life. Foetal testicular secretion is responsible for sexual differentiation of male external genitalia. The role in humans of early postnatal androgen secretion remains unclear. Post-pubertal testicular secretion is responsible for adult virilisation.

In adult life, a single well functioning testis is sufficient to achieve and maintain the virilisation of extra-testicular tissues. Consequently, in males with disorders of the testis itself, virilisation is usually unaffected with involvement, or even loss, of a single testis if the remaining testis is healthy. Impaired (inadequate) virilisation usually implies defects in the remaining testis with inadequate androgen production and/or androgen insensitivity of target tissues.

4.3.1. *Early onset of defective virilisation*

This timing produces distinctive clinical features, such as hypospadias and eunuchoidism (disproportionately long limbs due to delayed epiphyseal fusion) which reflect the severity of defects in pre-pubertal androgen action. For example, in an androgen insensitive genetic male, the severity of hypospadias is the best available clinical index of reduced tissue androgen sensitivity. The spectrum of androgen receptor abnormalities is from complete androgen insensitivity to minor degrees of hypospadias. Similarly, eunuchoidism reflects pre-pubertal oestrogen deficiency due to concomitant androgen deficiency because testosterone is the steroidogenic precursor of oestradiol, the gonadal steroid responsible for epiphyseal fusion.

4.3.2. *Later onset of defective virilisation*

This represents failure to partly or completely progress through puberty. Most disorders of virilisation evident during adolescence reflect congenital defects in gonadotropin and androgen secretion, but also acquired conditions which disrupt hypothalamic or pituitary function or damage both testicles. The expected timing of completed male puberty during adolescence provides the opportunity to identify such disorders.

5. Sexuality

Adolescent acquisition of adult gender role, identity and attraction is a critical outcome catalysed by the testosterone surge of puberty. While the biological determinants of these pivotal aspects of gender remain virtually unknown, the equally speculative social constructions are often assumed as self-evidently axiomatic. While the patterns of teenage sexual activity are well described, their driving influences remain an incompletely understood mixture of psychosocial and biological determinants. During adolescence, sexual activities characteristic of manhood, such as masturbation, curiosity about sex, and sexuality, become established and integrated into the young man's personality. Less frequent forms of sexual activity such as homosexuality and trans-gender are also often first encountered during adolescence, although often much later than first apparent to the individual. Sensitive and thoughtful handling when these arise in other medical contexts is a fundamental part of empathetic management of the adolescent's emerging sexuality.

References

Bojesen A, Juul S, Gravholt CH. (2003) Prenatal and postnatal prevalence of Klinefelter syndrome: A national registry study. *J Clin Endocrinol Metab* **88**(2): 622–626.

Crowne EC, Shalet SM, Wallace WH, Eminson DM, Price DA. (1990) Final height in boys with untreated constitutional delay in growth and puberty. *Arch Dis Child* **65**(10): 1109–1112.

Duke PM, Carlsmith JM, Jennings D, Martin JA, Dornbusch SM, Gross RT, Siegel-Gorelick B. (1982) Educational correlates of early and late sexual maturation in adolescence. *J Pediatr* **100**(4): 633–637.

Finkelstein JS, Klibanski A, Neer RM. (1996) A longitudinal evaluation of bone mineral density in adult men with histories of delayed puberty. *J Clin Endocrinol Metab* **81**(3): 1152–1155.

Gajdos ZK, Hirschhorn JN, Palmert MR. (2009) What controls the timing of puberty? An update on progress from genetic investigation. *Curr Opin Endocrinol Diabetes Obes* **16**(1): 16–24.

Gluckman PD, Hanson MA. (2006) Evolution, development and timing of puberty. *Trends Endocrinol Metab* **17**(1): 7–12.

Houchin LD, Rogol AD. (1998) Androgen replacement in children with constitutional delay of puberty: The case for aggressive therapy. *Baillieres Clin Endocrinol Metab* **12**(3): 427–440.

Lewis K, Lee PA. (2009) Endocrinology of male puberty. *Curr Opin Endocrinol Diabetes Obes* **16**(1): 5–9.

Mobbs EJ. (2005) The psychological outcome of constitutional delay of growth and puberty. *Horm Res* **63**(1): 1–66.

Patton GC, Viner R. (2007) Pubertal transitions in health. *Lancet* **369**(9567): 1130–1139.

Plant TM. (2008) Hypothalamic control of the pituitary-gonadal axis in higher primates: Key advances over the last two decades. *J Neuroendocrinol* **20**(6): 719–726.

Quigley CA, De Bellis A, Marschke KB, El-Awady MK, Wilson EM, French FS. (1995) Androgen receptor defects: Historical, clinical, and molecular perspectives. *Endocr Rev* **16**(3): 271–321.

Sisk CL, Schulz KM, Zehr JL. (2003) Puberty: A finishing school for male social behavior. *Ann N Y Acad Sci* **1007**: 189–198.

Chapter 52

Cardiovascular Risk Factors and Atherosclerosis

Marc S Jacobson and Michael R Kohn

1. Introduction

The consequences of atherosclerosis, including myocardial infarction, stroke, and peripheral vascular disease are delayed until adulthood. The process begins in early childhood. In this chapter, the pathophysiology of atherosclerosis is considered with the role of lipids, and other risk factors, and the transition between adolescence and young adult life. Assessment and management of risk is outlined and practical strategies for lifestyle modification, medical nutritional therapy, and pharmacotherapy are emphasised.

2. The Process of Atherosclerosis

Atherosclerosis is a pathologic process that develops in the arterial wall over some decades. The initial stages of plaque accumulation, infiltration of lipid-laden macrophages and proliferation of smooth muscle cells in the intimal layer at susceptible locations in the arterial tree, can be seen even in the aorta and coronary arteries of infants. During adolescence, these initial changes accelerate and ultimately in adulthood result in altered endothelial architecture and function as atheromatous plaques which expand and calcify, causing clinical symptoms and eventually occlusion following a cascade of inflammatory and clotting events.

The development of atherosclerotic lesions has been extensively studied in adolescents using autopsy material combined with pre- and post-mortem risk factor assessments. The commonly described adult risk factors, elevated low-density lipoprotein cholesterol, low high-density lipoprotein cholesterol, high triglycerides, hypertension, obesity, diabetes, and smoking, are all associated with the prevalence and extent of arterial lesions in adolescents and young adults in a dose-response fashion. Therefore, one can be reasonably confident that risk factors easily assessed in office practice will correlate with development of atherosclerotic plaque, and therefore of cardiovascular disease risk in the patient. Non-invasive *in vivo* imaging of arterial structure and function have shown that early vascular stiffening and intimal thickening can be measured in adolescents at risk, and improvements in observed risk factors such as elevated LDL cholesterol and body mass index are correlated with improved vascular reactivity. These techniques may soon be used in preventive cardiology clinics to evaluate individual patients. These techniques may also be employed in clinical trials for management of hyperlipidaemia and other risk factors.

3. Hyperlipidaemia

Heredity has an important role to play in vulnerability to atherosclerosis because lipid metabolism is affected by many genetically determined traits. The best-characterised form of genetic transmission of risk related to hyperlipidaemia is Familial Hypercholesterolaemia, although there are a number of additional diagnoses which are described in this section.

3.1. *Familial Hypercholesterolaemia*

FH is the phenotype resulting from mutation in the genes that encode for hepatic cell surface LDL receptors. Lessened receptor activity reduces clearance of LDL particles from the blood. This results in severely elevated LDL levels and subsequent accelerated atherosclerosis and early coronary artery disease. FH can be homozygous (which is rare) or heterozygous (which is common, occurring in 1:500 individuals in the United States). FH is inherited in an autosomal dominant fashion. Individuals with heterozygous FH have a 20% risk of myocardial infarction in their twenties, increasing to 75% by their fifties. Therefore it is critical to identify and treat FH by adolescence. Universal cholesterol testing is now recommended by age 10 years or following puberty in those missed earlier.

3.2. *Familial Combined Hyperlipidaemia*

FCH is characterised by mild elevation in total and LDL cholesterol, moderate to severe elevation in triglycerides, and reduced HDL cholesterol. In childhood and adolescence, this pattern is usually expressed in the presence of obesity. While significantly increasing cardiovascular risk at later ages, FCH is not associated with the same high risk of very early disease as is seen in those with FH.

3.3. *Mixed Environmental–Genetic Hyperlipidaemia*

This is a pattern of mild lipid abnormalities in individuals with a genetic sensitivity that is exacerbated by a diet high in saturated fat and cholesterol. No single gene is responsible, but genes encoding for the apolipoprotein E isoforms are known to impart variable sensitivity to dietary fat.

3.4. *Metabolic Syndrome*

Unlike the genetically linked types of hyperlipidaemia described above, the metabolic syndrome is a cluster of risk factors of unknown aetiology that impart an elevated risk of cardiovascular disease. With the rise in incidence of obesity in adolescents, metabolic syndrome could become the most frequent cause of lipid abnormalities. The lipid profile pattern associated with the metabolic syndrome includes normal to mildly increased total and LDL cholesterol levels, a moderate to severe increase in triglycerides and reduced HDL cholesterol.

There has been a heated debate over the past 30 years about whether cholesterol testing for atherosclerosis prevention should be universal, with a cholesterol test as part of health maintenance for every adolescent or selective, with only those adolescents with a positive family history or an associated risk factor such as hypertension being tested. One perspective suggests that all adolescents should know their cholesterol level along with their blood pressure, BMI percentile, and family history of cardiovascular disease. While there has been a modest lowering of mean cholesterol in adolescents over the past 20 years, the incidence of other risk factors such as obesity and diabetes is rising. Cholesterol testing is crucial to identify the one in 500 individuals with heterozygous FH who have a significant risk of myocardial infarct in their third or fourth decade. Furthermore, for males, who are at the highest risk for early heart disease, the adolescent visit may be the last preventive health care visit before their first heart attack, and half of all first heart attacks are fatal. Therefore, a random total cholesterol or preferably a fasting lipid profile should be part of routine care for all adolescents.

In adults, metabolic syndrome is currently diagnosed in individuals with three or more of the following: (1) elevated triglycerides, (2) low HDL cholesterol, (3) hypertension, (4) central adiposity, and (5) elevated glucose. In adolescents, the syndrome is less well defined. Numerous definitions have been proposed, with some more stringent than others. All definitions share the commonality of obesity, dyslipidaemia, insulin resistance, and hypertension.

4. Evaluation

In the US, the National Cholesterol Education Program guidelines for classification of lipid risk in children and adolescents have been in place since 1992. The NCEP guidelines were recently updated to include universal screening using lipid levels, and guidelines for triglycerides and HDL cholesterol, with age-based percentiles instead of single cut-off values. Adolescents with the metabolic syndrome have not been shown to have the very high 10 year risk of myocardial infarction that is characteristic of adolescents with FH. In addition, adolescents with metabolic syndrome are almost always overweight or obese, while those with FH are no more likely to be obese than the general population.

Evaluation of a lipid abnormality involves the patient's medical history, family history, physical examination, and a few simple laboratory studies, including the fasting lipid profile. Other risk factors for early cardiovascular disease, such as obesity, hypertension, smoking, and insulin resistance and diabetes need to be identified and managed. If hypercholesterolaemia and/or hypertriglyceridaemia are present, less common secondary causes of high cholesterol or triglycerides should be excluded. In adolescents, this would include primary hypothyroidism by measuring TSH, and AST and ALT to exclude any hepatic inflammatory process. The nephrotic syndrome is accompanied by significant elevations of total and LDL cholesterol, so a random urinary protein assay is also indicated. Type 2 diabetes mellitus and other forms of insulin resistance, such as polycystic ovary syndrome, are associated with hypertriglyceridaemia and low HDL cholesterol. Other conditions commonly associated with lipid abnormalities in adolescents are not likely to be missed on history and physical examination and thus do not warrant routine laboratory screening. These include connective tissue disorders, anorexia nervosa, and drug toxicity from oral corticosteroids, isotretinoin or antiretrovirals.

5. Identifying Adolescents at Risk: Case Scenarios

Evidence of a lipid problem that emerges during an unrelated evaluation presents an important opportunity to intervene early in the disease process. These case studies illustrate typical scenarios and suggest appropriate interventions.

5.1. *Incidental Finding*

Lipid issues are identified in an otherwise healthy adolescent male when a non-fasting blood test ordered as part of an acute illness workup reveals a total cholesterol level of 5.5 mmol/L (215 mg/dl). Liver and kidney function tests are normal and the acute illness resolves. What should be done regarding his cholesterol?

If there is no family history of early myocardial infarct, stroke or peripheral vascular disease, then provide basic lifestyle advice about healthy diet and exercise habits and smoking as prevention counselling. Repeat his cholesterol in 3 to 6 months.

5.2. *Positive Family History*

As part of a routine medical check, a 15 year old boy with no significant medical history is found to have a parent with early significant atherosclerotic cardiovascular disease (myocardial infarct, stroke or peripheral vascular disease before the age of 55 in males or age 60 in females). His total cholesterol is 6.2 mmol/L (240 mg/dl). What is your approach?

He should have a fasting lipid profile. If his LDL cholesterol is above 4.1 mmol/L (164 mg/dl) on two occasions he has presumptive heterozygous FH. His target LDL cholesterol is < 3.4 mmol/L (< 130 mg/dl) and he should be managed with therapeutic lifestyle changes as discussed below. If TLC fails to bring his LDL within target range within 1–2 years, he is a candidate for cholesterol-lowering medication.

5.3. *Secondary Dyslipidaemia*

A 15 year old female complains of fever, malaise, joint pain and an evanescent facial eruption. Her workup for a rheumatologic condition reveals an abnormal lipid profile: total cholesterol 5.7 mmol/L (220 mg/dl), triglycerides 4.7 mmol/L (275 mg/dl), LDL cholesterol 3.5 mmol/L (135 mg/dl), and HDL 0.9 mmol/L (35 mg/dl). She has no family history of early cardiovascular disease. How should this patient be managed in terms of her lipids?

This patient's dyslipidaemia is likely to have a secondary cause. Consider disorders affecting the thyroid, liver, kidney, or the immune system. Serum measures of thyroid stimulating hormone, hepatic enzymes (ALT, AST), albumin, globulin, antinuclear antibody, and erythrocyte sedimentation rate or C-reactive protein will cover the important secondary causes of hyperlipidaemia and help rule in or out significant medical conditions which affect the lipid profile. Manage the patient's underlying disease first. Counselling to improve her diet (Section 6) is the first-line treatment of her dyslipidaemia.

6. Lifestyle Management

Once an adolescent is found to have hyperlipidaemia with or without other risk factors, management consists of prioritising the risk factors and intervening in a step-wise fashion. Diet needs to be explored with a prospective diet diary, a food frequency questionnaire or questions in the clinical interview about usual intake.

6.1. *Basic Elements of a Therapeutic Lifestyle Change Diet*

- Less than 7% of the day's total calories from saturated fat.
- No more than 25%–35% of the day's total calories from fat.
- Less than 200 mg of dietary cholesterol per day.
- Less than 2,400 mg of dietary sodium per day.
- Just enough calories to achieve or maintain a healthy weight and reduce blood cholesterol level.

These criteria are those recommended for adults by the NCEP of the National Institutes of Health, and should be followed together with an increase in physical activity and a reduction in sedentary pursuits (Chapter 23 for more detailed information on weight management).

6.2. *Follow-Up Procedures*

Within six weeks to three months of the initial intervention, a repeat evaluation and counselling session needs to be scheduled to record progress and make adjustments to the intervention. Repeat these sessions at 3–5 month intervals until the lipid goals are met. If after 1–2 years the LDL cholesterol goal of < 3.4 mmol/L (< 130 mg/dl) has not been met in an adolescent with heterozygous FH, consideration of pharmacotherapy is indicated. It is essential that lifestyle intervention is presented as an essential component to long term management and not just a prelude to pharmacotherapy.

7. Pharmacotherapeutic Challenges

There are effective lipid lowering agents available, many of which are now approved for those under the age of 18 years. The initiation of pharmacotherapy in an adolescent or young adult is generally a commitment to lifelong therapy, and the cost to benefit ratio must be carefully assessed (Table 1).

Table 1: Important considerations and counselling points before initiating statin therapy in adolescents.

Either

1. An LDL cholesterol >4.9 mmol/L (190 mg/dl) plus the presence of xanthomas or xanthelasma (these skin lesions indicate familial hypercholesterolaemia).

Or

2. The history should reflect all of the following:
   - Patient over 8 years of age.
   - A Tanner stage greater than two in males or menarche in females.
   - LDL cholesterol >4.9 mmol/L (190 mg/dl) without other risk factors or 4.1 mmol/L (160 mg/dl) if risk factors such as hypertension, smoking, or obesity are present.
   - Careful monitoring of TLC for six months to two years by a registered dietitian experienced in working with adolescents and lipid abnormalities.
   - Failure to achieve significant LDL cholesterol lowering (15% or greater) with TLC.
   - Positive family history for early cardiovascular disease in an expanded first degree pedigree.

In addition

3. The adolescent and family should be clear about the low risk of muscle and liver side effects.
4. The adolescent and family should understand pregnancy risks including statin teratogenicity and the need for continued TLC, and smoking prevention.
5. There should be a commitment to come in at six weeks, three months, six months, and then yearly so that lipids, CK, ALT, and AST can be monitored.

7.1. *Failure of Therapeutic Lifestyle Change*

An 18 year old female comes to the clinic for a check up. Her medical history is unremarkable. She is sexually active and on a low-dose oral contraceptive. Her family history includes a father with hypercholesterolaemia on medication and a paternal grandfather who died of a myocardial infarction at age 50. Her lipid profile reveals total cholesterol 6.6 mmol/L (255 mg/dl), triglycerides 2.1 mmol/L (125 mg/dl), LDL cholesterol 4.9 mmol/L (190 mg/dl), and HDL cholesterol 1.0 mmol/L (40 mg/dl). Once TLC is given a sufficient chance to work (1–2 years) and her lipids are unchanged, what is the next step?

This patient meets the family history and LDL cholesterol criteria for heterozygous familial hypercholesterolaemia. She should have pharmacotherapy with a low dose of statin. Before prescribing, her clinician should make her aware of the low risk of muscle and liver side effects and the risks to a developing foetus. The need for continued TLC, including smoking prevention, should be emphasised. Her lipids, creatine phosphokinase, ALT, and AST should be followed at recommended intervals of six weeks, three months, six months, and then yearly. The contraindications of statins during pregnancy should be stressed and appropriate follow up ensured.

7.2. *Multiple Lipid Abnormalities in an Overweight Adolescent*

A 16 year old girl with a BMI = 90th percentile, the polycystic ovary syndrome and normal fasting glucose level comes to your clinic. Her mother is on a statin medication. Fasting lipid profile: total cholesterol 4.3 mmol/L (166 mg/dl), triglycerides 2.3 mmol/L (203 mg/dl), LDL cholesterol 2.5 mmol/L (98 mg/dl), HDL cholesterol 0.7 mmol/L (27 mg/dl). Her diet includes chicken, fish, pasta, rice, cereal, and skim milk. How would you approach dietary management in light of the elevated triglycerides, and which medication(s) might be considered?

This is a case of FCH in an adolescent with the polycystic ovary syndrome. Some carbohydrates (for example white rice, white bread, sweets, sugar-sweetened beverages) and alcohol are known to raise triglycerides, which in turn lower HDL cholesterol. These foods and beverages are also associated with insulin resistance, a feature of the polycystic ovary syndrome and metabolic syndrome. Even a small weight loss can normalise the lipid profile in this setting. For these reasons, dietary recommendations should begin with limitations on refined carbohydrate consumption, both in terms of portion size and frequency, and an increase in lean protein, vegetables and whole grains. Counselling should stress the importance of making lifestyle changes that increase overall physical activity levels. Lipid-lowering medications for this type of dyslipidaemia are the fibric acids and extended-release niacin. These drugs are not FDA-approved for use below age 18. Referral to a lipid specialist, endocrinologist, or cardiologist is the next step if medication is needed. Statins are not indicated because the LDL cholesterol is not elevated.

7.3. *Dyslipidaemia in a Thin Adolescent*

This patient is a 17 year old girl whose fasting lipid profile is: total cholesterol 3.9 mmol/L (152 mg/dl), triglycerides 2 mmol/L (175 mg/dl), LDL cholesterol 2.6 mmol/L (101 mg/dl), HDL 0.5 mmol/L (22 mg/dl). She has a positive family history of hypercholesterolaemia and early myocardial infarction. The patient is sexually active and wants to begin an oral contraceptive. She is thin, menstruating regularly, normotensive, and non-smoking. Would you suggest using a statin, and if so, at what dose?

Her lipid pattern is that of FCH. Total and LDL cholesterol are within normal limits making statins a poor choice of medication, but her combination of high triglycerides and low HDL cholesterol put her at risk for premature cardiovascular disease. Statins are also contraindicated in pregnancy, so must be used with caution in sexually active adolescent females. HDL levels may rise slightly in response to the oestrogen in the oral contraceptive and routine exercise and the latter should be recommended. If TLC fails to improve her lipids, the best choice of medication would be extended-release niacin or a fibric acid derivative as in Case 7.2. Lipids should be monitored six weeks after initiation of the oral contraceptive in case this exacerbates the hypertriglyceridaemia, and then twice yearly once stable.

8. Non Pharmacological Agents

The first line of treatment for hyperlipidaemia is TLC. Studies consistently report LDL cholesterol lowering of 10%–15% with this alone. Additionally, many young people are interested in 'natural' methods to lower cholesterol. If this is the case, work with them and do not dismiss their ideas out of hand.

8.1. *Cholesterol Lowering Products*

Some products have small effects on total and LDL cholesterol of the order of 3% to 5% and work best when used to replace foods high in saturated fat. These include:

- Soluble fibre-containing foods: oatmeal (regular not instant), beans, apples, citrus.

- Soy-based foods: tofu, soy milk or soy beans.
- Fish: salmon, herring, oysters, halibut, tuna.
- Foods high in unsaturated oils: walnuts, almonds, avocados, olive oil.

If additional LDL cholesterol lowering is needed, supplemental *plant stanols and sterols*, which are derived from non-food plant-based sources, may be indicated. These products, generally margarines, yoghurts and salad dressings, are available and clearly labelled in supermarkets. These products can also be obtained in tablet form over the counter. When ingested at a dose of 3 gm per day, plant stanols and sterols interfere with cholesterol absorption in the gut and inhibit the enterohepatic re-circulation of cholesterol. This, in turn, stimulates the liver to upregulate LDL receptors and lower plasma LDL cholesterol. Up to 10% LDL cholesterol lowering is seen in clinical trials in adolescents and adults.

8.2. *Triglyceride Lowering Products*

If the TLC approach is not enough to reach target triglyceride values, omega-3 oils derived from marine sources can be given. A dosage of 1–3 gm per day of combined eicosapentaenoic acid and docosahexaenoic acid in capsule or liquid form has been shown to be effective in reducing hypertriglyceridaemia and inflammatory markers.

9. Conclusion

Hyperlipidaemia and its management provide a unique opportunity to practise prevention with adolescent patients in an area that is less emotionally charged than sexuality and drug use, but which is every bit as important in terms of long term morbidity and mortality. All teens and their families should be made aware of their risk status and the ways to reduce their risk. This necessitates a focused family history, a random cholesterol test or fasting lipid profile when indicated, and counselling based on the findings. TLC is an effective approach to lipid management that accommodates opportunities for other types of health risk counselling. In a patient with heterozygous FH, if lipid levels are not controlled by TLC after a period of 1–2 years, pharmacotherapy may be initiated. Milder types of lipid disorders can be followed longer (into adulthood) without drug treatment.

References

The American Academy of Pediatrics. (2007) Cardiovascular risk reduction in high-risk pediatric populations: A scientific statement from the Heart Association Expert Panel on Population and Prevention Science. Executive summary. *Pediatrics* **119**(3): 618–621.

Belay B, Belamarich PF, Tom-Revzon C. (2007) The use of statins in pediatrics: Knowledge base, limitations, and future directions. *Pediatrics* **119**(2): 370–380.

Charakida M, Masi S, Luscher TF, Kastelein JJP, Deanfield JE. (2010) Assessment of atherosclerosis: The role of flow-mediated dilatation. *Eur Heart J* **31**(23): 2854–2861.

Jacobson MS, Kohn M, Neinstein L. (2007) Cardiovascular risk factors and hyperlipidemia. In: Neinstein L (ed.), *Adolescent Medicine*, 5th ed. Williams and Wilkins, Baltimore.

McCrindle BW, Urbina EM, Dennison BA, Jacobson MS, Steinberger J, Rocchini AP, Hayman LL, Daniels SR. A scientific statement from the American Heart Association Atherosclerosis, Hypertension and Obesity in Youth Committee, Council of Cardiovascular Disease in the Young with the Council on Cardiovascular Nursing. (2007) Drug therapy of high-risk lipid abnormalities in children and adolescents. *Circulation* **115**(14): 1948–1967.

Reiner Z. (2010) Combined therapy in the treatment of dyslipidemia. *Fundam Clin Pharmacol* **24**(1): 19–28.

Zimmet P, Alberti G, Kaufman F, Tajima N, Silink M, Arslanian S, Wong G, Bennett P, Shaw J, Caprio S, International Diabetes Federation Task Force On Epidemiology & Prevention of Diabetes. (2007) The metabolic syndrome in children and adolescents. *Lancet* **369**(9579): 2059–2061.

Abbreviations

17OHP	17 hydroxy-progesterone
21OHD	21-hydroxylase deficiency
ABAS	Adaptive Behaviour Assessment System
aBMD	areal Bone Mineral Density
ACE	Angiotensin-Converting Enzyme
ACR	Albumin:creatinine ratio
ACTH	Adrenocorticotropic Hormone
ADA	Americans with Disabilities Act
ADH	Antidiuretic hormone
ADHD	Attention Deficit Hyperactivity Disorder
ADPKD	Autosomal Dominant Polycystic Kidney Disease
AIDS	Acquired Immune Deficiency Syndrome
ALD	Adreno-leucodystrophy
ALL	Acute Lymphoblastic Leukaemia
ALT	Alanine Aminotransferase
AMH	Anti-müllerian hormone
AML	Acute Myeloid Leukaemia
AMN	Adreno-myeloneuropathy
AN	Anorexia Nervosa
ANA	Antinuclear Antibodies
ANCA	Antineutrophil Cytoplasmic Antibody
AND	Allow a Natural Death
APLS	Antiphospholipid Syndrome
APOE	Apolipoprotein E

APTT	Activated Partial Thromboplastin Time
AR	Allergic Rhinitis
ARB	Angiotensin II Receptor Blockers
AS	Alport Syndrome
AS	Ankylosing Spondylitis
ASD	Atrial Septal Defect
ASD	Autism Spectrum Disorder
ASOT	Antistreptolysin O Titre
AST	Aspartate Aminotransferase
AYA	Adolescents and Young Adults
BCNU	Bis-chloroethylnitrosourea
BDNF	Brain Derived Neurotropic Factor
BED	Binge Eating Disorder
BGLs	Blood Glucose Levels
BiPAP	Biphasic Positive Airway Pressure
BMD	Bone Mineral Density
BMI	Body Mass Index
BMT	Bone Marrow Transplant
BN	Bulimia Nervosa
BSL	Blood Sugar Level
CAH	Congenital Adrenal Hyperplasia
CAM	Complementary and Alternative Medicine
CAMHS	Child and Adolescent Mental Health Services
CARI	Caring for Australasians with Renal Impairment
CCB	Calcium Channel Blockers
CBT	Cognitive-Behavioural Therapy
CCNU	1-2-Chloroethyl-3-Cyclohexyl-1-Nitrosourea
CCP	Cyclic Citrullinated Peptide
CCSS	Childhood Cancer Survivor Study
CD	Conduct Disorder
CD	Constitutional Delay
CD	Crohn's Disease
CDC	Centers for Disease Control
CDGP	Constitutional Delay of Growth and Puberty
CDP	Constitutional Delay of Puberty
CF	Cystic Fibrosis

CFS	Chronic Fatigue Syndrome
cGvHD	chronic Graft versus Host Disease
CHARGE	Coloboma, Heart defects, Choanal Atresia, Retardation (growth and intellectual) and Genital and Ear defects
CHD	Congenital Heart Disease
CI	Cranial Irradiation
CIT	Conventional Insulin Therapy
CK	Creatinine Kinase
CKD	Chronic Kidney Disease
CMP	Comprehensive Metabolic Panel
CMV	Cytomegalovirus
CNS	Central Nervous System
COL1	Type I Collagen Gene
CP	Cerebral Palsy
CPAP	Continuous Positive Airways Pressure
CPP	Central (gonadotropin dependent) precocious puberty
CRH	Corticotropin Releasing Hormone
CRPS	Complex Regional Pain Syndrome
CRS	Congenital Rubella Syndrome
CSF	Cerebrospinal Fluid
CSI	Craniospinal Irradiation
CT	Computed Tomography
CVID	Common Variable Immune Deficiency
CXR	Chest X-ray
D9THC	Delta Tetra Hydrocannabinol
DBP	Diastolic Blood Pressure
DCCT	Diabetes Control and Complications Trial
DHA	Docosahexaenoic Acid
DHEA/S	Dehydroepiandrosterone/sulphate
DIP	Diffuse Idiopathic Pain
DKA	Diabetic Ketoacidosis
DMD	Duchenne Muscular Dystrophy
DNA	Deoxyribonucleic Acid
DNR	Do Not Resuscitate
DS	Down Syndrome
DSH	Deliberate Self-harm

DSM-IV	Diagnostic and Statistical Manual of Mental Disorders
DSPD	Delayed Sleep Phase Disorder
DT	Diphtheria Toxoid
DTI	Diffusion Tensor Imaging
DUB	Dysfunctional Uterine Bleeding
DXA	Duel X-ray Absorptiometry
EBV	Epstein–Barr virus
EC	Emergency Contraception
ECG	Electrocardiograph
EDNOS	Eating Disorder not Otherwise Specified
EEG	Electroencephalograph
EEN	Exclusive Enteral Nutrition
EoE	Eosinophilic oesophagitis
EPA	Eicosapentaenoic Acid
EPG	Electrophoretogram
ERA	Enthesitis Related Arthritis
ES	Ewing's Sarcoma
ESKD	End Stage Kidney Disease
ESR	Erythrocyte Sedimentation Rate
ESWL	Extracorporeal Shock Wave Lithotripsy
EURORDIS	European Organisation for Rare Disorders
FA	Food allergy
FAO	Food and Agriculture Organization
FAP	Familial Adenomatous Polyposis
FBC	Full Blood Count
FBE	Full Blood Examination
FCH	Familial Combined Hyperlipidaemia
FDA	Food and Drug Administration
FGFR1	Fibroblast Growth Factor Receptor 1
FGIDs	Functional Gastrointestinal Disorders
FH	Familial Hypercholesterolaemia
FSGS	Focal Segmental Glomerulosclerosis
FSH	Follicle Stimulating Hormone
FT3	Free Triiodothyronine
FT4	Free Thyroxine
GAD	Glutamic Acid Decarboxylase

GBM	Glomerular Basement Membrane
GCS	Glasgow Coma Scale
GCTs	Germ Cell Tumours
GH	Growth Hormone
GHB	Gamma-hydroxybutyrate
GHD	Growth Hormone Deficiency
GIT	Gastrointestinal Tract
GJB2	Gap Junction Beta-2
GN	Glomerulonephritis
GnRH	Gonadotropin Releasing Hormone
GORD	Gastro-oesophageal Reflux Disease
GPR	G Protein-Coupled Receptors
HAV	Hepatitis A Virus
Hb	Haemoglobin
HBV	Hepatitis B Virus
HCG	Human Chorionic Gonadotropin
HCM	Hypertrophic Cardiomyopathy
HCV	Hepatitis C Virus
HDL	High-density Lipoprotein
HDM	House Dust Mite
HDT	Hormonal Development Therapy
HELENA	Healthy Lifestyle in Europe by Nutrition in Adolescence
HEV	Hepatitis E Virus
HGSA	Human Genetics Society of Australasia
HH	Hypogonadotropic Hypogonadism
HIV	Human Immunodeficiency Virus
HLA	Human Leukocyte Antigen
HPO	Hypertrophic Pulmonary Osteopathy
HPV	Human Papillomavirus
HRT	Hormone Replacement Therapy
HSP	Henoch-Schönlein purpura
HSV	Herpes Simplex Virus
HT	Hypertension
hTRAb	human Thyrotropin Receptor Antibody
I131	Radioactive Iodine
IA	Insulin Antibody

IBD	Inflammatory Bowel Disease
ICD	International Classification of Diseases
ICEC	International Consortium for Emergency Contraception
ICSD	International Classification of Sleep Disorders
ICSI	Intracytoplasmic Sperm Injection
ID	Intellectual Disability
IGF-1	Insulin-like Growth Factor
IIT	Intensive Insulin Therapy
IL	Interleukin
IPT	Interpersonal Therapy
IPV	Inactivated Poliovirus Vaccine
IQ	Intelligence Quotient
IRBs	Institutional Review Boards
ITB	Intrathecal Baclofen
ITP	Immune Thrombocytopenic Purpura
IUCD	Intrauterine Contraceptive Device
IUGR	Intrauterine Growth Restriction
IVIG	Intravenous Gammaglobulin
JDM	Juvenile Dermatomyositis
JE	Japanese Encephalitis
JHS	Joint Hypermobility Syndrome
JIA	Juvenile Idiopathic Arthritis
JLN	Jervell and Lange-Nielsen Syndrome
JME	Juvenile Myoclonic Epilepsy
JPS	Juvenile Polyposis Syndrome
KS	Klinefelter Syndrome
LA	Left Atrium
LAIV	Live Attenuated Influenza Vaccine
LARC	Long Acting Reversible Contraceptives
LDL	Low-density Lipoprotein
LFT	Liver Function Tests
LH	Luteinising Hormone
LNG-IUS	Levonorgestrel-releasing Intrauterine System
LSD	Lysergic Acid Diethylamide
LV	Left Ventricle
MAS	McCune Albright Syndrome

MDIs	Multiple Daily Insulin Injections
MDMA	3,4-methylenedioxymethamphetamine
MDS	Myelodysplastic Syndrome
menC	meningococcal C
MMR	Measles, Mumps and Rubella
MMS	Multi-media Messaging Service
MPGN	Membranoproliferative Glomerulonephritis
MRI	Magnetic Resonance Imaging
MRSA	Methicillin Resistant *Staphylococcus aureus*
MSLT	Multiple Sleep Latency Test
MTA	Multimodal Treatment of ADHD
MTOR	Mammalian Target of Rapamycin
NAAT	Nucleic Acid Amplification Testing
NAFLD	Non-alcoholic Fatty Liver Disease
NCEP	National Cholesterol Education Program
NCS	Nerve Conduction Study
NHBPEP	National High Blood Pressure Education Programs
NHL	Non-Hodgkin's Lymphoma
NHMRC	National Health and Medical Research Council
NMDA	N-methyl D-aspartate
NREM	Non-Rapid Eye Movement
NSAIDs	Non-Steroidal Anti-Inflammatory Drugs
NTD	Neural Tube Defects
OAS	Oral Allergy Syndrome
OCD	Obsessive-Compulsive Disorder
OCP	Oral Contraceptive Pill
ODD	Oppositional Defiant Disorder
OECD	Organization for Economic Cooperation and Development
OGTT	Oral Glucose Tolerance Test
OI	Osteogenesis Imperfecta
OPV	Oral Polio Vaccine
OS	Osteosarcoma
OSA	Obstructive Sleep Apnoea
PAH	Pulmonary Hypertension
PAS-ADD	Psychiatric Assessment Schedule for Adults with Developmental Disability

PCD	Primary Ciliary Dyskinesia
PCOS	Polycystic Ovary Syndrome
PCR	Polymerase Chain Reaction
PCV	Pneumococcal Conjugate Vaccines
PDA	Patent Ductus Arteriosus
PDGF	Platelet Derived Growth Factor
PEIR	Prevention and Early Intervention
PET	Positron Emission Tomography
PFO	Patent Foramen Ovale
PID	Pelvic Inflammatory Disease
PJS	Peutz–Jegher Syndrome
POEMS	Polyneuropathy, Organomegaly, Endocrinopathy, Monoclonal Gammopathy, Skin changes
PPI	Proton Pump Inhibitor
PPV	Pneumococcal Polysaccharide Vaccine
PSGN	Post Streptococcal Glomerular Nephritis
PSSR1	Serine Protease 1
PT	Prothrombin Time
PTSD	Post Traumatic Stress Disorder
PUJ	Pelviureteric Junction
PUVA	Psoralen+Ultraviolet A
PVFS	Post-Viral Fatigue Syndrome
QOL	Quality of Life
RAP	Resourceful Adolescent Project
RBC	Red Blood Cell
REM	Rapid Eye Movement
RF	Rheumatoid Factor
RMS	Rhabdomyosarcoma
RP	Retinitis Pigmentosa
RPR	Rapid Plasma Reagin
RV	Right Ventricle
SB	Spina Bifida
SBP	Systolic Blood Pressure
SD	Standard Deviation
SHBG	Sex Hormone Binding Globulin
SI	Spinal Irradiation

SIB	Self-Injurious Behavior
SLE	Systemic Lupus Erythematosus
SMN	Subsequent Malignant Neoplasms
SMS	Short Message Service
SPECT	Single Photon Emission Computed Tomography
SPINK1	Serine Protease Inhibitor
SPRM	Selective Progesterone Receptor Modulator
SSA	Same-Sex Attracted
SSRI	Selective Serotonin Reuptake Inhibitors
STIs	Sexually Transmitted Infections
STS	Soft Tissue Sarcomas
SVC	Superior Vena Cava
T1DM	Type 1 Diabetes Mellitus
T2DM	Type 2 Diabetes Mellitus
TAFE	Technical and Further Education
TBI	Total Body Irradiation
TCAs	Tricyclic antidepressants
TD	Tardive Dyskinesia
TENS	Transcutaneous Electrical Nerve Stimulator
TFR	Teenage Fertility Rate
TFT	Thyroid Function Tests
TG Ab	Thyroglobulin Antibodies
TIA	Transient Ischaemic Attack
TIN	Tubulointerstitial Nephritis
TIV	Trivalent Inactivated Influenza Vaccine
TLC	Therapeutic Lifestyle Changes
TNF	Tumor Necrosis Factor
TOVA	Tests of Variables Attention
TPO Ab	Thyroperoxidase Antibodies
TRH	Thyrotropin Releasing Hormone
TS	Turner Syndrome
TSH	Thyroid Stimulating Hormone
TSI	Thyroid Stimulating Immunoglobulin
TTY	Telephone Typewritten
TU	Testosterone Undecanoate
TV	Television

UC	Ulcerative Colitis
UEC	Urea, Electrolytes and Creatinine
UKMEC	UK Medical Eligibility Criteria
UNCRC	United Nations Convention on the Rights of the Child
UNU	United Nation University
US	Usher Syndrome
VDRL	Venereal Disease Research Laboratory
VLED	Very Low Energy Diets
VPD	Vaccine Preventable Diseases
VRS	Video Relay Service
VSD	Ventricular Septal Defect
VTE	Venous Thromboembolism
VV	Varicella Vaccine
VWD	Von Willebrand Disease
VWF	Von Willebrand Factor
WHO MEC	World Health Organization Medical Eligibility Criteria
WHO	World Health Organization
WISC	Wechsler Intelligence Scale for Children
WS	Waardenburg Syndrome
XRT	X-ray Therapy
YF	Yellow Fever

Index